The Guide to
WOMEN'S HEALTH
and WELLNESS

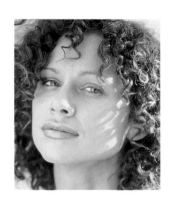

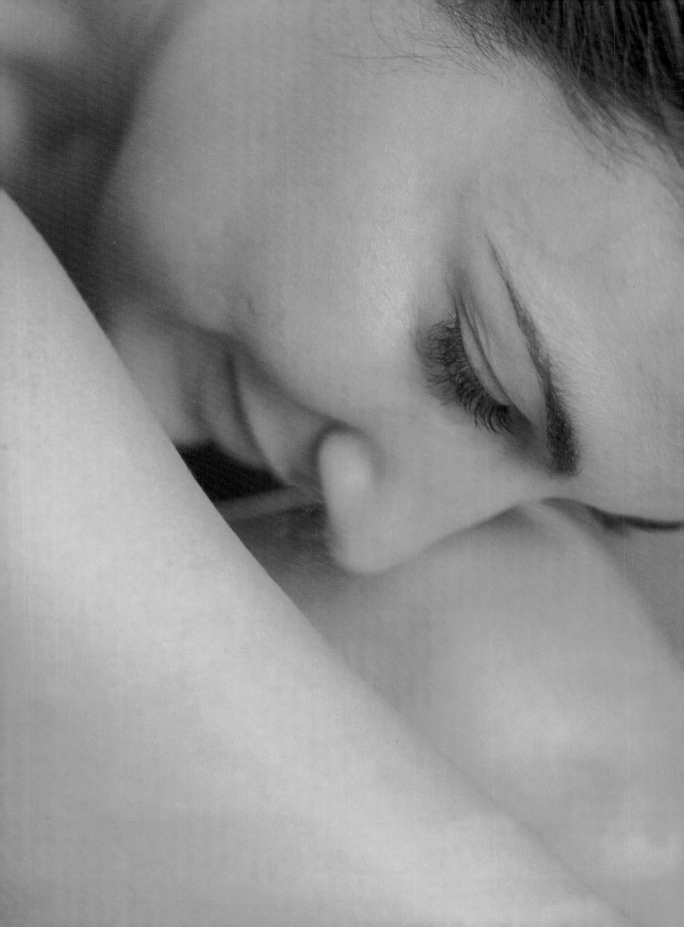

The Guide to
WOMEN'S HEALTH
and WELLNESS

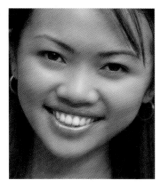
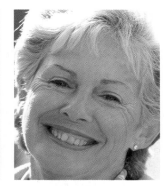
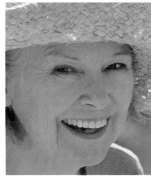
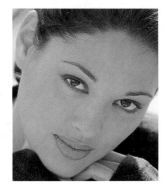

General Medical Editor

DR. LESLEY HICKIN

MARSHALL PUBLISHING • LONDON

A Marshall Edition
Conceived, edited and designed by
Marshall Editions Ltd, The Orangery
161 New Bond Street, London W1S 2UF

First published in the UK in 2001 by Marshall Publishing Ltd

ISBN 1-84028-250-9

Originated in Singapore by Master Image
Printed and bound in Portugal by Printer Portuguesa
10 9 8 7 6 5 4 3 2 1

Project Editors Wendy James, Anna Fischel
Editors Ros Highstead, Sue Harper
Art Editors Hugh Schermuly, Nick Buzzard
Designer Phil Gamble
Photoshoot Art Director Tania Volhard
Managing Editor Anne Yelland
Managing Art Editor Helen Spencer
Picture Editor Antonella Mauro
DTP Editor Lesley Gilbert
Editorial Coordinator Gillian Thompson
Editorial Director Ellen Dupont
Art Director Dave Goodman
Production Nikki Ingram
Indexer Hilary Cooper
Proofreader Emma Fischel
Complementary Health Consultant Professor P. Pietroni

CONTRIBUTORS Anne Charlish, Sue George, Victoria Goldman,
Sue Hubberstey, Jan Hurst, Chris McLaughlin, Nigel Perryman,
Dr Jenny Sutcliffe, Patsy Westcott, Belinda Whitworth
ILLUSTRATIONS Richard Tebbitt

Note: Every effort has been taken to ensure that all information in this book is
correct and compatible with national standards generally accepted at the time of
publication. The information and recommendations given are not intended to be
a substitute for medical advice. The author and publisher disclaim any liability,
loss, injury or damage incurred as a consequence, directly or indirectly, of the
use and application of the contents of this book.

CONTENTS

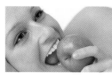

CHAPTER 1
BEING A WELL WOMAN

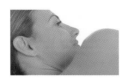

CHAPTER 2
SEX AND SEXUALITY

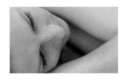

CHAPTER 3
GENERAL HEALTH ISSUES

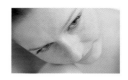

CHAPTER 4
HORMONAL HEALTH

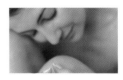

CHAPTER 5
ILLNESSES AND EMERGENCIES

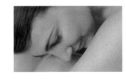

CHAPTER 6
TREATMENTS AND THERAPIES

INTRODUCTION

Thanks to much recent medical research, there is more information than ever before on women's health. It is now known that women respond differently from men to illnesses and their treatment. This is the first book to give you the unbiased facts in a clear, straightforward way so you know how to help yourself and what to do when things go wrong.

There is so much information in the media about your health that it's hard to sort out what is important and what is less so. Added to that, opinions differ and reports on medical theories and treatments can confuse and worry rather than reassure. Is smoking even more dangerous for women than for men? Is butter good or bad for you and your family and is it better or worse than margarine? Which cancers are hereditary and which are more prevalent in women than men? Such topics make headline news one day but disappear—or are not updated—the next, leaving you uneasy, your fears awakened.

This book cuts a swathe through the fog of opinion to present the results of the most up-to-date medical advances. It sums up the latest research into good and bad health specifically from the point of view of women. Some problems affect everyone equally but others are more relevant to women. Naturally, reproductive issues and illnesses such as breast lumps, ovarian cysts, contraceptive choices and infertility are covered in detail, but there are also

HEALTHY MIND AND BODY
Find an exercise plan you enjoy so you carry on with it (pages 22–23). Feeling good about yourself helps give you the confidence to communicate clearly at home and at work (pages 26–29).

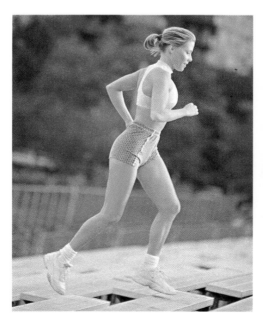
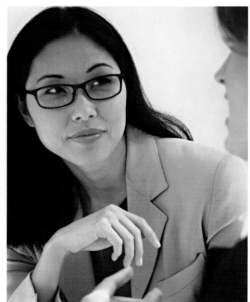

pages on depression and anxiety, panic and phobias, written from a female slant as neurotic illness is more common in women. As well as such emotional topics, occupational hazards like repetitive strain injury (RSI) are dealt with, since many women suffer from problems relating to long hours at a computer or other tasks requiring repeated similar movement. Above all, this book aims to inform you correctly and relevantly so you have the tools for good health. It enables you to communicate effectively with your doctor or specialist and take an active part in your mental and physical health, treatment and recovery.

CONVENTIONAL AND HOLISTIC

Many health books tackle the subject solely from the disease angle. We take a long look at how you can preserve the gift of your health through your lifestyle—and instil good habits in your children, if you have them, or in those around you by example.

If you are suffering from a diagnosed disease, you are probably receiving conventional medical treatment, and this book explains what you can ask and expect and what the aims and outcome may be. Drugs are improving all the time, and we give you the most up-to-date information on what they are and what they can and can't cure. If you are well, or suffer from sporadic minor symptoms such as occasional headaches, holistic (treating the whole person rather than isolated parts of the mind or body) treatments offer an alternative approach. Complementary therapies such as yoga are excellent stress-relievers, and help both your mental well-being and physical suppleness. A directory on pages 312–314 gives the addresses of women's health sources, whether you are keen to explore a new therapy, or you are a sufferer or carer.

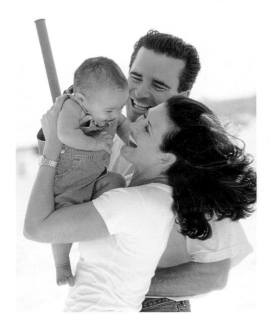

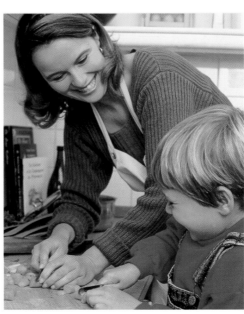

HAVING CHILDREN
Watching a child develop from a helpless baby to an independent teenager is one of life's great joys (pages 178–179).

How to use this book

The book is divided into six chapters. Every chapter is broken down into sections with double or single pages devoted to each topic, shown in headings at the top of the page for handy reference if you are flicking through. When you want to find a specific entry, look at the contents list on page 5 or the index at the end on pages 315–319.

BEING A WELL WOMAN

Chapter 1 studies ways in which you can achieve your optimum good health—allowing for a little indulgence—through diet, exercise, sleep, coming to terms with your looks and asserting your rights in the workplace. Look at the section on female body systems if you wish to know how your body works in good health. The pages on a healthy mind help you beat stress, act positively and assertively and cope when things are hard to handle.

SEX AND SEXUALITY

Chapter 2 starts with a frank look at your sexual self—it includes discovering your own sexuality, relationships, intimacy, fantasy and abuse. The section on choosing contraception surveys all your options, followed by what to do in the event of an unwanted pregnancy. The pages on sexual problems steer you through the pain or embarrassment to find a sympathetic solution, while a chart on sexually transmitted diseases (STDs) makes it clear exactly what to do if you suspect or realize you have a sexual infection.

TAKING UP EXERCISE
Whatever your age, taking up a new sport will improve your body shape, as well as being a pleasure. Load-bearing exercise is particularly good to combat the effects of progressive diseases such as osteoporosis (page 90).

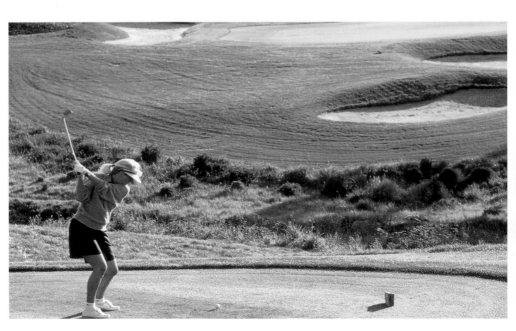

GENERAL HEALTH ISSUES

Turn to chapter 3 to read the female perspective on conditions that affect men and women. Skeletal, circulatory and heart disease are included, as well as a detailed section on problems of the mind such as alcohol, smoking and drug abuse, eating disorders and anxiety-related disorders including obsessions, fears, post-traumatic stress and how to rate your stress levels.

HORMONAL HEALTH

Chapter 4 explains all about menstrual disorders and the menopause, breast care, cervical, uterine and ovarian problems as well as endocrine system problems such as diabetes and thyroid disorders. Look at this chapter, too, for advice on pregnancy, motherhood and problems with conception.

ILLNESSES AND EMERGENCIES

Read chapter 5 to find out what happens when the body systems stop working perfectly. This is the place to look up diseases, whether it's gallstones or appendicitis, irritable bowel syndrome (IBS) or eczema, Alzheimer's or asthma, psoriasis or deafness. Turn here if you're confused about the difference between bacteria and viruses. The emergency first aid section on pages 252–259 is a must if there's an accident at home or in your workplace.

TREATMENTS AND THERAPIES

Finally, find charts detailing tests, which specialists do what, and drug types and uses in chapter 6. As well as conventional treatments, holistic mind and body medicine and complementary therapies are discussed.

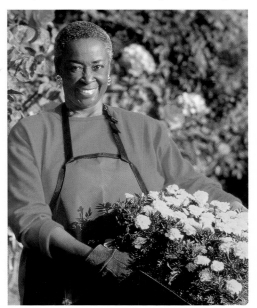 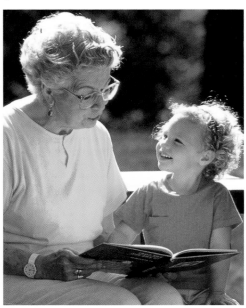

GROWING OLDER GRACEFULLY
Seeing your age in a positive light helps you enjoy its benefits: leisure to enjoy hobbies such as gardening, and the fun of grandchildren without all the responsibilities of parenthood (page 15).

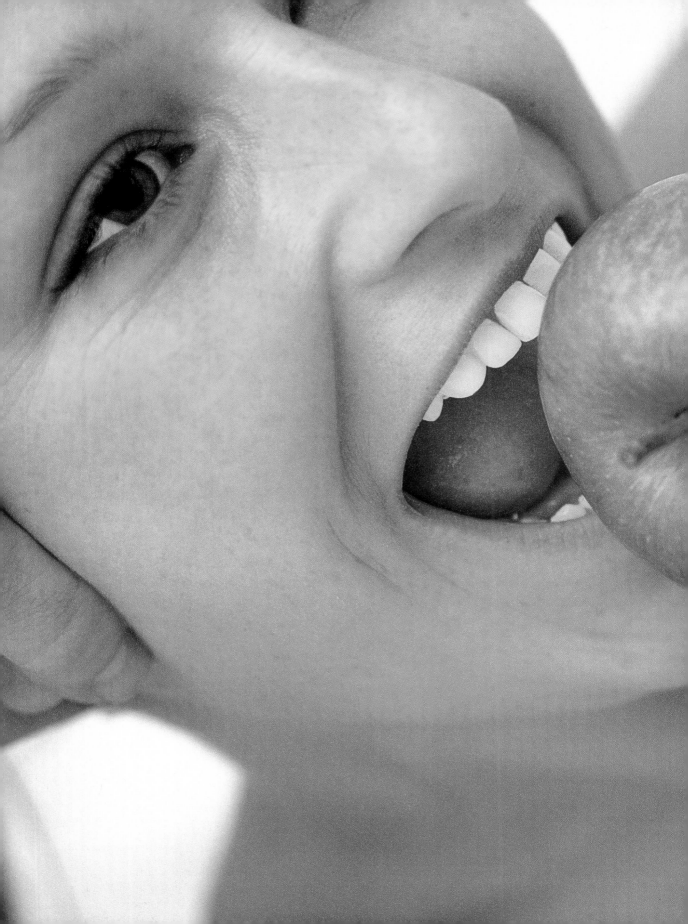

BEING A WELL WOMAN

What is wellness? It is a state of being that makes you feel healthy, happy and full of vitality. It is what makes you look forward to each new day, the surge that carries you through times of crisis and gives your life energy and purpose. Women's approach to wellness is distinct—different from men's in subtle but important ways. Once it was thought women and men reacted similarly, but now the search to find the precise mechanisms for these differences has accelerated. Knowing how to sustain a state of well-being starts with understanding what makes us the way we are, how the workings of our body systems reflect the effects of hormones and genetics.

SEASONS OF A WOMAN'S LIFE

As a woman, you will experience many changes, both physical and emotional, during your lifetime. They are often slow, sometimes even barely perceptible, with one stage blending into another like the seasons, and you may be aware only in retrospect that there has been a transition. Nevertheless, each stage has its own features and the health issues you may face will vary with each stage.

Early adulthood

THE EMERGING WOMAN
As you develop from a child into a teenager and a young woman, your friends, body, learning and lifestyle will provide a strong base for your future health and achievements.

When you emerge from adolescence, you move gradually away from your parents' influence. You become ready to take on some of the responsibilities of the adult world, while still retaining the energy of youth. Physically you are ready to have babies, but you are under far less pressure than your mother was to find a husband, settle down and start a family.

You are more likely to choose to delay having a child until your late 20s or early 30s, to concentrate on your career, studies or travel. You may be reluctant to relinquish your freedom and strive to achieve the same economic independence as your male friends.

As a young adult woman, you can expect to have good health but this does not mean forgetting the need for sound nutrition, exercise and regular health checks such as cervical smear tests. At this age you may not fully grasp the importance of good health and consequently take risks. You may spend hours at the gym but smoke and drink more alcohol than you should. You may be tempted to go on crash diets and then have weeks when you eat nothing but junk food. A hectic social life may mean you also go without sleep on a regular basis. You may occasionally use illegal drugs.

Early womanhood is also a time when emotional problems can dominate your life and may perhaps give rise to eating disorders or chronic fatigue syndrome. If you have left your parents' home to live by yourself, it is important to have the support of close friends.

You may seek a sexual partner without necessarily having commitment in mind. Indeed, you may have had several sexual partners before you begin a long-term relationship. This has become acceptable behaviour in Western cultures, but carries its own risks. You need to be aware of the importance of contraception to prevent an unwanted pregnancy and of practising safe sex, not just because of the small but real risk of becoming HIV positive, but to avoid more common sexually transmitted diseases such as herpes, gonorrhoea and chlamydia. All or any of these could be detrimental to your future well-being and happiness.

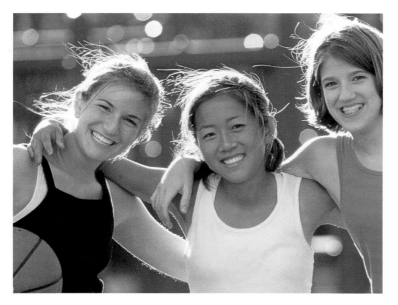

The prime of life

Like many women, you may find that your 30s are a time when your confidence has grown and you feel happy to be yourself, relieved to have left the uncertainties and peer pressures of early adulthood behind. You are well established in your career and know what you want out of life.

For many women there comes a time when they want to have a child. Reliable contraception has made it possible to put parenthood on hold until you and your partner believe the conditions are right. Alternatively, you may decide that you don't want a co-parent, and choose to go it alone. You should be aware of the importance of good health before conception and get your body into peak form before trying to become pregnant. However, you may choose to pursue your career or interests instead of having a child, or you may find that a partnership is fulfilment enough without feeling the need for motherhood as well.

MOTHERHOOD AND CAREERS

Most women are able to conceive naturally and have healthy babies which give them great pleasure in the years of nurturing. You may be surprised by the intensity of the love you have for your child; alternatively, bonding with the baby may take time to develop.

Your relationship with your partner, if you have one, will change with the arrival of the baby. It can be enriched by your mutual joy in the child, especially if you parent together and accept equal responsibility. However, the relationship may be put under pressure by the new demands. Relationships with both sets of parents will also change and need to be balanced. Equally, if you continue to work, particularly if you have a successful and demanding career, you may find that managing a job and a family is more difficult than you had anticipated, even if you have help at home. It may be a struggle to establish a routine that allows you to be a person as well as a mother.

The woman who has unrealistic expectations of what motherhood involves may feel the loss of freedom deeply. Some mothers may even experience depression. Prolonged depression after the birth of a baby should not be dismissed as merely "baby blues" and should always be

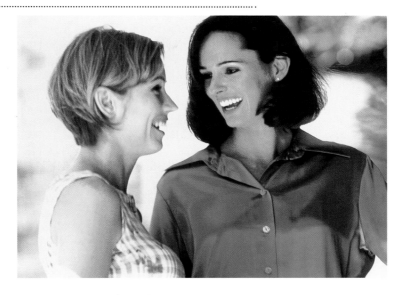

taken seriously. As a new mother, you may be alarmed by the demands the new baby makes on you. Some new mothers who do not have an extended family to turn to at this time can feel lonely and isolated if they have chosen not to return to work. They may want to look to other mothers in their community for company and support. Physically, parenting becomes easier after the first couple of years, but the demands of raising children still pose important challenges of this stage of life.

Equally, for those without children, career pressures or life crises such as redundancy or separation from a partner can trigger depression and anxiety. If you don't wish to lean on your friends and family—or if they are the cause of your misery—seeing your doctor, a counsellor or psychotherapist can be a great help.

BECOMING A PARENT
When you have a baby, you no longer think of yourself first, but of the child who gives you a new sense of purpose and direction.

FREEDOM OF CHOICE
Many women nowadays choose to delay motherhood, giving them the chance to pursue a career and enjoy a carefree social life.

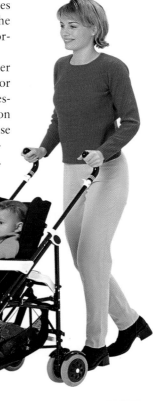

The middle years

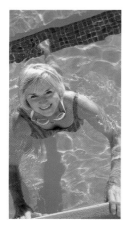

KEEPING FIT
Keep your figure in trim by taking regular exercise such as swimming, which calms the mind as well as toning the body.

For many women, their 40s and 50s can be a rich stage of life. At work, your career may have developed to give you wider scope and responsibilities. Your emotional life may be more settled than the turbulent earlier years, either in a relationship or with single status. The 40s are also a hugely varied time: you may be childless, whether from choice or not, or looking after babies or toddlers, or your children may be becoming independent, leaving you with time to take up new interests.

If you have not become pregnant as planned—you have at most a 25 percent chance every month—by the age of 40 you will be conscious of your biological clock ticking. If motherhood is delayed, the cause may take longer to identify but, whereas past generations accepted infertility as something they had to live with, modern advances in medical science mean that there are a number of options available to women who have difficulty in conceiving. These—often costly—methods range from in vitro fertilization (IVF), sometimes using donor eggs or sperm to, in rare cases, finding a surrogate mother to carry and give birth to a child.

At the other end of the scale, you may suffer from the "empty nest syndrome", a feeling of loss when your children leave home. Occupying yourself with new, absorbing interests or taking up a sport may help fill the gap. Bear in mind that their love for you has not necessarily altered because your role in their lives has changed. Adult children can become good friends and confidantes and never really grow out of needing the support of their parents. Having reared your children and enjoyed watching them become independent through good and not-so-good times may have given you the confidence to take on any challenge that comes your way. Now is your chance to transfer the skills acquired during your years of raising children to the work world or, if you have always done paid work, to branch out and up.

The middle years do not necessarily bring problems with health, but regular screening to rule out or identify illnesses such as breast cancer becomes important. Increased responsibilities at work may cause stress and a woman will find that her body loses the elasticity of youth and often tends to put on weight. It is important in these years to take regular exercise and enjoy plenty of fresh air.

CHANGES OF THE MENOPAUSE

The end of fertility can bring great relief. At last, there is no longer the fear of an unwanted pregnancy, and this can have a positive effect on your sex life and your attitude toward embarking on new interests. If you were one of the unlucky few who wanted a child and did not have one, this is the time to adjust to the fact. The passage through the menopausal years will be marked by physical and emotional changes, some of which can be difficult, but sensitivity and the right kind of medical help will bring a new understanding of the way the body changes and what is important to ensure well-being for the rest of your life.

THE INNER WOMAN
Discovering new talents, or reviving those that were set aside due to lack of time, ensures that the mind is exercised and can be immensely satisfying. It can result in new friendships with those who share the same interests.

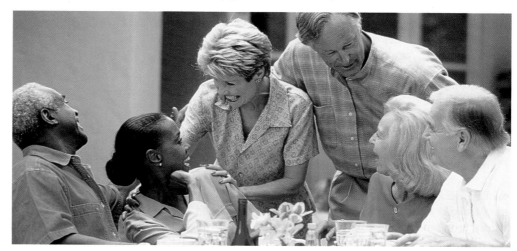

The "golden" years

With good health and vitality on your side, you can hope to live life to the full for 20–30 years after the age of 60. An optimistic approach to life after retirement can allow you to discover great happiness as a role model to the young, be an inspiration to your children and grandchildren, if you have them, and a valued companion to your friends.

If you understand yourself and are realistic about the hazards of later life that inhibit mobility and threaten independence, you will be able to take the best steps to help yourself. While medical advances can help—improved surgery provides new joints, such as hip replacements, and can give hearts new life with by-pass operations—prevention remains better than cure.

STAYING ALERT AND ACTIVE

The older woman is best fortified by a healthy lifestyle and positive attitude. It is never too late to stop smoking or to cut back on alcohol intake. Make sure that you continue to eat nutritious meals and exercise regularly. Exercise may need to be modified to suit your state of mobility, but a brisk walk every day keeps both body and mind stimulated. You should consult your doctor about what sort of exercise is suitable for you. Older women can have a session with a personal trainer just as well as younger ones, to find out their optimal exercise plan.

Exercising the mind is as important as exercising the body and now is the chance to make up for lost educational opportunities. Learning can open doors to many creative and productive hours. The marketplace is just realizing the potential of the older age group so take advantage of preferential rates on courses.

It may be that an older woman is increasingly confined indoors: it is now important to have the support of family, if possible, or medical or social workers. A network of more mobile friends will also help to keep you stimulated by visits, sharing books or videos and ensuring that you do not feel lonely or bored. There is generally no reason why the mental faculties should not function as well as they have ever done and many older women take great pleasure in reading and writing. A local history group may value your memories and compiling records can be an enjoyable activity.

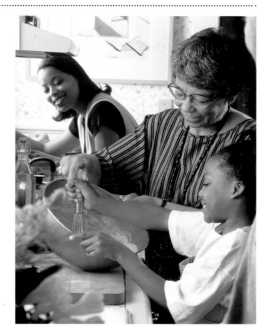

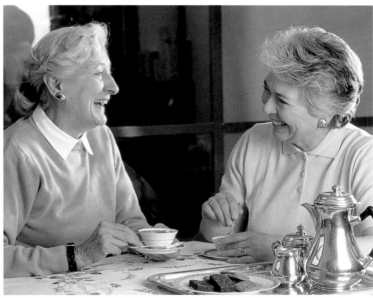

One inevitable part of growing older is the loss of loved ones. The death of a lifelong partner may seem like an irrecoverable blow. The sadness and depression that follows bereavement is a natural part of the mourning process. But if you can't move on—and many women hide their feelings and find it difficult to talk about their grief—your doctor should be able to refer you to someone who can help with this psychological impasse.

THE PLEASURES OF AGE
Having opportunities to keep in touch with the young enables a woman to pass on knowledge and experience. A sense of purpose may help her to find peace of mind.

SUPPORT AND FRIENDSHIP
Chatting to friends is one of the best tonics. In later years, women of the same age can share past experiences and provide mutual practical and moral support.

ESSENTIALS OF GOOD HEALTH

The earlier you establish good habits in terms of your general health, the more likely it is that well-being will be natural to you and your predisposition to certain illnesses may be decreased. There are some things you can't change, but there are others you can do something about.

See also:

3/GENERAL HEALTH ISSUES
Osteoporosis pp. 90–93

5/ILLNESSES & EMERGENCIES
Digestive system problems
pp. 190–203

Healthy nutrition

Nutrition is an art. To get the balance right, you need to ensure that your diet is varied, provides the nutrients your body needs and is both enjoyable and satisfying without placing you at risk of developing illnesses.

To find an approach to nutrition that will be sustainable, you should forget all about diets and dieting, which may cause you to feel stressed and will usually be abandoned. Your own nutritional plan can be established gradually from a basis of understanding why your body needs different types of foods and why too much of some do you no favours. Women often derive a third or more of their calorie intake from fat and this increases their susceptibility to cancer of the colon and breast, diabetes, high blood pressure and other disorders. Sugar, salt and alcohol may also affect women's health.

PROTEIN

From the time a child is conceived, it is protein that ensures the body's growth and good health. It is the body's building material, playing an essential role in making tissue and repairing it after damage through wear and tear.

Animal sources of protein are poultry, meat, fish, cheese, milk, yogurt and eggs. Vegetable sources are soy products, legumes (peas and beans), nuts and bread. Most people who eat meat consume more protein than the body needs and the excess is stored in the muscles and liver as glycogen. It can be converted for use as energy when there is not enough sugar circulating in the blood. The aim of healthy eating is to keep the blood sugar level balanced and to have little glycogen or fat stored.

CARBOHYDRATES

The body turns starches and sugars, known as carbohydrates, into glucose, which circulates in the blood to meet your energy needs. Nutritionally, carbohydrates should be the greatest part of a day's eating (as in the food pyramids, p. 19). There are, however, two categories.

Complex carbohydrates, which provide starch and fibre, are found in bread and wholegrain cereals, rice and pasta, vegetables and fruits. These release energy slowly and steadily. Simple carbohydrates are found in sugar and honey and in refined products such as biscuits, desserts, pies, ice creams and some breakfast cereals. They release energy quickly, but contain no essential nutrients. In healthy eating, simple carbohydrates should be taken as sparingly as fats.

FAT

Most people obtain dietary fat from eating protein foods, in which it is present naturally, through adding it when cooking and through eating foods in which it is not obvious. Studies have shown that while saturated fats are harmful, monounsaturated and polyunsaturated fats have health benefits.

Fat that you can see—on poultry, lamb, pork, beef or ham, for example—should be ▶

CARBOHYDRATE POWER
Provide yourself with energy by eating more pasta, rice, bread and cereal—foods high in carbohydrates. But be sparing with fatty sauces or spreads.

VITAMINS

Your body cannot function without vitamins, which are substances that provide the biochemical trigger for nerves, muscles, hormones, energy and waste production. The body can make some vitamins, but most come from foods. Those transported from the digestive tract in fat (called fat-soluble vitamins) can be stored by the body, but an excess of those vitamins soluble in water is generally excreted in the urine. Antioxidant vitamins counteract the damaging effect of molecules called free radicals, which are a by-product of energy production and are thought to trigger the ageing process.

Vitamin	Action	Sources
Vitamin A (fat soluble)	A major antioxidant, it keeps eyes and skin healthy and protects linings of respiratory, digestive and urinary tracts.	Liver, eggs, full-fat milk, butter, margarine and green, yellow and orange vegetables.
Vitamin B1 (thiamine)*	Assists in processing carbohydrates, protein and fats for energy.	Wholegrain cereals, milk, lean pork, soya beans and other pulses.
Vitamin B2 (riboflavin)* and B3 (niacin)*	Essential for energy and growth.	Lean offal, milk, cheese, cereals, enriched bread and flour, soya beans and green leafy vegetables (especially broccoli).
Vitamin B5 (pantothenic acid)*	Required for metabolism, the nervous system and sex hormones.	Most vegetables, eggs, wholegrain cereals, salmon, nuts and offal.
B6 (pyridoxine)*	Necessary for making red blood cells and antibodies.	Meat, fish, egg yolks, sweetcorn, bananas, avocados, nuts and wholegrain cereals.
B12 (fat soluble)	Vital for growth, red blood cells and the central nervous system.	Meat, offal, fish, eggs and dairy products.
Folic acid (folate)*	Crucial to the development of foetal nervous system during pregnancy.	Liver, kidneys, eggs, wholegrain cereals, peas, beans, nuts and green leafy vegetables.
Vitamin C (ascorbic acid)*	An antioxidant, it prevents infections, heals wounds, helps absorption of iron and controls blood cholesterol.	Fruit (especially citrus), green vegetables, potatoes, tomatoes and peppers.
Vitamin D (fat soluble)	Works with calcium to make healthy bones and is manufactured by the action of daylight on the skin.	Milk, oily fish and egg yolks; it is added to margarine, flour and some bread.
Vitamin E (fat soluble)	Reduces the risk of heart disease and can relieve menstrual cramps and PMS.	Most vegetable oils, eggs, nuts, lettuce, seeds, soya beans, seafood and offal.
Vitamin K (fat soluble)	Helps in blood clotting, bone formation and kidney function.	Green leafy vegetables, beef, liver, green tea, cheese and oats.

* water soluble

Fat facts

Fats have many functions. They absorb fat-soluble vitamins (p. 17), promote childhood development, help to produce sex hormones and regulate the metabolism. Fat has nine calories a gramme, over twice that of protein and carbohydrates, so a diet high in fat can cause a weight problem.

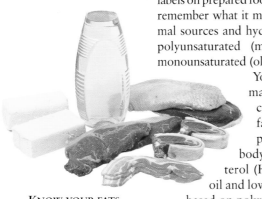

KNOW YOUR FATS
Saturated fats, such as butter or that found on meat, are hard at room temperature. Fats that are polyunsaturated are from vegetable sources, such as sunflower and corn, and oily fish. Olive oil and avocados contain monounsaturated fats.

See your doctor

Calcium, vitamin A, and iron supplements should be taken with care. As the condition of your bones and blood is essential to health, your doctor may prescribe calcium and vitamin D for women at risk of osteoporosis and iron for women with anaemia. You should not take either without first discussing it with your doctor. You may want to consult a nutritionist about substitutes for foods you don't eat, which provide essential vitamins and minerals.

trimmed before cooking or eating. Hidden fats are the biggest problem—they are included in processed foods such as pies, cakes and biscuits, in fast foods, and in many prepared, convenience dishes. Always read the labels on prepared foods; note the fat content and remember what it means—saturated (from animal sources and hydrogenated vegetable oils), polyunsaturated (most vegetable oils) and monounsaturated (olive and rapeseed oils).

You need to be careful in making choices. Foods that contain good fats—essential fatty acids that help transport vitamins around the body and benefit good cholesterol (HDL)—are oily fish, olive oil and low-fat spreads and dressings based on polyunsaturated vegetable oils. All contain linolenic acid which works with vitamin E to protect the heart. To reduce intake of bad fats, avoid eating block margarine, lard or dripping, french fries, pastries, doughnuts and croissants.

Some products may not necessarily be low in fat—the fat content could simply be "reduced" compared to the regular version of the product. Check the calorie values of a normal serving and a lower fat one. Foods can be labelled "reduced" or "low" fat and still have a high calorie count because of added sugar.

Fat substitutes such as Olestra, a synthetic compound, may be used in some snack foods (potato snacks, biscuits and "energy" bars) though it may not be listed among the ingredients. Eating foods containing fat substitutes may cause cramps and diarrhoea, and this in turn may cause important fat-soluble vitamins as well as other nutrients to be lost from the body.

VITAMINS AND MINERALS

Together, vitamins and minerals are called micronutrients and unlike the macronutrients—protein, carbohydrates and fats—they are only needed in trace amounts. With few exceptions, the body does not manufacture micronutrients: you must get them from a varied and balanced diet that includes dairy foods, fruits,

vegetables, nuts and seeds. Vitamins (p. 17) work in tandem with minerals to keep you mentally and physically healthy.

The antioxidants—vitamins A, C and E—are partnered by selenium, a mineral thought to be important in preventing heart disease and cancer. All minerals have a role, but calcium and iron are especially pertinent for women. Calcium builds bones and teeth, assists in normal blood clotting and in transmitting nerve impulses. Along with magnesium and phosphorus, also essential to bone building and muscle activity, it is found in milk, cheese, yogurt, tofu, green leafy vegetables and canned fish, such as sardines and salmon.

To make use of calcium the body needs vitamin D, which may come from the diet (p. 17) or through sunlight on the skin. Bone and teeth formation continues through your teens and 20s and, as calcium deficiency can lead to osteoporosis later in life, calcium should be part of your daily diet.

Iron is needed to make haemoglobin, which gives the blood its red colour and carries oxygen to all the cells. If you are deficient in iron you may feel tired, depressed and lack energy. This may happen if you suffer from heavy menstrual periods or if you are not obtaining enough vitamin C for your body to use the mineral efficiently. Iron is found in red meat (beef, lamb, liver), seafood, eggs, broccoli, brussels sprouts, peas, spinach and wholemeal bread.

LIQUIDS

About 70 percent of your body is water; it is in the bones, blood and every cell. Every day about 2½ litres (4¾ pints) leaves the body in sweat, breath, urine and faeces—and you need to drink plain water to make up for this loss. On a cold day, six to eight 225ml (8 oz) glasses are recommended; in hot weather you may need twice that. If you drink too much, you will simply urinate the excess. If you drink too little, your skin will dry out and

MOISTURE LEVELS
Sipping water throughout the day ensures that your body gets enough to make up for natural loss.

How much is a serving?

The amount of food you eat is measured as calories (also called Kcalories and kilojoules) which the body turns into energy. The aim is to eat the number of calories that meets your energy needs and provides you with healthy proportions of the right foods. Women's needs vary depending on age, activity level and whether pregnant or not.

Carbohydrates should form the basis of your day's eating. One serving: 1 slice wholemeal bread, 1 wholemeal pitta bread, 75 g (3 oz) cooked rice or pasta or kidney beans, 175 g (6 oz) baked potato, 120 g (4 oz) cooked peas, beans, lentils or sweetcorn, 25 g (1 oz) cooked broccoli, spinach or carrots, 1 tomato, 1 apple, pear, peach, nectarine or orange, 2 apricots or plums, 120 g (4 oz) berry fruits.

Calcium-rich foods, important for women, are in the next, protein, layer. One serving: 50 g (2 oz) hard cheese, 300 ml (half pint) semi-skimmed milk, 150 g (5 oz) yogurt, 75 g (3 oz) almonds or canned sardines, mackerel or salmon. Other protein servings: 75 g (3 oz) red or white meat, 1 egg, 120g (4 oz) fish.

you will become constipated. Tea and coffee should not be substitutes for plain water; more than three or four cups a day can inhibit the absorption of iron and keep you from sleeping well. In moderation, alcohol can be part of a nutritious diet.

HEALTHY EATING

What is known as an 80/20 plan is a good way to start. The plan recognizes that overconsumption of fats is the major problem in bad nutrition, regardless of the type of fat, and that fat is often accompanied by sugar. If you ensure that 80 percent of what you eat is healthy, low-fat food based on the wider bands of any of the pyramids (right), then you can allow yourself to eat sensible amounts of favourite foods containing fat/sugar for the other 20 percent. The 80 percent should include proteins (skinless chicken, lean meats, pulses, soya products), carbohydrates (fresh fruits, vegetables, grains, breads, cereals, potatoes and pasta) and little fat (low-fat dairy foods).

The changeover can be tackled gradually by substituting lower fat foods for high fat foods.

THE FOOD PYRAMIDS

All have the same purpose: to help you eat well and healthily. Choose foods from the wider, lower bands and eat less of the foods in higher bands. With all pyramid plans regular daily exercise is a recommended accompaniment.

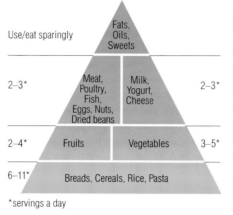

OPTIMAL WESTERN DAILY DIET

The first food pyramid was devised in the United States by nutritional scientists to increase intake of complex carbohydrates and reduce fats, saturated in particular, and simple sugars in the daily diet. Recommended servings balance vitamins and minerals needed for health, and provide fibre.

TRADITIONAL MEDITERRANEAN DIET

High in plant foods, particularly tomatoes, onions and garlic, and cheese, yogurt and olive oil every day. Fish, poultry, eggs and sweets can be eaten a few times a week. Red meat is optional once every 10 days and alcohol intake, typically red wine, is moderate, 2 glasses a day.

OPTIMAL ASIAN DIET

Traditionally rich in wholegrain, complex carbohydrates. Small servings of dairy products and fish can be taken daily, but sweets, eggs and meat are best restricted to once a week or even once a month. The balance goes awry in the Western world if too many sweets are eaten at the expense of grains.

Dieting and your weight

Women are bombarded with images of waif-like models—in magazines, movies and on television—presented as the ideal of beauty. These images can be a powerful force, especially for the young, who may come to accept that losing weight and "being on a diet" are a fact of life. The word "diet" in this context does not mean medically advised weight loss programmes designed for severely obese patients (see box, below right). The doubtful "diets" are those which promise miraculous transformation in the short term.

A hundred or more years ago women would not have had time to be as preoccupied with weight. The everyday preparation of food took energy and there was little opportunity to overeat. Their daily lives required constant energy, for almost non-stop work in the house and looking after a family. Their metabolism was attuned to burning up calories, with little to spare. Women today have more sedentary lifestyles and endless options for saving, rather than using, energy. But two important points remain true for women who lived then or now: food is good for you, and if you eat more than your body can use the excess will be stored as fat. For your metabolism to work at optimal speed, there needs to be a combination of chemical and physical processes.

DIETING MAKES FOOD AN ENEMY
Diet plans favouring grapefruits, cabbage soup, food combinations or even low-fat regimes are not the answer to losing weight. If you have been considering dieting because you think you ought to, give some thought to this fact: the vast majority of dieters eventually go back to their pre-diet weight, or become heavier than they were before. Most people who start dieting will continue to do so, on and off, for the rest of their lives. If a range of foods are designated as forbidden, dieters feel guilty if they transgress, which makes them feel worse about themselves.

Dieting makes food an enemy, not a source of sustenance and well-being. So called yo-yo dieting—losing weight, putting it back on, losing it again and so on—is bad for your health. If you suddenly reduce your food intake, your body, because it is designed for survival, will slow down your metabolic rate in order to store energy more efficiently. This is why people on a diet crave snacks like chocolate, which gives a quick boost to their energy levels, and why

Obesity and weight loss

Obese women have an excessive amount of body fat, which may affect them medically and psychologically. Dieticians work with doctors to devise and supervise a weight-loss programme which allows weight to be lost over time while re-educating eating habits. Basic to this is LEARN—an acronym for Lifestyle, Exercise, Attitudes, Relationships and Nutrition—which tracks these significant factors in the woman's life and gives her both reasonable goals and understanding of why each can influence her weight.

Low- and very low-calorie diets, under medical supervision, are designed to cause rapid weight loss while maintaining nutritional needs. Energy comes from stored fat, encouraged by prescribed exercise based on the health status of the woman and how overweight she is. In some cases medication may also be prescribed.

CHOOSE FOODS WELL
To reach and maintain a reasonable body weight you need a balanced diet full of nutrients to prevent disease and to ensure optimal energy and psychological well-being.

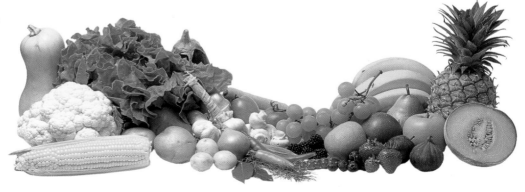

weight loss slows down dramatically after the first couple of weeks.

Weight loss in the early weeks of crash dieting is not, as many women believe, made up mostly of unwanted fat. First you lose those carbohydrates stored in the muscles and liver as glycogen. This is why you feel tired on such a diet and have less strength for lifting and running—because you are losing muscle power. You also lose a lot of water, which may make you feel less bloated and slimmer, when in fact you are still carrying the same amount of fat on your body.

REASONS FOR WEIGHT INCREASE

The way you feel about yourself, and your life, plays a part in weight build-up. It is quite common for people to report that when they are happy they stop overeating and their body weight stabilizes. Others say they gain weight when they are miserable. But both of these may be too simplistic. There are various factors that are known to play a part in being overweight. Keeping a daily diary of thoughts, feelings and events may help you understand which of the factors relate to you.

An unbalanced diet Good nutrition is all about balance and variety. You may not be aware how frequently you opt for types of foods, particularly those that are high in fat or sugar. In your diary make a note of everything you put in your mouth over a period of two weeks, then look at your notes carefully. How many days did you have pizza or a burger or other takeaway? How many days did you not have milk or fruit or vegetables? How many days did you have sweet snacks or a drinking session with friends? How many days did you not eat wholegrain cereals or breads?

Not enough exercise Many people genuinely feel that they do not eat more than friends and family but they put weight on more easily. Perhaps your body is just not expending enough energy. From the mid-30s on, about 225 g (8 oz) of muscle can be lost each year in women, usually replaced by fat. What is called your "fat-free mass" determines your resting metabolic rate (RMR) which gets on with the job of converting about 75 percent of your daily calories for the body to use. The larger your frame and the more toned your muscles the greater your RMR. The most effective way of improving this is to exercise regularly.

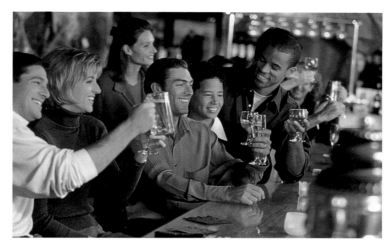

Boredom and depression Note the time you ate, along with what you ate, and how hungry you felt, in your food diary. Note the reason you ate, too, such as because you were offered food, it was a mealtime, you were putting off doing something else you didn't want to do or you were upset. Eating for comfort may be satisfying in the short term, but if you are really depressed or unhappy with your circumstances, eating will aggravate your problem. It would be better to seek help from your doctor.

Poor self image If you have low self-confidence, for whatever reason, you may subconsciously believe your body is not worth respecting, that you deserve to feel fat and unattractive because no one, including yourself, thinks that you're worth anything. This then becomes self-perpetuating. If you let yourself put on excess weight, you are less likely to feel at your best and you will despise yourself more for not being able to control what you eat.

Poor eating habits How and when you eat may be part of your problem, especially if you do not have established mealtimes. Do you feel pressured to eat and drink more than you should when out with friends? Do you grab a chocolate bar or fast food when you don't have time for a meal? Do you eat when you have nothing to do or are feeling stressed? Do you finish up food left on your child's plate? Your food diary will help you to identify these habits.

Genetic links If your parents were overweight, you may have inherited the tendency (though this is the least common cause). It can be difficult to differentiate whether you have inherited poor eating habits or possess a real disposition to store fat. Either way, there is no need to accept being overweight as a way of life.

WOMEN AND ALCOHOL
The social pressure of drinking may be hard to resist and having too much too often can cause weight gain. However, a moderate amount of alcohol, taken with food as part of a considered eating plan, may be beneficial to health.

An exercise plan

Today most people do not get as much exercise going about their daily life as they used to—increasingly, jobs and shops are some distance from home so it is impossible to walk to and from them. As well, labour-saving devices have taken much of the exertion out of housework, we spend too much of our working lives sitting in front of computers and our leisure time watching television.

It remains a fact, however, that the route to good health is a combination of regular exercise, nutritious eating, maintaining an ideal weight and enjoying plenty of restful sleep. Lifelong adherence to this may prevent some of the disorders that primarily affect women, including premenstrual syndrome (PMS), constipation and osteoporosis, as well as, in recent years, diabetes and coronary artery disease which were once predominantly male problems. The effect of regular exercise provides other benefits, such as relieving stress, helping to slow the effects of ageing and reducing the symptoms of debilitating diseases like osteoarthritis.

Before deciding on an exercise plan, consider your reasons for getting fit. You may want to be fitter to play a sport, to fulfil an ambition, such as running a marathon, or to lose weight and stop it returning. You may simply want to feel better, have energy left at the end of the day, be emotionally stable and enjoy activities which entertain and reward you. Exercise should never be a punishment or boring.

To change your shape, you need a programme that combines aerobic and strength training. Fitness training can make you a better sports player, tone your muscles and cut down your body fat. There are three components to an overall fitness programme: aerobic endurance, muscle strength and flexibility. Aerobic exercise is vital for a strong heart and efficient lungs. Muscle strength and endurance mean good support for your skeleton and better posture. Flexibility keeps you mobile as you age, minimizing any risk of straining or pulling muscles in daily life.

The aim of exercise

Women should aim to reach from 75 to 85 percent of the average maximum heart rate for their age group during aerobic exercise. You calculate the rate by deducting your age from 220. So, if you are 35, your average maximum rate is 185 beats per minute; when exercising, your heart rate should be 138 to 157. If you are a beginner, start slowly. Gradually increase session frequency and length until your heart rate is 92 to 111 beats per minute, 50 to 60 percent of the maximum.

WOMEN AND EXERCISE

Varying what exercise and how much you do challenges your body. But it should never be overdone. Excessive exercise can alter a woman's body fat to lean muscle mass ratio. This can lead to menstrual irregularities and can be a problem for athletes and performers, such as gymnasts and skaters, and women with eating disorders who use exercise as a method of burning calories. What is called exercise-induced amenorrhoea may be reversed, but during the time the body does not ovulate it lacks oestrogen, which can cause calcium to leach out of bones, and bone thinning, leading to osteoporosis later in life.

It is not the exercise that is at fault, but the strenuousness of it. At and after the menopause women can reduce their risk of osteoporosis with weight-bearing exercises which help the bones. Walking, hiking, jogging, dancing, step aerobics, tennis and cross-country skiing all improve bone mass, agility and balance. Add training with weights to this and you increase bone density and muscular strength as well.

SETTING YOUR GOALS

Take into account the amount of time you have and plan accordingly. Flexibility exercises should be done daily—stretching helps to lengthen the muscles and tendons. You should warm up first with slow, smooth and rhythmic movements, and cool down with the same movements after your session is over.

To increase fitness levels, at least three times a week you should do 20 minutes of aerobic exercise to the point of being nearly breathless—sustained running and swimming, for example. This makes you breathe harder, and the heart beat faster to supply the muscles with extra oxygen. At this level of activity you should be able—just—to keep up a conversation.

Exercise specialists suggest an activity formula of 70 to 80 percent aerobic to 20 to 30 percent anaerobic (not requiring extra oxygen). The combination increases the ratio of muscle to fat more effectively than either approach on its own. If you wish to lose weight you can work up to the aerobic level, having first of all checked with a doctor that the programme you are beginning will be right for you and your health. Remember that pain is a sign that you should stop. If your joints start to hurt as a result of walking or running, change to swimming, in which the water cushions the joints, so that you can maintain aerobic fitness without placing further strain on your body.

CHOOSE YOUR ROUTINE

There is a variety of ways in which to motivate yourself to regular exercise.

Exercising on your own If you plan to work out to a fitness video or buy home exercise equipment be sure, before spending too much, that you have the self-discipline to go it alone. Goal: at least three days a week.

A structured approach At a gym you will receive the benefits of a tailor-made programme and guidance from experts, but you can go at times that suit you and exercise at your own pace. Investigate weight training using special-ized equipment such as Nautilus or Bodymaster, or free weights. You must use a trainer's help to learn the right techniques and to prevent injury. Do not do more than an hour at a time and don't exercise the same muscle group on two consecutive days. Goal: three times a week, for 45 minutes each time (build up to 60).

If you are sociable Aerobic, aqua aerobics or Stairmaster classes are a good choice. In a class you will feel motivated by other members. The qualified instructors are trained to ensure your movements don't do more harm than good. Goal: two 60-minute classes a week. If possible, a weekly swim or yoga session as well.

Take up a sport Badminton can be enjoyed at all levels; squash can too, but it is faster and more competitive. Basketball and tennis are routes to aerobic fitness and bone strength. Golf has the added advantage of combining fresh air and walking. Country and ballroom dancing are good for bones, and for training the memory. Goal: two or more sessions a week.

Be flexible Even if you are resolutely against gyms, classes or playing a sport you can improve your fitness by incorporating more walking into your daily routine and increasing the pace gradually. Goal: a brisk 30-minute walk five times a week, but build up to this.

> **! Caution**
> Do not attempt too much too soon. Always warm up by gentle stretching. Muscles that are not used to exercise can be easily strained or damaged. Never exercise if you have a weight-bearing joint that is swollen, painful or has a reduced range of movement. You should not work out every day. Your muscles need time to recuperate between sessions. After exercise, even at rest, lean muscle burns calories.

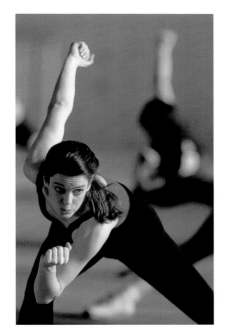

CLASSES CAN BE FUN
In a gym you will have the support of exercise physiologists who can give you guidance on a range of activities which will strengthen your muscles, increase bone mass and density, and burn up calories so fat doesn't have time to be stored.

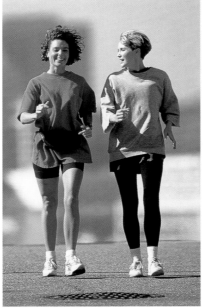

KEEP ON THE MOVE
Jogging, running or brisk walking will get you out into the fresh air, raise your spirits and keep the muscles of your legs, arms and trunk well toned. Always wear the right type of shoes to protect your feet and prevent damage to tendons.

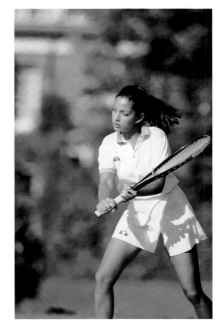

BECOME A TEAM PLAYER
Racket sports, played outdoors and indoors, allow you to meet people and to keep fit at the same time. Tennis and badminton are especially good for women as the movements stimulate the bone marrow, helping bone strength.

The rewarding pattern of sleep

Sleep is a basic need, as essential for mental and physical health as nutrition and exercise. It allows your body to rest and recuperate so it can function efficiently and energetically during the waking hours.

On average you spend one-third of your life asleep, although this varies through the years, and less is needed in later life. A year-old baby will sleep for about 14 out of 24 hours but most adults need just seven or eight hours a night. Some say they manage on as few as four hours; others need 11 or 12 to be at their best.

The occasional sleepless night will do no harm, though it can make you feel awful next day. Continuous sleep deprivation, however, may affect the way you work, your moods and your physical well-being, for without sleep the body does not have the chance to repair itself. Going without sleep for as little as three days can lead to confusion, serious mental problems and may even cause hallucinations.

Through research on volunteers attending sleep laboratories, scientists now know what happens to the body while you sleep. A normal sleep pattern has been identified that has two parts to it: REM (rapid eye-movement sleep, when your brain is most active and you dream) and NREM (non-rapid eye-movement sleep, when you don't dream).

Volunteers, linked to an electroencephalogram (ECG) that measures brain waves, are woken when electrical activity indicates REM and confirm that they were dreaming. People tend not to remember a dream unless they wake up during or immediately after it.

During sleep your brain remains active, analysing the past day's events and storing and processing information. Sleep may also be a time of mental healing, because dreaming is thought to help you come to terms with any emotional problems.

HOW SLEEP HAPPENS

Once you are comfortable in bed, your eyes close and you begin to doze; your body twitches as nerves and muscles relax. During this phase, called shallow sleep, you can be wakened easily by the slightest disturbance because you are still aware of your surroundings. After half an hour or so, sleep becomes deeper: you relax, your heart beats more slowly and you become oblivious to your surroundings. Truly deep sleep follows, during which you are completely relaxed. You remain in one position, your heart rate slows right down and your breathing is slow and regular.

It was once thought that this deep sleep continued until you woke naturally, but scientists have discovered that each of the three stages lasts about half an hour, and that the 90-minute sleep cycle repeats itself through the night. On average, four cycles are needed for a good night's sleep. Toward morning, sleep is more shallow than deep as brain waves speed up again, the heart rate increases, breathing is more rapid and you become more restless. You can seem on the verge of waking and may even open your eyes, but in fact you are asleep.

YOUR BIOLOGICAL CLOCK

The natural sleep pattern is regulated by your biological clock, synchronized by the 24-hour, or circadian, cycle of light and dark. It oversees all body functions, from digestion and waste disposal to sleeping and cell repair.

One of the clock's influences is the so-called third eye, the pineal gland at the front of the brain. As daylight fades, the gland secretes the hormone melatonin into the bloodstream, which makes you sleepy. Melatonin works with another hormone, cortisol. The cortisol level

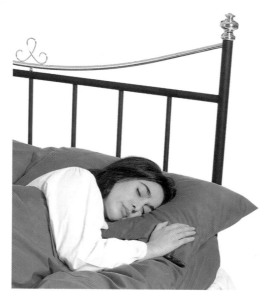

SLEEPING AND DREAMING
Scientists in sleep laboratories use a device called an electroencephalogram (ECG) to record the volunteer's electrical brain activity. During dreaming, characterized by rapid eye movements (REM), the activity is much the same as when a person is awake.

CIRCADIAN RHYTHM
During a 24-hour period, the rise and fall of the hormones cortisol and melatonin tell you when to wake up and when you are tired and need sleep.

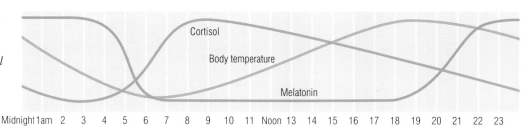

Cortisol

Body temperature

Melatonin

Midnight 1am 2 3 4 5 6 7 8 9 10 11 Noon 13 14 15 16 17 18 19 20 21 22 23

falls gradually and is at its lowest point after you've been asleep for several hours, when your body temperature is also low. At this stage the hypothalamus in the brain prompts the pituitary to direct the other endocrine glands into action to stimulate your metabolism. Your body temperature rises along with the cortisol level and eventually this wakes you from sleep.

WHEN REST IS DISTURBED

If you suffer from sleep disturbance, the balance of these biological processes is upset. In many instances the effects may only be short term. Periods of sleeplessness occur during pregnancy, and parents may end up feeling exhausted after weeks or months of night-time feeds after a child is born. Long-distance air travel across several time zones can also play havoc with the body's clock so that night and day lose their meaning.

When sleep disturbance is ongoing, it may need attention. Working mothers who don't get enough rest may be stressed from trying to balance the demands of career, home and children. The most common symptoms of lack of sleep are irritability and loss of concentration, which can have serious consequences. It is estimated that one in five car accidents is caused by sleepiness or sleep disorders, and people who work with machinery put themselves at risk. For safety, people who work night shifts have to establish a pattern that forces the body to adapt to sleeping by day.

CAUSES OF INSOMNIA

Most women experience sleep disturbance at some point in their lives, but you should consult your doctor if you can't remain asleep for an adequate length of time, and you do not wake feeling refreshed. This is medically known as insomnia and may be treated by drugs which establish good sleeping habits and reduce brain activity. Insomnia is not unusual at the menopause, and may also be a symptom of migraine, stress, anxiety or depression. For all of these medical help should be sought.

The most unfortunate are those who suffer from chronic insomnia, which means that they are either unable to fall asleep, or that they fall asleep immediately they put their head on the pillow but wake not long after and stay that way for much of the night. This may affect their metabolism which relies on being stimulated in the hours before waking by deep breathing.

If your body is showing signs of oxygen starvation—rapid shallow breathing, interspersed with frequent sighing, yawning and erratic breathing rates—deep breathing exercises, in which you take a lot more oxygen into your lungs, may improve your situation. Over time this type of shallow breathing results in emotional distress and physical exhaustion.

> **! Caution**
> If you believe you sleep well and wake naturally but still feel tired all the time, you should consult your doctor. Any number of conditions may be the cause, including anaemia, poor thyroid function or night sweats caused by the onset of the menopause. Your place of work may be the culprit if there is a serious lack of light and circulating fresh air. Too much of the day spent in this environment can affect both your biological clock and your metabolism.

Tips for a good night's sleep

♀ Try to keep to a regular bedtime routine, even at weekends. Going to bed and getting up at roughly the same time every day can programme your body to behave as you wish.

♀ Avoid stimulants such as coffee or tea several hours before bedtime. Have a warm, caffeine-free drink instead.

♀ Have your last meal several hours before retiring and avoid too much alcohol—this may help you fall asleep initially but may make you restless later.

♀ Try some relaxing techniques before getting into bed. Have a warm—but not hot—bath, listen to restful music or do gentle and reflective exercises, such as yoga or meditation.

♀ Make your bedroom conducive to rest and relaxation. The ideal temperature for sleep is 15–18°C (60–65°F). Make the room as dark as possible—light can come in through closed eyelids. This is particularly important for shiftworkers, who will find it easier to sleep during daylight hours if night-time conditions can be simulated.

♀ Check that your bed is as comfortable as it should be, particularly if you are waking with a stiff neck or back. Ideally, you should buy a new bed every 10 years or so, during which time you will have spent on average 29,000 hours in it. If you sleep with a partner, the bed should be big enough for you both to move easily without disturbing each other. Both of you should check the bed's size in the store.

♀ If you can't get to sleep, don't lie there worrying about it. Get up and do something else until you feel tired enough to try again.

The look of well-being

Too often women can be affected by negative thought structures. They might have picked them up from their families as children, from the society they live in or from the media. One of the most powerful of these is your perception of the way you look, but it spills over into behaviour patterns such as parenting, relationships and work, if the accompanying unspoken message exhorts you to "be perfect". Difficulties then arise when there is so much in your daily life that you feel you fail if you can't do it all. Living up to demands and expectations of you as a girlfriend, wife, mother and working woman may force you to set impossibly high goals which are counterproductive to mental and physical health.

BE POSITIVE

Researchers have found that being good to yourself has physical health benefits that show on the outside. The healthiest people seem to be those who love, seek and create pleasure. Positive moods and emotions delight the senses and directly affect the immune, nervous and cardiovascular systems. Taking time for yourself, seeking beautiful sights, melodious sounds, delicious smells, delectable tastes and warm touch, enhances well-being and is self-nurturing.

This may be the first move you need to take if you feel you are being compromised mentally and physically by the way you are living. When you make the decision to embark on changes you have been considering for a while and discover how cheerful and well you feel the benefits will start to show. You will find you are thinking more clearly and are more optimistic. Self-nurturing is a positive step to reduce risks for illness.

You may not experience an overnight change to glowing skin and shining hair after starting a healthy eating and exercise programme. You can, however, be heartened by the fact that what you put into your body in terms of nutritious food and how actively you engage in strength- and stamina-promoting exercise will show up eventually. All changes take time.

Your determination to succeed will be helped by setting realistic and achievable goals. There are no miracle shortcuts. You need to work at losing weight or maintaining an ideal weight and the support of an exercise physiologist or group with similar interests will encourage you to get the best perspective and boost you if you are not progressing as well as you had hoped. Concentrate on what you have achieved, and make sure you get a good night's sleep and sensible rest periods between activities.

INVEST IN SELF-ESTEEM

Self-confidence has nothing to do with youth or money, but it is an attractive quality to foster. It is possible to achieve it by committing yourself to a lifestyle in which you take time for your own pleasure (it need not be expensive or complicated, but should bring you joy). Don't base your sense of worth on other people's approval or gratitude toward you, don't feel you have to give in order to get praise and don't think of yourself only as a caretaker of others.

Finding time to care for yourself, to build your self-esteem, has a good effect on your physical health. If there are things you feel need some correction—facial hair or skin problems, for example—you'll have the confidence to seek the right help from professionals.

HOW DO YOU FEEL ABOUT YOUR BODY? *Most women probably have something they want to change about their size or shape. Having the confidence to invest in health and fitness will enhance self-acceptance and self-esteem.*

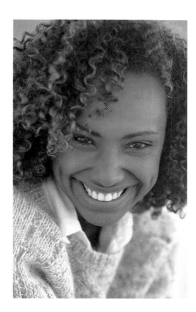

EXUBERANCE OF YOUTH
The world is your oyster—there are so many opportunities to seize and you have a positive view of your future development. Being surrounded by family and friends helps you to have a sense of your own individuality and worth.

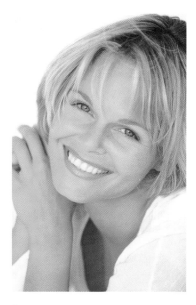

STRENGTH OF PURPOSE
Concentrating on career and burgeoning relationships can bring a sense of contentment with self. You are aware that things do not always turn out the way you had anticipated, but with this realization comes the ability to deal with unforeseen events.

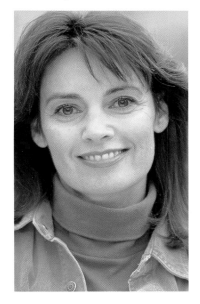

THE CERTAINTY OF MATURITY
Growing confidence comes from knowing yourself and what you want to achieve, and the best ways to do it. If you find you are unable to choose or have difficulty in making decisions, it may be that you need to reassess your priorities.

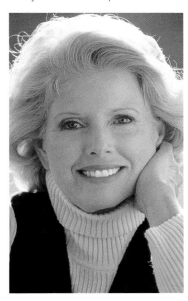

AT HOME IN THE PRESENT
Being happy with the age you are shows for all to see. It's not a matter of looking back or forward, but enjoying all that the present offers. Accepting that changes can and do occur can help you cope with twinges of anxiety such changes can cause.

Cosmetic surgery: the questions to ask

Many people today have cosmetic surgery. It has come to be regarded as a procedure performed not only for vanity—although that does still occur—but also to correct pronounced features that may be causing a person distress. If, for example, you feel so self-conscious about your nose (despite friends' reassurances) that it is interfering with the way you lead your life, your doctor may refer you to a cosmetic surgeon who can reshape it.

Having cosmetic surgery is a big undertaking and not to be embarked on lightly. Consider the following:

♀ Is it really the offending feature that causes you grief or are you troubled by other aspects of your life, such as a recent divorce, bereavement or crisis of self-confidence? Why not seek help for these problems and then see how you feel?

♀ Are your expectations realistic? Don't proceed with surgery expecting to come out looking like a model. Bear in mind, too, that you may in fact have become so used to the feature you are going to have changed that you find it difficult to adjust to the new one or, worse still, that you end up not liking the result.

♀ Do you know what such surgery entails? How many operations are involved, and over what length of time?

♀ Are you fearful of growing old? Cosmetic surgery will not delay signs of ageing forever, and you may have to repeat the procedure after a few years. In the long term, healthy eating and exercise are better.

If you decide to go ahead with surgery, seek the best, but not through advertisements. Take recommendations from your doctor or friends. See more than one surgeon, if necessary, before you commit yourself. It is important that you like and trust a prospective surgeon, that she or he will happily show you extensive before and after pictures of work done and is willing to answer all your questions, and at length.

Make a list of questions you want to ask before the appointment. You need to know whether you should take time off from work, whether there will be bruising or scarring and what after-care is involved. Make sure you understand the answers.

A safe place to work

See also:

3/GENERAL HEALTH ISSUES
Skeletal system problems
    pp. 84–89

5/ILLNESSES & EMERGENCIES
Respiratory problems
    pp. 213–221
Problems of the senses
    pp. 236–243

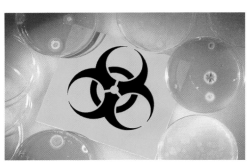

KNOW THE DANGERS
Wherever you work, you should be aware of anything that may be a hazard to your health. Substances that are dangerous should be labelled and well displayed for all to see.

People can suffer ill health or injury as a direct result of their jobs. Employers have a duty to ensure that the working conditions of all employees are compatible with their safety, health and well-being.

As women make up such a large part of the workforce and work in a wide variety of jobs, it is important that they know what the minimum requirements are. Workplaces are not all the same and you should know what you should expect from yours, and what can be done about it if conditions are not satisfactory.

All parts of the working areas should be cleaned regularly, have good ventilation and be well lit. You should be provided with the correct equipment or furniture to carry out your work properly. There should be separate and easily accessible toilets for men and women (which should not lead directly from a workspace), with hand washing and drying facilities. Women should be provided with an efficient and hygienic way to dispose of sanitary protection. There should be a safe place for staff to keep personal belongings secure against theft.

Buildings need not be old and run-down for working conditions to be poor. Sometimes the most modern and attractive working environment can have an inefficient ventilation system and the lack of fresh air can cause headaches, respiratory conditions, sleep disturbance and other health problems.

Some types of work involve hazards that need specific rules. Many workplace accidents happen because employees have not been given proper training. Where there are dangerous substances involved, for example, labels should be large and clear—easily recognizable by the words "irritant", "corrosive", "toxic" or "poisonous". You should receive proper instructions about these substances, including action that should be taken if you come into contact with one or if fumes are escaping into the work area.

An employer should routinely carry out an assessment of such substances, making sure they

Assessing your risks

Your health is important, obviously, but it is important to keep a sense of proportion about your work and workplace. There may be many rewards from the job you do that you would be reluctant to lose. It's a matter of balancing the risks and benefits.

You certainly don't want to run any risk which could cause you to become long-term unemployable. Accepting that hazards are a part of everyday life—for example, that you are much more likely to be run over by a bus than have a blood clot when taking the oral contraceptive pill—will help you see your workplace from a rational perspective.

If allergies start appearing or you are constantly getting colds, backache or headaches, these may be symptoms of an unsuitable environment and a job you are not enjoying. Try focusing on what you can change—the chair you sit on, the air you breathe, the number of breaks you take—and see if that makes a difference. If it doesn't, looking for a new job may be the best solution.

are not putting anyone at risk. People working in laboratories or as cleaners or caretakers are particularly vulnerable, but any member of staff can touch or inhale a substance that has not been stored securely or labelled correctly.

Some potentially harmful substances are not so obvious and protective clothing or masks may be needed. In a garment factory, the large amount of fluff and dust in the air may get into your lungs; or working with paper and inks can result in cuts and irritated skin. People working with flowers can get rashes from pesticides and from the plants themselves.

TAKE A BREAK
Regular breaks are necessary for those whose work involves repetitive hand and arm movements to prevent the development of serious upper limb disorders. These disorders are characteristic of a wide range of occupations (food and clothes production, assembly line manufacturing, cleaning, hairdressing and using computers) and account for a large percentage of occupational poor health in women, who are

mostly employed in these jobs. Constant pressure to meet tight deadlines, lack of regular breaks and badly designed seating and equipment can all affect the body.

Short frequent breaks—5 to 10 minutes every hour or so—are better than longer, occasional breaks. These breaks are most effective if you can walk away from your immediate workspace to refresh yourself. Getting some fresh air into your lungs during the course of the day—a brisk walk in the lunch break, for example—is the best antidote to workplace air.

If you experience any pain, swelling, pins and needles or numbness in the arms or legs you should report it immediately to your supervisor or employer so that action can be taken to find out what is wrong.

SPEAKING OUT

Whether it is about pregnancy or another issue, you may not know your rights and feel daunted at the thought of approaching your employer to discuss it. Talking problems over with colleagues to get their views and then speaking to your line manager could be the best solution. If this worries you, you could ask a trade union representative to speak to the employer on your behalf. You could also investigate assertiveness training to learn to put your point of view.

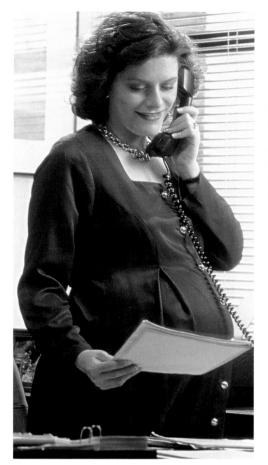

WORK WHILE YOU WAIT
In some types of employment, work that is normally safe may become hazardous if you are pregnant. You should express your concerns and see if you can move to a safer job within the company for the duration of the pregnancy.

SAFE WORKING AT A SCREEN

♀ Make sure your desk is at the correct and comfortable height for you.
♀ You should have an adjustable and stable chair, preferably with a foot rest.
♀ You need sufficient space in front of the keyboard to provide support for hands.
♀ There should be enough space for you to change position and vary your movements.
♀ Your desk should be large enough to hold all of the documents that you are working from.
♀ The screen should not have light shining on it directly and should have an anti-glare surface. It should be able to be moved.
♀ Your neck and shoulders should not be under stress.
♀ Blink often to prevent your eyes becoming dry or use eye drops to moisten them.

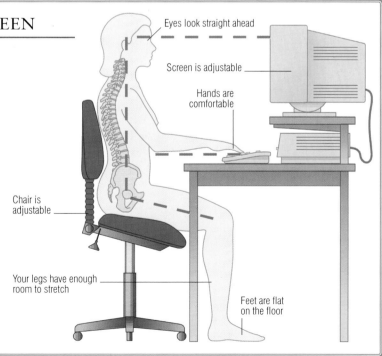

Eyes look straight ahead

Screen is adjustable

Hands are comfortable

Chair is adjustable

Your legs have enough room to stretch

Feet are flat on the floor

HEALTHY BODY SYSTEMS

There are many differences between the male and female body systems, related to the various functions needed. Knowing about all the parts that make up your body can help you be alert to changes that may need to be dealt with.

See also:

1/BEING A WELL WOMAN
Essentials of good health
pp. 16–29

3/GENERAL HEALTH ISSUES
Skeletal system problems
pp. 78–93

The skeletal system

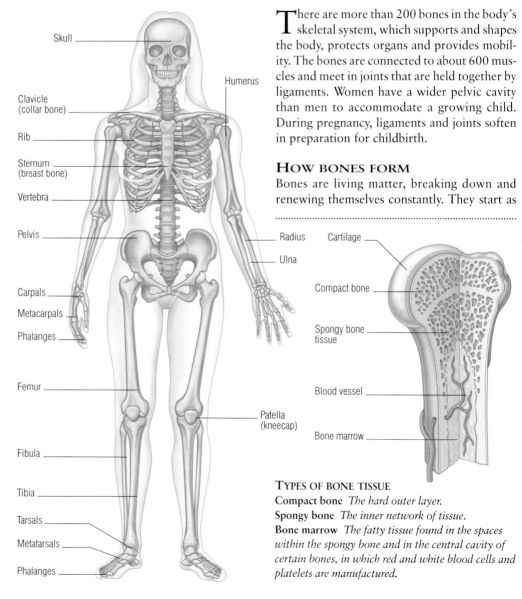

Skull

Humerus

Clavicle
(collar bone)

Rib

Sternum
(breast bone)

Vertebra

Pelvis

Radius

Ulna

Carpals

Metacarpals

Phalanges

Femur

Patella
(kneecap)

Fibula

Tibia

Tarsals

Metatarsals

Phalanges

Cartilage

Compact bone

Spongy bone
tissue

Blood vessel

Bone marrow

TYPES OF BONES
Long bones *These consist of a shaft with a knob at each end and are found in legs, arms and ribs.*
Short bones *Found in, for instance, the ankles and wrists, these are box shape, and are sited in places where extra strength is required.*
Flat bones *Found in the skull and shoulder blades, and similar in construction to short bones.*
Irregular bones *These include pneumatic bones, found in the nasal cavities and the middle ear, which contain aircells; sesamoid bones, like the kneecap, which are embedded in cartilage; and accessory bones, extra bones that did not fuse during development and are sometimes found in the feet.*

There are more than 200 bones in the body's skeletal system, which supports and shapes the body, protects organs and provides mobility. The bones are connected to about 600 muscles and meet in joints that are held together by ligaments. Women have a wider pelvic cavity than men to accommodate a growing child. During pregnancy, ligaments and joints soften in preparation for childbirth.

HOW BONES FORM
Bones are living matter, breaking down and renewing themselves constantly. They start as

TYPES OF BONE TISSUE
Compact bone *The hard outer layer.*
Spongy bone *The inner network of tissue.*
Bone marrow *The fatty tissue found in the spaces within the spongy bone and in the central cavity of certain bones, in which red and white blood cells and platelets are manufactured.*

cartilage and harden as you grow. This process is continuous and is particularly important around puberty, when hormones stimulate the mix of protein (collagen) and minerals to strengthen and thicken the bones. By the age of 25, bone has reached its maximum length.

Cartilage remains only at the end of weight-bearing bones in joints and between vertebrae in the spine, where it acts as a shock absorber; cartilage also gives shape to the end of the nose, the ears and the trachea. Bone thickness continues to increase until you are in your 30s, after which it declines gradually. The fastest decline is in the first year following the menopause, because of loss of oestrogen, and continues for a decade. By the age of 70, bone density is reduced by as much as one-third.

Bones are hard on the outside but soft and spongy inside. Bone marrow, which manufactures blood cells and is stored in bone cavities, is red at birth. Later, most of it becomes yellow fatty tissue. In adults, red blood cell production—about 200 billion cells a day— takes place in the spine, breastbone (sternum), ribs, collarbones, hip bones and skull bones.

WHAT CAN GO WRONG

The human skeletal system has to work hard to meet all the demands made upon it. The weight-bearing joints—the spine, hips and knees—are the most vulnerable. All bones are susceptible to fractures if they are twisted or have excessive strain placed on them. Frequent fractures may indicate bones are more fragile than normal.

Osteoarthritis—long-term damage to the cartilage-covered surface of the joints—is common in older people as a result of wear and tear; it affects twice as many women as men. Osteoporosis, in which the total bone mass is reduced and the bones become brittle, is the most common bone disorder affecting women. Preventive measures can minimize bone loss.

TYPES OF JOINTS
Hinge *In the elbows, fingers and toes.*
Gliding *In the spine, wrists and ankles.*
Ball and socket *In the shoulders and hips.*
Saddle *In the thumbs.*

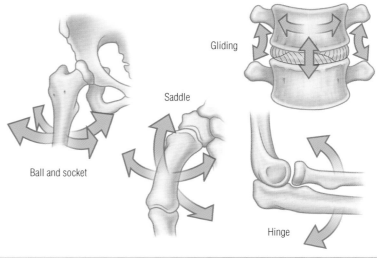

Gliding

Saddle

Ball and socket

Hinge

MUSCLE POWER

Bones can go nowhere without muscles, which make up between 30 and 40 percent of the weight of a woman's body. It may take 20 or 30 muscles working together to move you around, yet keep you balanced. The muscles lift and rotate bones, enabling you to carry out physical actions such as pulling, pushing, squeezing, stretching, walking, running and jumping. They work as opposing pairs. One is known as an agonist and the other as an antagonist—as one contracts, the other relaxes automatically under the direction of the brain. Only when learning new physical skills do you become aware of the complex coordination of this partnership. The skeletal muscles—in the legs, arms, neck, chest and face—are joined to bones by tendons: bands of tough, elastic protein fibres called collagen. Ligaments are also made of collagen and act to support the joints. Muscles carry their own store of fuel that is used to meet the demands of increased physical effort. The more you exercise, the more the muscles call for oxygen and blood glucose. The everyday actions of the skeletal muscles, heart, liver and brain, use about 70 percent of your total energy.

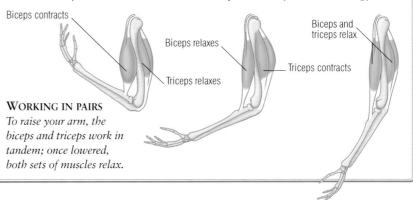

Biceps contracts

Biceps relaxes

Triceps relaxes

Biceps and triceps relax

Triceps contracts

WORKING IN PAIRS
To raise your arm, the biceps and triceps work in tandem; once lowered, both sets of muscles relax.

The nervous system

See also:

3/GENERAL HEALTH ISSUES
Skeletal problems pp. 88–89

5/ILLNESSES & EMERGENCIES
Nervous system problems
pp. 210–212

All parts of the body are kept in touch with each other by its communication and command network—the nervous system—which ope rates via several different and complex parts. The central nervous system consists of the brain and the spinal cord. Muscular movements, both conscious and unconscious, are controlled from the brain, which sends and receives messages via the spinal cord. The brain is the learning centre in which memory and decision-making operate. The central nervous system also mediates your senses of touch, sight, taste, smell and hearing. Through your eyes, ears, nose, tongue and skin sensitivity it controls your balance, ability to judge distance and to feel pain, pressure and cold. Such sensations are conveyed by sensory nerves to the brain, which instructs the motor nerves by electrical signals to enable the body to react appropriately. The left side of the brain usually controls the right side of the body and vice versa.

The peripheral nervous system connects the central system with other parts of the body. Pairs of nerves, 31 pairs in all, link the spinal cord to the muscles. The peripheral system includes the autonomic nervous system, which controls the body's unconscious functions, like the heart and the digestion. This system has two sets of nerves—the sympathetic, which works while you are active, and the parasympathetic, which takes charge when you are at rest.

Each individual nerve consists of a bundle of nerve cells, called neurons, with long branch-like extensions along which signals travel fast. Neurotransmitters are chemicals that carry the signal across the synapse—the gap between the sending neuron and the receiving neuron or muscle. Each neuron is protected by a sheath which, if damaged, disrupts the message network and affects the body's functions.

WHAT CAN GO WRONG?

The most common neurological disorder is dementia, which largely happens in old age, but is a feature of both Parkinson's and Alzheimer's diseases. Stroke happens when the blood supply to the brain is cut off by an artery being blocked, and the body systems controlled by the damaged area are impaired. In multiple sclerosis (MS) the protective sheath of the nerves is damaged, resulting in visual or mobility problems. Women are twice as susceptible as men. Motor neurone disease is a rare disorder in which the motor neurons become damaged. In the spinal cord, nerves can become trapped between the vertebrae. In sciatica, acute pain in the buttocks and sides of the legs is caused by pressure on the sciatic nerve.

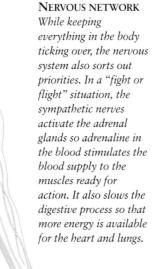

Brain

Cerebellum

Medulla

Spinal cord

Nerve

Sciatic
nerve

NERVOUS NETWORK
While keeping everything in the body ticking over, the nervous system also sorts out priorities. In a "fight or flight" situation, the sympathetic nerves activate the adrenal glands so adrenaline in the blood stimulates the blood supply to the muscles ready for action. It also slows the digestive process so that more energy is available for the heart and lungs.

NERVE CONNECTIONS
Neurons vary in length from a few millimetres to a metre. Chemicals (neuro-transmitters) carry the signals across gaps between nerve endings (synapses).

Nucleus

Myelin sheath

Direction of
nerve impulse

Cell body

Synapse

The endocrine system

See also:

4/HORMONAL HEALTH
Endocrine system problems
pp. 136–143

In the endocrine system, glands produce the hormones that govern various functions of your body that are not under conscious control. The major glands are the thyroid, parathyroids, pancreas, adrenals and gonads (sex glands: the ovaries in women, testes in men). The hormones—chemical messengers—travel in the blood to designated organs, carrying messages that maintain the organ's activities. They are crucial for the correct functioning of every body cell and play a central role during puberty, menstruation, pregnancy and menopause.

The endocrine system is governed by the hypothalamus in the centre of the brain via hormones that it produces, although it is not in itself a gland. The hypothalamus is vital to factors such as sleeping and waking, temperature regulation, stress and excitement.

A short stalk connects the hypothalamus to the master gland, the pituitary, which is the size of a pea. Hormones flow from the hypothalamus to the pituitary, which then stimulates or represses hormone production in the other major glands according to the body's needs.

WHAT CAN AFFECT IT?

Pituitary hormones oversee growth rates, bone growth, sexual development (the ovaries and testes make increased levels of sex hormones at puberty) and fluid levels within the body. The butterfly-shaped thyroid gland is positioned across the voice box in the throat. Thyroxine secreted by this gland governs energy levels and your metabolic rate. Next to the thyroid are the parathyroid glands. They make parathormone, which combines with vitamin D and calcitonin from the thyroid to ensure the blood has the correct balance of calcium and phosphorus to build strong bones.

At the top of the kidneys are the adrenals, which are both sex and stress glands producing androgens (male sex hormones—in women as well as men) and adrenaline, which has a direct effect on blood pressure, heart rate, the lungs and digestive system, to enable the body to handle stress. Other important hormones are secreted by cells in the kidney. These include renin, which helps to control blood pressure, and erythropoietin, which stimulates production of red blood cells in bone marrow.

The pancreas, a long, thin gland lying behind the stomach, makes the hormones insulin and glucagon, which work together to keep blood sugar levels balanced. Insulin is produced after you have eaten to help the cells absorb glucose (made from carbohydrates and, sometimes, fats); it is this function that is impaired in diabetes. Any excess glucose is converted to glycogen for storage in the liver and muscles. When the blood sugar level starts to fall, glucagon stimulates the liver to convert the glycogen back into glucose to bring the levels back to normal.

Other hormones, like prostaglandins, are made by tissues and body fluids in response to a local trauma to help control, for example, inflammation, fever, circulatory disorders and stomach secretions.

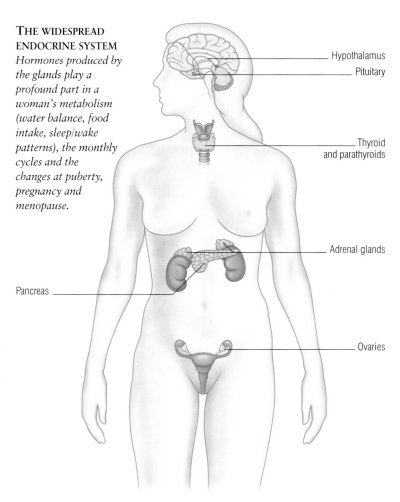

THE WIDESPREAD ENDOCRINE SYSTEM
Hormones produced by the glands play a profound part in a woman's metabolism (water balance, food intake, sleep/wake patterns), the monthly cycles and the changes at puberty, pregnancy and menopause.

Hypothalamus
Pituitary
Thyroid and parathyroids
Adrenal glands
Pancreas
Ovaries

Blood and the circulatory system

See also:

3/GENERAL HEALTH ISSUES
Blood and the circulation
pp. 116–133

The blood delivers oxygen and nutrients to—and removes waste from—all your organs and tissues. The average healthy adult woman has about 4 litres (9 pints) of blood constantly circulating. It is a sticky red fluid that carries hormones from the glands, oxygen from the lungs and nutrients from the digestive system to most cells of the body. It also transports waste matter—carbon dioxide (CO_2), lactic acid—to organs to be excreted. The liquid part, plasma, accounts for 55 percent of the blood mass. Suspended in the plasma are solids, mostly red blood cells, which make up the other 45 percent. White blood cells, which defend the body, and platelets or thrombocytes, which help the blood to clot, each make up less than 1 percent.

There are two blood circulation systems. The systemic blood system carries oxygenated blood from the heart to the organs and limbs and deoxygenated blood back to the heart. The pulmonary system is a loop from heart to lungs and back. Bright, scarlet blood is oxygen rich; the darker red it is the less oxygen it is carrying.

HOW IT WORKS

The power behind the system is the heart, a pump about the size of a clenched fist, which sits in the lower chest, left of centre. When the muscular heart wall contracts, deoxygenated blood is sent from the right side into the lungs where its tiny capillaries surround small air sacs called alveoli. Carbon dioxide moves from the blood to the alveoli. It is then expelled from the body during breathing. Oxygen is picked up by haemoglobin in the red blood cells; it is the oxyhaemoglobin molecule that makes blood bright red. The oxygenated blood returns to the left atrium of the heart, which contracts to pump it into the ventricle and out into the main artery, the aorta. This then sends branches to the organs.

Arteries have elastic walls, and expand and contract according to changes in the volume of blood. This is the "pulse" you can feel in any artery close to the surface of the body. Branching off are the smallest blood vessels, the capillaries, which take oxygen to the tissues. Blood laden with waste carbon dioxide enters very small veins, then larger veins as it returns—mostly "uphill"—to the heart. The two main veins are called venae cavae. Muscles squeeze the thin-walled veins to force the blood on and up, and valves open and shut en route to prevent it flowing back. The entire systemic circuit takes about half a minute to complete.

Blood tests are widely used to diagnose many disorders and infections. A sample is generally easy to obtain and can provide information on chemicals that may be present, such as glucose, salts or drugs; the amounts of different hormones in circulation; and microorganisms such as bacteria and viruses.

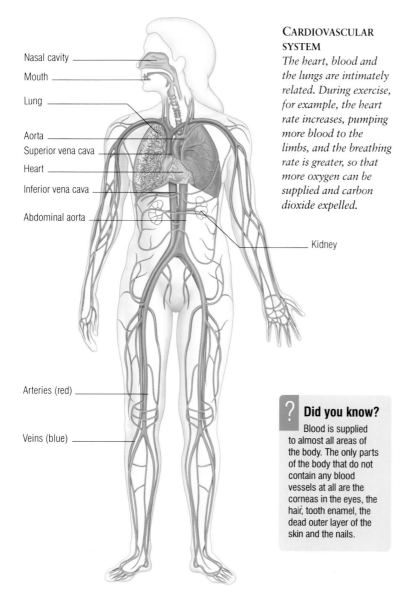

CARDIOVASCULAR SYSTEM
The heart, blood and the lungs are intimately related. During exercise, for example, the heart rate increases, pumping more blood to the limbs, and the breathing rate is greater, so that more oxygen can be supplied and carbon dioxide expelled.

Nasal cavity
Mouth
Lung
Aorta
Superior vena cava
Heart
Inferior vena cava
Abdominal aorta
Kidney
Arteries (red)
Veins (blue)

? Did you know?
Blood is supplied to almost all areas of the body. The only parts of the body that do not contain any blood vessels at all are the corneas in the eyes, the hair, tooth enamel, the dead outer layer of the skin and the nails.

The respiratory system

See also:

5/ILLNESSES & EMERGENCIES
Respiratory problems
pp. 213–221

Providing the body with life-giving oxygen to maintain the health and efficient functioning of all the organs and cells is the sole purpose of the respiratory system.

An adult woman at rest needs about 6 litres (13 pints) of air a minute. During an aerobic exercise session, almost six times that amount is needed. The respiratory system is designed to cope with this increased demand without conscious control on your part.

The respiratory system is divided into two tracts. The upper tract includes the nose, the sinuses, the mouth and the pharynx—the cavity behind the nose and mouth that connects them to the oesophagus (gullet). The lower respiratory tract consists of the larynx (voice box); the trachea (windpipe); the bronchi (airways) and the lungs. The lungs are not in fact identical—the right has three lobes, the left two—but they perform the same function.

Every time you breathe in through your nose or mouth, the upper respiratory tract filters, warms and humidifies the fresh air. From the trachea, the air enters either the right or left bronchus and goes into one of the lungs. The airways divide into bronchioles (ever-finer branches), the finest of which end in alveoli. These little air sacs within the lungs take oxygen from the inhaled air and convey it into the bloodstream. At the same time, carbon dioxide is transferred from the blood to the alveoli to be exhaled along with some water vapour. There are about 350 million alveoli in each lung and the total area available for exchange of gases is about 5.4 sq m (600 sq ft).

The lungs are surrounded by a continuous membrane called the visceral pleura and the chest cavity is lined with a similar membrane called the parietal pleura. The narrow space in-between is filled with moisture, which, as the lungs move with each breath, provides the necessary lubrication.

The air you breathe is packed with minute particles such as smoke, dust and other environmental toxins, which can cause health problems. The respiratory tract has impressive defence mechanisms to combat such invasions—many of the immune system cells are located here. Some of these cells envelop and destroy incoming bacteria or viruses; others

THE POWER OF LUNGS
Alveoli are like miniature bunches of grapes. They are so small that 40 alveoli would have to be placed side by side to make a bunch 1 mm wide. The alveoli secrete a detergent-like substance called surfactant to keep them inflated during breathing. Infants born prematurely, with their lungs not fully developed, sometimes have to be given artificial surfactant.

Bronchus

Alveolus

Bronchiole

Air enters alveoli

Oxygenated blood goes to the heart to be carried around the body

Blood carrying CO_2 from the heart to the lungs

Alveolus

ALVEOLI CLOSE-UP
Each tiny alveolus is surrounded by a large number of thin-walled capillaries ensuring fast and efficient oxygen and gas exchange into the bloodstream.

CO_2 transfers from blood to air in the lungs

Oxygen transfers from air in the lungs to the blood

manufacture antibodies, which are secreted into the mucous lining of the respiratory tract and provide a continuous wash through it. The mucus also contains other substances that can deactivate or kill bacterial or viral organisms.

WHY YOU COUGH

Another protective mechanism is provided by the cilia. These are numerous very fine hairs that line the airways and move in waves to push the mucus, including particles that it may have trapped, up from the bronchioles. The coughing reflex is activated to force secretions and any inhaled particles out of the lungs. Smokers produce more sputum because of inflammation of the airways and therefore cough more.

The digestive system

See also:

3/GENERAL HEALTH ISSUES
Problems of the mind pp. 102–103

5/ILLNESSES & EMERGENCIES
Digestive system problems
pp. 190–203

All the food and drink you consume is broken down by the digestive system into a form that your body can make use of or expel if it can't be used.

Digestion takes place in a long muscular tube called the alimentary canal, which runs all the way from the mouth to the anus. The first stage of the food's journey occurs when it is cut up into manageable pieces by the teeth. Saliva moistens the food and begins to break down starch, helping the process of swallowing. The masticated food, in the form of a round lump or bolus, is prevented from entering the windpipe by the epiglottis at the back of the throat, and travels down the oesophagus aided by peristalsis (muscle contractions). The bolus then enters the stomach, a J-shaped reservoir with a mucous membrane lining. Glands within the lining manufacture gastric juice—a mixture of hydrochloric acid and digestive enzymes—which, combined with churning movements of the muscular stomach, breaks food down to a pulp, much as a food mixer does. It is at this stage that some drugs (for example, aspirin and paracetamol) and water are drawn through the stomach walls. The rest of the food, now liquefied and called chyme, passes into the duodenum at intervals when the pyloric valve at the base of the stomach opens. It only allows a certain amount through before shutting again.

The duodenum—the first part of the small intestine—contains bile, which is manufactured in the liver and stored in the gall bladder. It also receives enzymes from the pancreas that digest proteins (changing them into amino acids), fats (which have been emulsified by bile) and carbohydrates. Some nutrients are taken straight into the bloodstream through the duodenum walls, while the rest moves on to the next section, the jejunum, then to the ileum.

The hepatic portal veins lead to and from the liver. Here glucose is extracted from the blood arriving from the intestine, converted to glycogen and stored for use as energy. The liver breaks down drugs, toxins, poisons and pollutants and produces pigments from old red blood cells, which give colour to bile, urine and bowel motions. It also stores vitamins A, D, K and B_{12}, makes lipoproteins and cholesterol and helps to make vitamin A from betacarotene. Any amino acids not required by the body are changed into urea to leave the body in urine, and their residues are stored as glycogen.

THE INTESTINES

Continuing its journey, the watery chyme, which remains after the nutrients have been absorbed in the small intestine, is pushed along by contractions of the bowel walls. Digestion is almost complete by the time chyme reaches the large intestine, but water is reabsorbed here. The chyme turns into a thick paste. Finally, the indigestible fibrous residues and the intestinal bacteria become faeces, which stay in the rectum until ready to be excreted through the anus.

The intestinal bacteria perform a useful function in synthesizing vitamins K and B_{12}, but it is their activity that also produces wind.

DIGESTIVE PROCESS
Food spends a minute or less in the mouth, four hours each in the stomach and duodenum, two hours in the lower small intestine and about 14 hours in the large intestine.

Parotid gland

Mouth

Salivary gland

Oesophagus

Liver

Gall bladder

Small intestine

Appendix

Stomach

Colon

Rectum

The urinary system

See also:
4/HORMONAL HEALTH
Endocrine problems pp. 136–143

5/ILLNESSES & EMERGENCIES
Urinary system problems p. 188
Acute infections pp. 244–246

About 70 percent of your body weight is water, and the urinary system plays its part in keeping the balance right while getting rid of soluble waste. It is designed to safeguard the health of the blood and to ensure the consistency of the body's water balance, its temperature, acidity and alkalinity. Most important to this function are the kidneys, two bean-shaped organs behind the lower part of the rib cage. They are like fine sieves through which all the body's blood passes many times a day to remove toxins and maintain the correct volume and chemical composition of the blood.

The kidneys process about 8 litres (14 pints) of fluid every hour. Only about 1 percent becomes urine and the rest—including salts, glucose and minerals—returns to the circulation. Urine is almost all water. Only 4 percent is waste such as urea—a product of the breakdown of protein—which gives urine its colour. Urine travels through the ureters, which descend from each kidney, to the bladder for temporary storage. The bladder's wall stretches to hold about 700 ml (1¼ pints) of urine to be expelled through the urethra. Up to 2 litres (3½ pints) of urine are passed in 24 hours.

Thirst is a late warning sign that the body, and the blood in particular, is lacking water for its needs. The body has only to be 10 percent dehydrated for the pulse rate to increase and blood pressure to fall. The kidneys, to maintain blood pressure, respond to an instruction from a pituitary hormone and reabsorb water rather than releasing it as urine. Dehydration can occur as a result of insufficient fluid consumption, exercising, heat, sweating, caffeinated drinks, alcoholic beverages or medications.

URINARY PROBLEMS

The shortness of the female urethra and its position close to the anus cause several urogenital conditions affecting women at different times of life, such as infection of the urethra (urethritis) or of the bladder (cystitis).

When a woman is pregnant, she has more fluid in her body and may pass urine more often. The hormone relaxin, in preparing the body for birth, relaxes the bladder and other pelvic muscles. As the uterus enlarges and presses on the bladder, frequency of urination increases. This is not normally a problem but sometimes it can indicate gestational diabetes, infection or pre-eclampsia. Later in life, stress incontinence can occur, usually as the result of vaginal delivery.

At and after the menopause, lack of the hormone oestrogen can also result in urinary problems such as incontinence.

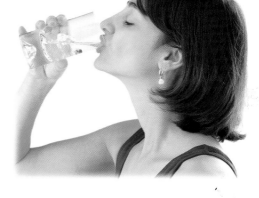

THIRST IS A WARNING
The pressing desire to drink water is a very late response to the body's needs. When the body senses a lack of water, it rations it for essential parts (like the blood and brain), so the skin, hair and the urinary system suffer.

THE URINARY SYSTEM
The kidneys are the body's filters and remove excess fluid and waste materials from the blood. This passes, as urine, into the ureter and then into the bladder, where it can be stored for some time. From the bladder, urine passes into the urethra and out of it during urination. The process is not under conscious control until the urine reaches the external urethral sphincter, a ring of muscle that can be contracted to hold back urine.

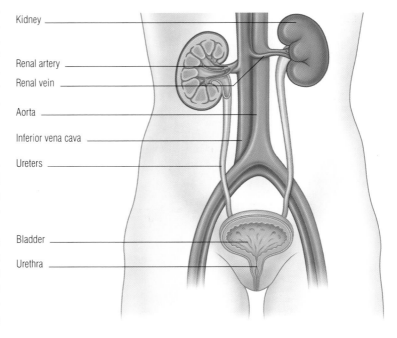

Kidney

Renal artery

Renal vein

Aorta

Inferior vena cava

Ureters

Bladder

Urethra

See also:

2/SEX & SEXUALITY
Your sexual self
pp. 52–55

4/HORMONAL HEALTH
Reproductive problems
pp. 146–149
Pregnancy pp. 170–179
Conception problems pp. 180–185

5/ILLNESSES & EMERGENCIES
Acute infections pp. 244–246

The reproductive system

A woman's reproductive system is designed to produce eggs, receive sperm and nurture the unborn child. The system is made up of the uterus (womb), two ovaries and two Fallopian tubes, all of which reach adult size between the ages of 10 and 15. They lie in the abdominal cavity, partly covered by the peritoneum—the lining of the abdomen—and are held in place by the pelvic floor muscles.

The uterus is a hollow, thick-walled muscular sac with a lining (endometrium), which is able to receive and nurture a fertilized egg. Before a woman becomes pregnant for the first time the uterus is about the size and shape of a pear, but after childbirth it does not revert to its previous size. Usually, it tilts slightly forward, but in some women it may tilt slightly backward (known as retroverted). The ligaments attached to the uterus allow it to shift a little as the rectum and bladder empty and fill.

On each side of the uterus is a walnut-sized ovary. From the start of her life, a woman stores many thousands of immature eggs (oocytes), in the ovaries. During the reproductive years, only about 400 of them will be released and ripen under the influence of luteinizing hormone and follicle stimulating hormone.

Each month the process ripens at least one egg (ovum), then causes it to burst out of its follicle on the ovary in a process known as ovulation. It travels down the 10 cm (4 in) long Fallopian tube to the uterus where the lining has been prepared to nurture it. If the egg isn't fertilized by a sperm in the Fallopian tube, becoming an embryo, the lining is shed 14 days after ovulation as menstrual blood. The first period at puberty is the menarche (pronounced *menarkey*). Periods cease at the menopause although, as they usually first become irregular, menopause is defined as occurring when a woman has not had periods for a year.

The neck of the uterus (the cervix), is narrow and leads to the vagina, a thin-walled, muscular tube about 7.5–10 cm (3–4 in) long, between the bladder and the rectum. It provides the entrance for sperm and is the passageway through which a baby is born and through which menstrual blood leaves.

The vagina, which stretches considerably during sexual intercourse and childbirth, in a virgin is covered by the hymen, a membrane that may bleed when ruptured during first sexual intercourse. It is, however, just as likely to be broken from tampon insertion.

A WOMAN'S GENITALS

The external genitalia (the vulva) surround the vagina. The labia majora are two large folds of skin, shaped like lips, which in the reproductive years contain lots of fatty tissue. They join together in the pad of fat on the pelvic bone, known as the mount of Venus, which is covered with pubic hair. Protecting the entrance to the vagina are the labia minora: delicate, less fatty

A WOMAN'S LIFE CYCLES
From pre-puberty (at about 12 years) to menopause (about 50) the female sex hormones have an influence on the reproductive system. Changes in the levels and activity of the hormones vary according to major life happenings. On average the monthly cycle for most women continues for 38 years, excluding pregnancy.

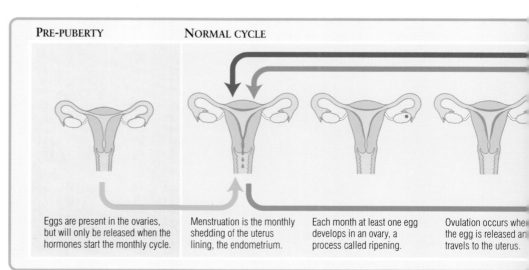

PRE-PUBERTY

NORMAL CYCLE

Eggs are present in the ovaries, but will only be released when the hormones start the monthly cycle.

Menstruation is the monthly shedding of the uterus lining, the endometrium.

Each month at least one egg develops in an ovary, a process called ripening.

Ovulation occurs when the egg is released and travels to the uterus.

A WOMAN'S BODY
The reproductive system is protected inside. Two ovaries which store and release eggs for fertilization are situated at the end of the Fallopian tubes. The tubes connect to the uterus, the neck of which—the cervix— leads to the vagina. It is the vagina through which semen (carrying sperm) enters and travels toward the uterus. If a sperm meets an egg in a Fallopian tube and the embryo implants there instead of in the uterus this is called an ectopic pregnancy.

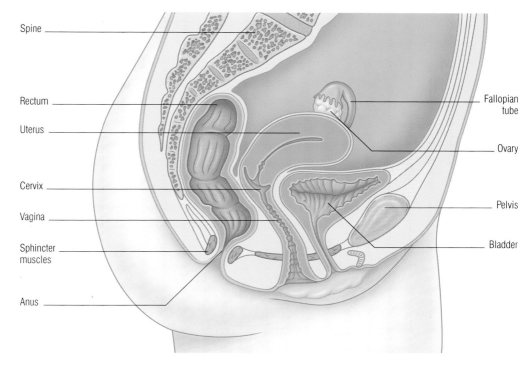

Spine

Rectum

Uterus

Cervix

Vagina

Sphincter muscles

Anus

Fallopian tube

Ovary

Pelvis

Bladder

folds of skin, which become more prominent as a woman ages and fatty tissue decreases. Glands around the vaginal opening release mucus to keep the vagina moist and lubricated so that it can easily accommodate the penis.

The clitoris is a small protruding structure— the female equivalent of the penis—which mainly consists of erectile tissue (as do the nipples). It is highly sensitive to the touch and becomes swollen with blood when a woman is sexually aroused.

A woman is usually at her most fertile in her late 20s. For fertilization to take place, sperm travelling upward from the cervix must make satisfactory contact with the egg in the Fallopian tube within 24 hours of its release from the ovary. A healthy woman has a 25 percent chance of conceiving a child in an average month. Most women who want to do so will conceive naturally within a year of trying. If they do not, they can be referred to an infertility specialist by their doctor.

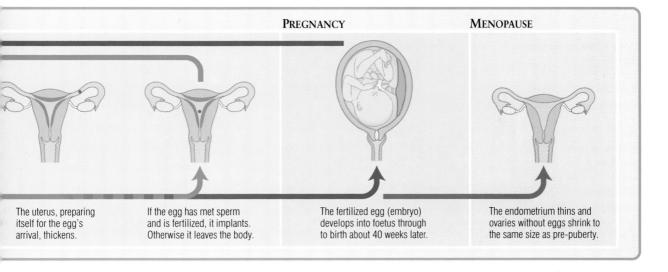

PREGNANCY

MENOPAUSE

The uterus, preparing itself for the egg's arrival, thickens.

If the egg has met sperm and is fertilized, it implants. Otherwise it leaves the body.

The fertilized egg (embryo) develops into foetus through to birth about 40 weeks later.

The endometrium thins and ovaries without eggs shrink to the same size as pre-puberty.

See also:

4/HORMONAL HEALTH
Breast care pp. 154–157

5/ILLNESSES & EMERGENCIES
Immune system problems
pp. 204–209
Acute infections pp. 244–251

6/TREATMENTS & THERAPIES
Conventional treatments pp. 278–281
Complementary therapies
pp. 292–293

The immune system

Also known as the lymphatic system, the immune system is an intricate network that protects the body from infection and illness. It collects and drains the fluid that is forced out of the bloodstream to bathe and nourish tissues, picking it up from the spaces between cells. The fluid moves into the lymphatic capillaries and through the system until it is returned to the bloodstream. Defence mechanisms—the spleen, thymus gland, the tonsils and lymph nodes—are positioned at strategic sites around the body and perform different functions.

Lymph fluid is similar to blood but it has no red cells. All body tissue, except the brain and heart, is bathed by lymph. It circulates throughout the body, like the blood, but does not have a central pumping mechanism. Instead, the fluid is moved along by the muscular action of the lymphatic vessels and is also squeezed by the body's skeletal muscles during movement.

Along the lymphatics are small bean-shaped nodes that contain leucocytes (white cells). One sort, the lymphocytes, recognize foreign matter (antigens) and produce antibodies (immunoglobulins), which in turn stimulate another sort, the phagocytes, to engulf and destroy the invaders. The nodes are concentrated in certain areas—the neck, armpits and groin, and in the deeper tissue around the lungs and liver.

When the body is fighting a bacterial infection, the lymph nodes swell. Swollen glands in the neck, under the arms and in the groin are

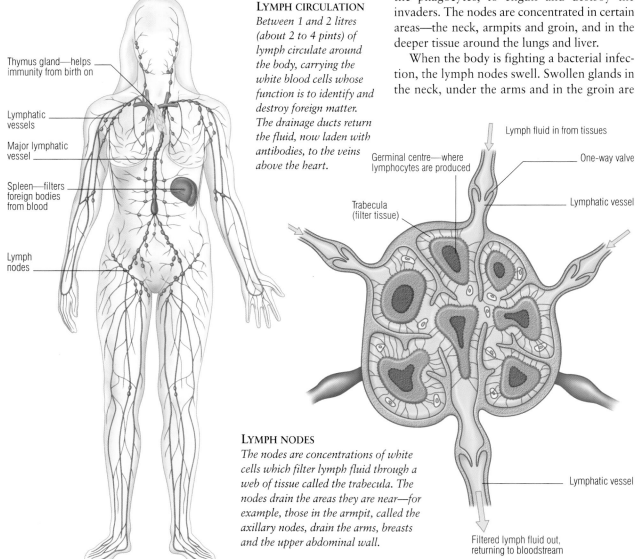

Thymus gland—helps immunity from birth on

Lymphatic vessels

Major lymphatic vessel

Spleen—filters foreign bodies from blood

Lymph nodes

LYMPH CIRCULATION
Between 1 and 2 litres (about 2 to 4 pints) of lymph circulate around the body, carrying the white blood cells whose function is to identify and destroy foreign matter. The drainage ducts return the fluid, now laden with antibodies, to the veins above the heart.

LYMPH NODES
The nodes are concentrations of white cells which filter lymph fluid through a web of tissue called the trabecula. The nodes drain the areas they are near—for example, those in the armpit, called the axillary nodes, drain the arms, breasts and the upper abdominal wall.

Lymph fluid in from tissues

Germinal centre—where lymphocytes are produced

One-way valve

Lymphatic vessel

Trabecula (filter tissue)

Lymphatic vessel

Filtered lymph fluid out, returning to bloodstream

the most telling sign that your body is fighting an infection. The antibodies are also passed into the blood to be transported around the body to provide immunity.

Babies already have some natural immunity. This can be increased by the antibodies and other substances present in breast milk, which is why health professionals advocate breast-feeding infants. Throughout childhood, you come into contact with a host of infections which, by provoking your body's immune system to react, provide you with immunity to those particular diseases later in life.

With some infections, the immunity lasts a lifetime; with others, resistance is only for the short term. This is why children and adults in certain circumstances receive boosts to the immune system through inoculation, also called vaccination or immunization, when they are given a modified strain of the organism causing the disease.

What is administered depends on what is thought necessary and safe at the time; measles, whooping cough, tetanus, polio, rubella, mumps, diptheria and now haemophilus and meningococcus C are the ones most routinely offered, particularly in early life. People travelling to places where contagious illnesses are a risk are also immunized so that the body is stimulated to produce protective antibodies.

Viruses and bacteria can enter the body in various ways. At obvious entry points—such as the mouth and nose in the upper respiratory tract—lymphoid tissue is present to fight invaders. However, as some illnesses are caused by different strains of a virus, you cannot have the total immunity necessary to resist every infection. The common cold is a prime example.

As adults, the efficient working of our immune system can be quite seriously affected by stress and exhaustion. Disorders of the immune system can occur when cells of the immune system are specifically attacked by a virus, as in HIV/AIDS, or sometimes when the immune system turns on itself to attack the tissues of the body, as in rheumatoid arthritis.

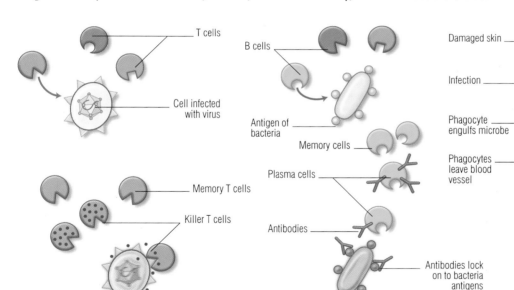

T cells

Cell infected with virus

Memory T cells

Killer T cells

B cells

Antigen of bacteria

Memory cells

Plasma cells

Antibodies

Antibodies lock on to bacteria antigens

Damaged skin

Infection

Phagocyte engulfs microbe

Phagocytes leave blood vessel

SKIN RESPONSE

The skin is the immune system's first line of defence. Antigens breaching the surface are met and "eaten" by phagocytes, a type of white cell in blood, which activate T and B cells in lymph to recognize the invader.

T CELL LYMPHOCYTES

Certain lymphocytes called T cells are the fighting force of the immune system. They do not produce antibodies, but stimulate B cells and macrophages. Some T cells are killers, others helpers, suppressors or memory aids. Memory T cells act as a regulatory mechanism "remembering" invaders and ensuring that the body's own cells are not threatened. T cells come from bone marrow and proliferate in response to antigens in the lymph nodes.

B CELL LYMPHOCYTES

B cells are responsible for the "primary immune response", when antibodies are produced against an invading microorganism. The antibodies produced are then carried round the body in the blood and lymph to sites of infection where they attach to the antigens and cause their destruction with the help of the T cells. The body is able to make a seemingly unlimited number of antibodies, each of which has specific targets.

41

See also:

5/ILLNESSES & EMERGENCIES
Skin problems pp. 222–233
Problems of the senses
     pp. 236–243

6/TREATMENTS & THERAPIES
Conventional treatments
     pp. 286–289
Alternative medicine pp. 298–309

The skin and the senses

Most people are born with five senses—sight, hearing, smell, taste and touch. Each has specific functions. If you lose one sense your body attempts to compensate by heightening all or some of the others.

The skin—the organ of touch—is the largest organ of the body and has four layers: outer dead cells, the living epidermis, the dermis and the subcutaneous fat layer that provides warmth and insulation. Fine networks of nerves and blood vessels permeate the layers so that the brain registers temperature, pressure, pleasure and pain experienced on any part of the skin.

The epidermis, largely made up of a protein called keratin, provides the body with a protective suit. It prevents moisture loss from the skin (while allowing waste, such as sweat, to escape), is virtually impervious to harmful substances and has antibacterial properties. Cells grow, mature, age and die, moving upward to the outer skin where they are sloughed off by clothing or by rubbing or washing.

The next layer down, the dermis, contains the support structure of the skin, including collagen, the elastic tissue that keeps the skin springy. Collagen is a protein and responds directly to the hormone oestrogen to give skin a youthful, supple appearance. After the menopause, and with age, skin becomes thin and wrinkled through the loss of collagen, moisture and fat and as a result of long-term exposure to environmental pollution, including the sun's rays.

The sense of sight keeps you in touch with your surroundings. Behind the iris, the coloured part of the eye, is a lens controlled by a set of muscles and an array of nerves linked to the brain. The lens bends rays of light entering through the cornea so that an image of an object is focused on the retina, at the back of the eye. The two—slightly different—images from the eyes are sent to the brain, which interprets them as one three-dimensional object. A person who is colour blind (much more common in men than women) was born with a fault in the retina.

THE SKIN
The skin is a complex area, containing blood vessels, nerves, hair follicles and sweat glands. Its function is to protect and contain the body's organs, to release excess heat and fluid to the outer air and to serve as a warning system against dangers such as burning.

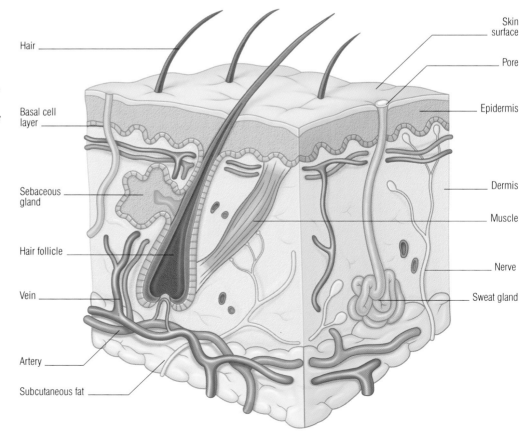

Hair

Basal cell layer

Sebaceous gland

Hair follicle

Vein

Artery

Subcutaneous fat

Skin surface

Pore

Epidermis

Dermis

Muscle

Nerve

Sweat gland

Bright lights and foreign bodies are kept out of the eyes by the eyelids and lashes. Lachrymal glands constantly secrete tears that bathe the eye with every blink and wash away any irritant that enters. Tears are also an emotional response to both happiness and sadness.

Hearing is the second of your vital senses, allowing you to tune into the world and sounds of danger. The external ear contains the eardrum, which passes sound waves to three tiny bones called ossicles in the middle ear, and then to the cochlea in the inner ear, which translate the sound wave into a nerve message that goes to the auditory part of the brain. Also in the inner ear are the semicircular canals, which maintain your sense of balance.

The sense of smell probably evolved to warn us when food is bad and of potential dangers such as smoke from fire. It is also used less consciously to detect pheromones (natural body scents), which are given off in response to sexual arousal or fear. The disappearance of this sense, along with memory loss, is the prime symptom of Alzheimer's.

Taste allows the enjoyment of food and it also warns about potential poisons. There are many thousands of "taste buds" in the mouth, mostly on the tongue but also at the back, responsible for distinguishing flavours.

TASTE
The tongue has over 10,000 receptors called taste buds, with different sections in which the tissue is sensitive to flavours such as sweet, sour, salty and bitter, and responds to sensations such as excess heat.

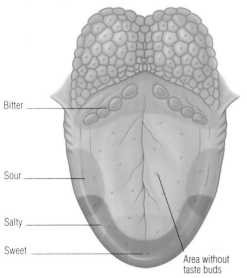

SIGHT
Light enters through the pupil and is focused by the lens on to the retina at the back of the eye, where the rod and cone cells are sensitive to light and colour.

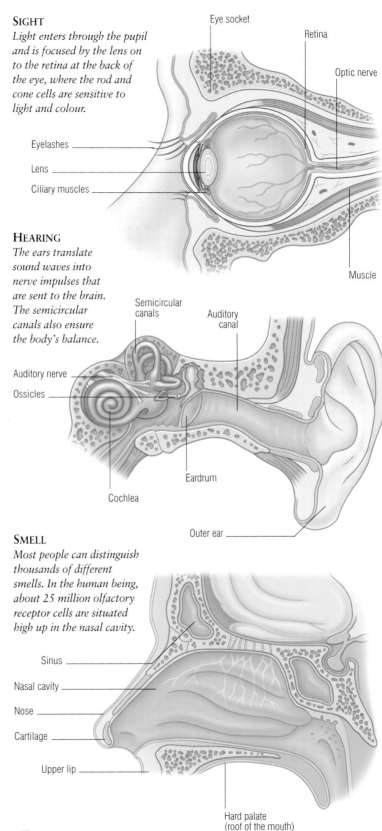

HEARING
The ears translate sound waves into nerve impulses that are sent to the brain. The semicircular canals also ensure the body's balance.

SMELL
Most people can distinguish thousands of different smells. In the human being, about 25 million olfactory receptor cells are situated high up in the nasal cavity.

A HEALTHY MIND

Being able to deal with events as they happen without getting too stressed, taking things in your stride and keeping emotions and relationships in perspective are all part of a healthy approach to life. Developing some skills will help you maintain your equanimity.

Beating stress

Any life-changing event, even a happy one such as the birth of a baby or a new job, can be the cause of stress. Stress is a normal response and a necessary reaction to physical or mental challenges. It is only when demands become too much that the stress can become harmful to the body and mind.

Individuals tolerate different levels of stress depending on temperament to a great extent, so there is no indisputable way of measuring when stress reaches the danger zone. What is known is that too much stress over a period of time may damage your health.

There are many symptoms of stress, including palpitations, digestive disorders, headaches, insomnia, increased urination and irritability. You may experience a reduction in sexual desire or your periods may become irregular. There can be even more serious health problems. One of the most common physical symptoms of stress is an increase in blood pressure. When you are challenged or feeling anxious, your blood pressure may rise and if this occurs on a regular basis the body may adjust the pressure to a higher level. An overstressed person may also smoke, drink too much alcohol or turn to illegal drugs, which cause other problems.

It is important that the symptoms of stress be distinguished from psychiatric disorders like depression and anxiety. Talk to your doctor about whether professional help is necessary. If this is not the case, you must decide what is making your life so stressful and then what steps you can take to change it.

PINPOINTING THE PROBLEMS

Are you trying to fit too much into each day so that you never feel on top of things? You may need to prioritize your workload. This may be easier said than done for many women who are juggling the needs of children or elderly parents and other domestic issues with the demands of a full-time job outside the home. If aiming for perfection is the problem, it is worth trying to strike a balance. You may take pride in having a spotless house, for example, but would it not give you more pleasure to spend time with someone you love rather than concentrating on the household chores? Perhaps you need to enlist some help. People may not realize how desperate you are feeling unless you tell them that

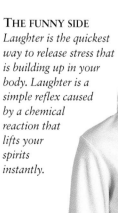

THE FUNNY SIDE
Laughter is the quickest way to release stress that is building up in your body. Laughter is a simple reflex caused by a chemical reaction that lifts your spirits instantly.

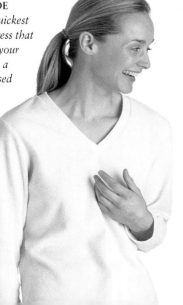

you are finding it difficult to cope. Ensuring that every member of the family shares the chores is a good first step. Even young children can make their own beds, put clothes or toys away or feed the cat.

If the care of elderly parents is making too many demands on you, it is time to discuss it with your family. Often this type of responsibility falls on the shoulders of only one sibling, and brothers and sisters need to know you are having difficulties. Also explore the possibility of getting help from volunteer groups. If this isn't available you may have to consider finding paid help—perhaps a house-cleaner or a nurse for a parent. You must decide whether the extra expense is better than putting your own health in jeopardy.

If it is your job that is causing you the most concern, don't brood on what you see as your failings but ask for help. Sometimes even a job you have been doing for years can suddenly become stressful, because there has been a change of personnel or there is a threat of reorganization or redundancy.

Approach your immediate superior or the human resources manager and tell him or her about your concerns. You may be surprised to hear that the company views you as a valued member of the workforce and that your fears have no foundation. It can be difficult to judge your own performance. If there seems to be a gap in your knowledge, perhaps with regard to new technology, request some training.

Too much stress does not always relate to excessive commitments. Having too little to do, as in the case of the unemployed or the elderly, can be stressful as well. Boredom and isolation both play a part. If you find yourself in this situation it is better to accept that paid work may not be an option, and to find out which organization would welcome your help as a volunteer and appreciate your contribution.

FINDING SOLUTIONS

One proven way of reducing anxiety and stress is talking and it helps if you are able to tell other people when you are feeling worried and upset. If you do not think you can confide in family or friends, seek out a trained counsellor or mental health professional.

Exercise is known to reduce stress and improve mood. Take a brisk walk every day; make a regular weekly time for a sport or a dance class. Above all, start being kind to yourself. Giving yourself treats can put pleasure back into your life.

Learn to breathe calmly

A good way of getting in touch with yourself in stressful situations is by controlling your breathing. When you are anxious, you breathe shallowly—inhaling and exhaling so fast that hardly any oxygen-rich air is getting into the lungs and therefore to the rest of the body. This state, called hyperventilation, makes you feel dizzy. Fear and anxiety can also cause you to hold your breath.

To calm yourself you need to slow your breathing to a rate of 12 even breaths a minute or less. The best form of relaxed breathing is diaphragmatic, using the muscular sheet to force air into the lungs.

Lie flat on your bed or floor and put your hands on your abdomen. Breathe in deeply through the nose, counting mentally to four and at the same time feeling your abdomen rise. Breathe out slowly through your mouth counting from four to one as your abdomen lowers. Repeat 10 times.

INNER PEACE
Meditation and yoga have been shown to increase the feelings of calm and well-being, both of which are antidotes to stress. You can learn the techniques in a class, but take time for yourself and practise relaxation at home.

FEEL YOUR BREATHING
Breathing deeply and rhythmically is a good route to relaxation. It brings more oxygen into your body and helps you feel calmer.

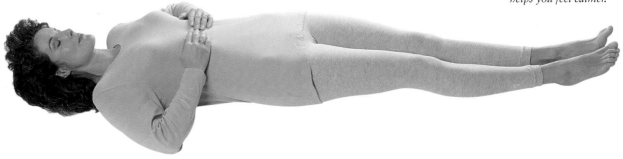

Developing a positive attitude

Women throughout their lives may be vulnerable to the attitudes and the needs of others. The influences come from their earliest years, the culture in which they grew up, the relationships they have and the society which puts a perceived value on them and their role.

The reactions you have to irritations and problems in your everyday life can be indicative of whether those influences were positive or not, whether you expressed your emotions without causing physical damage. If you take difficult situations in your stride and don't let them get out of proportion, you can feel assured that from childhood you were given the tools to deal with problems without them affecting

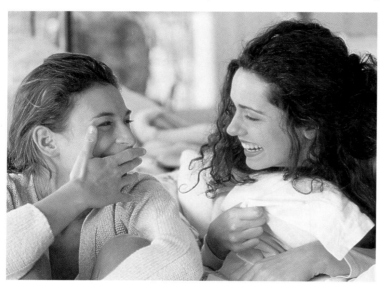

TALKING WITH FRIENDS
Being able to express yourself and explain your feelings and fears is a healthy trait. You can talk to a close friend or write your thoughts down to help you gain insight into your emotions.

you. Thoughts determine your emotional state, which in turn can influence your physical health. Holding back your emotions time after time increases your heart rate, blood pressure and muscle tension—all signs of stress.

COGNITIVE RESTRUCTURING

To help you uncover negative thought patterns that you may not know about, you can apply the principles of cognitive therapy. These principles enable you to reveal automatic thoughts that colour your life without you being aware of them. This method of discovery is especially applicable to women, as they are prone to socially conditioned negative thoughts—about their body or self-worth, for example. The first

step is to analyse these thoughts, to recognize where the downturn in your mood springs from and how you may possibly be creating your own lack of self-esteem. If, for example, you go for a job and don't get it, then say: "I'll never amount to anything", you are creating an ongoing problem. If you discover your lover is cheating on you and instead of getting angry with him you say: "I don't deserve to be loved", you are putting the blame on yourself.

KNOW YOURSELF

The aim of cognitive restructuring is to find out what lies behind these negative thoughts, to get rid of them and to replace them with ones that are truthful and empowering. If your problem stems from your early life—from the attitude of a parent, sibling or teacher—or from your own worst fears at the present time, you can set about trying to change it.

First, identify the negative thought, then ask yourself four questions:
Does this thought contribute to my stress?
Where did I learn this thought?
Is this thought logical?
Is this thought true?

Take time with your answers. You may want to try and help yourself by writing down your thoughts or ask the help of a close friend or therapist. You may prefer to join a small group where you can talk it through.

MOVING FORWARD

A lifelong habit of seeing everything negatively may not disappear immediately, but if you take steps to alter your attitude you will soon appreciate the results.

Start by making an honest balance sheet of the positive and negative things in your life. You may be surprised to find that there are many more things that you like or enjoy than you had anticipated. The negative side is that you may not have given them enough time to bring you pleasure. You can now put that right.

Identify all the negative things that you can do something about—getting into shape physically, finding new friends or interests, perhaps getting a new job. If none of these seems to offer solutions, you may be depressed and should see your doctor. Depression can be treated.

THE JOURNALLING ROUTE

Writing down your deepest thoughts and feelings can help you gain new insight into yourself. This process, called journalling, may help you release deep emotions, such as anger or fear, that lie frozen in your mind and body. It is a way of finding out whether something you

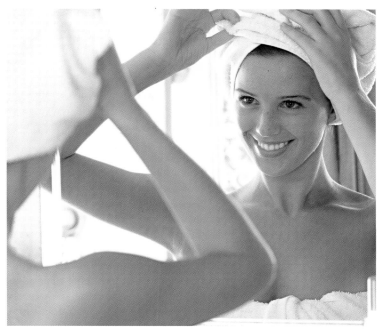

Assertiveness training

Learning to assert yourself, to use anger as an agent for change, especially in your relationships, is a positive process. It is the opposite of passivity but is not unbridled fury or aggression. It can be applied to coworkers, husbands and partners, children and parents, siblings and friends and people in medical and healthcare situations.

♀ Speak in the "I" language. Learn to say, "I think", "I feel", "I want" instead of "You are", "You don't". A true "I" statement says something about you without criticizing or blaming the other person and without holding the other person responsible for your feelings or reactions. Beware of falling into the trap of telling him or her, "I think you are controlling and self-centred".

♀ Recognize that each person is responsible for her or his own behaviour. Don't blame your mother-in-law because she seems to have a hold over your husband. If you are angry with your husband because of his closeness to her, find another way to make him aware of it. Your husband's behaviour is his responsibility, not his mother's.

♀ Resist telling another person what she or he thinks or feels or should think or feel. If someone gets angry in reaction to a change you make, it is not a time to criticize feelings or deny her or him the right to be angry. It is much better to say, "I understand that you are angry and if I were in your shoes I would be angry too. But I have thought it over and this is my decision".

♀ Remember that there are three ways to say no: 1, a simple "no"; 2, "no, because . . ." ; and 3, "no, but how about. . .".

These offer alternative ways to protect yourself from requests that impinge upon your needs, boundaries or energy reserves. Sometimes it may be difficult, but knowing the ways to say "no" won't inflict hurt or be devastating to relationships that you value and don't want to harm.

don't know about is plaguing you and preventing you from being positive about your life.

If you are physically healthy, write about the most stressful event or ongoing problem you face in your daily life. If you believe your current problems are the result of past events, write about the traumatic times in your past. Take 20 minutes to do it. Write about what happened and how you felt or feel about it. The facts and the emotions are equally important to help you understand the experience.

Repeat this process for at least three or four days, even a week, if you feel that you are gaining from the exercise. You can use it as a process of decision making too. If you have come to a crossroads in your life and need to deal with a relationship or a physical problem, writing down how you feel about it may help you make sense of it. You may find your way through your loneliness or unhappiness and gain the strength to make the decision that is right for you.

Anger is a powerful emotion which women with medical conditions commonly feel when their body appears to let them down. For example, they hate the way premenstrual syndrome makes them lose control. If they are infertile, they may feel fury with their body for not being able to produce a baby. At the menopause they are angered by the embarrassing symptoms. The way to move forward is to acknowledge the anger with journalling, then assertiveness (see box, left) to make the anger an ally.

TAKE A POSITIVE VIEW OF YOURSELF
Start in a small way and treat yourself well. Before you leave the house to go to work or to meet friends, breathe deeply, look in the mirror and smile. The act of smiling has a physical effect on your feelings.

Coping skills

Life cannot be lived free of emotional events which may threaten to overwhelm you. Knowing how to cope mentally when you experience personal upheaval can help prevent physical repercussions later.

BALANCING WORK AND FAMILY

Most women now spend the greater part of their life in paid work and an increasing number of young mothers continue to work during pregnancy and their child's infancy. Working full time while raising a family can be demanding on mind and body.

Survival tactics include learning to compartmentalize your life and being clear about your priorities. It would be rare if you were the only one at your workplace who didn't have similar domestic problems and discussing them with colleagues may reveal ways to help you deal with conflicts of interest. Having to take work home, for example, can be tricky if it eats into the time you spend with your children. Talk to your employer about the pressure this puts you under and seek another method of dealing with the work. Make sure you have established a good back-up system of friends, relatives or neighbours who can step in if there is a crisis with your children while you are at work.

If you work from home prioritizing your energies will be important. Isolation can be a problem when you are housebound with young children. Make sure you get to know other mothers in your neighbourhood, who you can spend time with when you are not working.

DEALING WITH ANGER

Anger is an emotion that can be both positive and negative. If it encourages you to try to improve things in the face of an injustice, anger can be positive. Negative anger, however, can be a destructive force, especially when it tips over into rage and even turns into physical violence. This type of rage is unacceptable. Venting feelings in this way indicates a complete loss of control. If it occurs in a personal relationship irreparable harm may be done.

Parents who feel exasperated by their children should relieve anger by punching a few cushions rather than risk lashing out. If you fear your aggression could harm your child or you

are in a relationship which is violent you should seek professional help. If you find that you are increasingly angry about everything, it may indicate stress levels that are too high.

Some people may not know what the real cause of their anger is. Simmering resentment or hostility may have built up for various reasons and the anger is transferred to something else, often another person. The most serious form of anger is that which is turned in on the self. This can lead to self-inflicted harm and needs immediate professional attention.

FACING UP TO DISEASE

Most people suffer ill health at some time in their lives, but usually they know that they will get better. Learning that you or a loved one has a serious illness that is life-threatening or will permanently impair physical or mental faculties can be devastating. You may become so preoccupied with the situation that you exclude other aspects of your life.

There is no easy way to cope with a serious illness of your own, but it does help if you have a good relationship with your doctor and other caregivers and are fully involved in your own care. You should keep yourself informed about the nature and implications of the condition so that you can participate in decisions about treatment and remain in control of your life as much as possible. Sometimes knowing what you are up against can remove some of the fear.

Contact with other people suffering similar illness or disability can be helpful and encouraging. Confronting the grief or anger you feel and finding ways to express it may be an important step in the healing process. Mental health back-up may be essential for the person suffering the disease and also for the caregiver.

BEREAVEMENT

It is inevitable that at some point in your life you will have to confront the death of someone very close. The most common first experience of such loss is when a grandparent or parent dies, but for some it may be the death of a friend of your own age, a young child, a partner or a sibling. It can leave you feeling stunned by the sense of finality and may cause you to face your own mortality, something you may never have

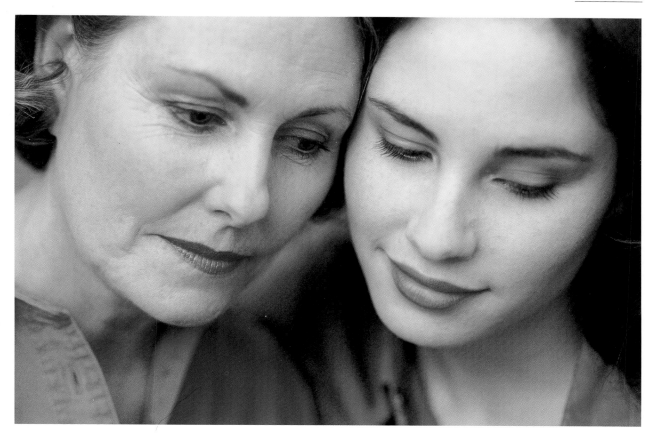

considered before. Whether you have a strong religious belief in an afterlife or see death as the end of any existence, the death of a loved one is always going to be painful.

Under whatever circumstances the death has occurred—shocking and sudden, or the result of a drawn-out terminal illness—the bereaved person must be allowed to go through the grieving process. Grief is a natural and healthy response to a death and helps you to come to terms with your loss, even though you may continue to miss the person all your life.

In some circumstances, a person who does not allow herself to grieve should be cause for concern. A woman who has had an abortion or miscarriage may want to put the experience behind her, but if she hasn't expressed her emotions it could be detrimental to her mental or physical health. The grieving process has merely been postponed and may surface, possibly years later, in a potentially more harmful way.

Sometimes a bereaved person may refuse to show her feelings for fear of upsetting others. This may be true of a mother who has lost her partner at an early stage but wishes to protect her young children from her distress. But chil-dren need to be allowed to grieve, too, to express their sadness. Crying together can be the beginning of the healing process. Take your own time. Don't allow yourself to be rushed into putting away photographs or disposing of your loved one's belongings. You can do this when you are ready. Having familiar reminders around you for a while can be comforting and strengthen your memories.

Working for a cause or campaign in the name of the person who has died may help you regain equilibrium. This can be true of parents who have lost a child through an accident or disease and find new resolution in trying to help prevent other parents suffering in the same way.

You may always have a sense of sadness at the loss of people you loved, but you will find yourself able to return to activities you once enjoyed after the hurt you feel lessens. If your unhappiness or depression isn't lifting, or you start getting symptoms such as migraine headaches, seek the help of a mental health professional or a bereavement counsellor who will understand your feelings. In some cases, medication may be the best way in the short term of dealing with grief that weighs you down.

CLOSE COMFORT

Sharing feelings at an emotional time can draw mother and daughter or friends closer together. You may not always understand why someone is so deeply affected, but you can sympathize—and literally provide a shoulder to cry on.

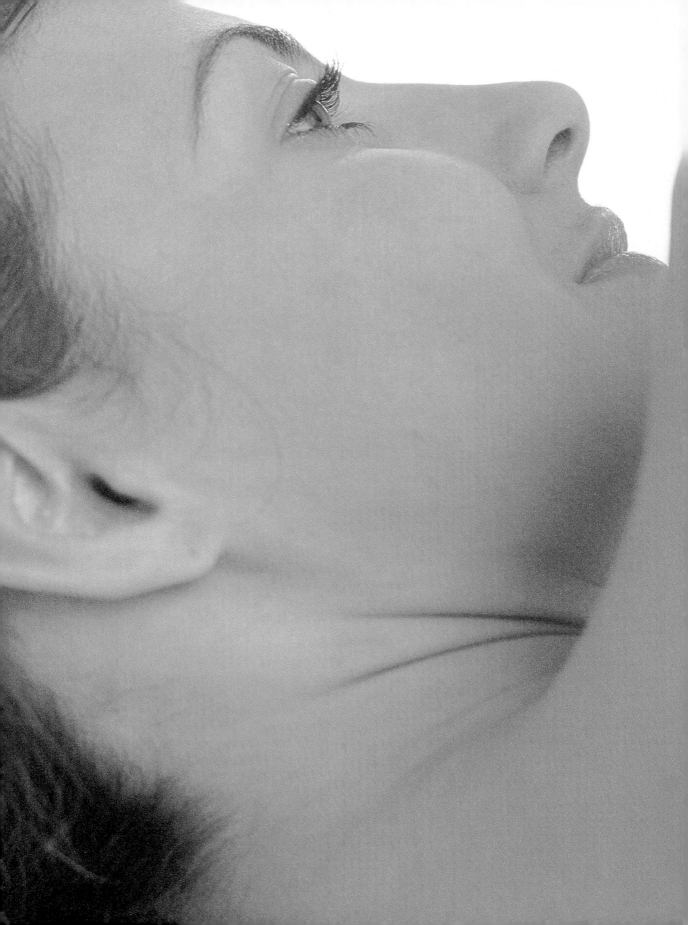

SEX AND SEXUALITY

Whether you are single or in a relationship, young or old, sexually active or celibate, sexuality is an important aspect of every woman's life. It is part of your personality. An element of your sexual identity and preferences will be formed by your genetic make-up; other parts will bear the influences of your environment—the events of your childhood and the years of growing up. From puberty, your personal feelings about sexuality, reproduction and sex roles evolve, helped by your own level of awareness and the parameters set by the society in which you live. The way you consciously view your sexual self can determine the outcome of relationships.

YOUR SEXUAL SELF

The essence of sexuality is the way a woman develops her sexual potential and becomes knowledgeable physically and emotionally. There are many issues that have a bearing on both, including what happened in the past and the way her feelings change through the years.

See also:

1/BEING A WELL WOMAN
Healthy body systems p. 38

2/SEX & SEXUALITY
Sexual problems pp. 69–71

Understanding your sexuality

The first step to having a happy and rewarding sexual relationship is to understand what sex and sexuality mean to you as a person. This means having clear knowledge of yourself and what makes you the way you are, knowing what influences came from your past and understanding their impact—good and bad—on you.

Becoming aware may be a long process, as the effects of some of those influences may have been subtle. They may now be so deep-rooted that they seem second nature, yet they may underpin the way you act in a relationship and be important to it. For example, do you depend on others to feel good about yourself? Do you fantasize about love and romance, about finding the lover of your dreams?

WHERE DO YOU COME FROM?
Like every woman, you have your individual history involving background, religion, cultural beliefs and personality. All combine to make you the sexual being you are today.

The way sexuality and relationships were viewed in your family will affect how you regard sex as an adult. This can be positive or negative. For instance, if your parents were loving to their children and to each other, the chances are that you will believe a close couple relationship will be rewarding for you. Not all people, however, experience such a background. If your parents argued a lot, for instance, you may find it hard to accept that loving relationships are possible. You may find

HOW FEELINGS MAY CHANGE
Many things can have an effect on your sexuality and they may differ throughout your life. Your relationships, whether you become a parent and whether you choose to remain single will all have different degrees of significance for you at different ages.

TWENTIES

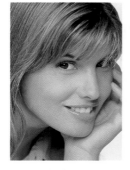

You probably form relationships easily with both sexes, enjoying the mix of fun and pursuit of a career. You may vacillate between wanting commitment and preferring freedom.

THIRTIES

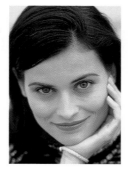

You will know yourself better by now and may be in a relationship. You may have embarked on a life of sharing, balancing work and play. Marriage and having a child may be issues at this time.

FORTIES +

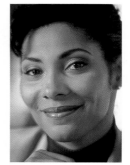

Your sexuality may be influenced by meeting the needs of your partner, your family and your own changing feelings about what the future may hold for you after the menopause.

OVER 60

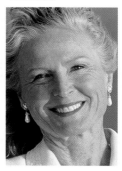

Sexuality does not stop and continues to have an effect on your attitude to relationships. But with maturity you may have a different perspective of your priorities and wants.

How to stop sexual harassment

There have been radical changes in women's sexuality as women's roles in society have altered. On occasions these changes may bring a woman into conflict with a man or perhaps another woman who has power over her, probably at work. Sexual harassment is when that person states or implies that if you provide him or her with sexual favours, he or she will give you something in return. Other tactics may have bullying undertones—intimidating you with behaviour involving sexual gestures, leering or discussing sexual matters in an over-personal or offensive manner. He or she may also imply that if you object in any way, your career will be damaged.

Everyone has the right to work or study in an atmosphere without harassment or pressure. Most workplaces and colleges have policies to prevent harassment, as well as methods of punishing the perpetrator if it takes place. If you find yourself in this position, you need to act assertively. You should tell the person that you find such behaviour offensive and that it must stop. Write down what has happened, together with the date, and keep it in a safe place. Take your colleagues or friends into your confidence. If the person continues to bully or threaten, write to him or her, reiterating what has happened and on what dates the incidents took place, and making it clear that you will take further action. Your copy of the letter will be evidence for your union or student representative or human resources manager to act on if the harassment persists.

you carry this behaviour into your own life, needing the tension that arguments bring in order to become sexually excited.

Your own individual relationship with your mother, your father, and how each regarded you as a person, can affect you. If you were brought up in an affectionate family, you will appreciate physical warmth and cuddling. If the body was seen as shameful in your family, the close physicality of lovemaking could present problems. Some people may have difficulty with sharing and intimacy. Others may have a strong sense of independence, which they are not willing to give up in a relationship.

One of the strongest influences on the sort of sex you have is the way you value yourself.

If you feel that your needs and desires are as important as your partner's, your sexual relationships—like other aspects of your life—will be equal, honest and loving. Women who have been sexually, physically or emotionally abused as children may find it difficult to experience warm and loving sexual relationships. Untangling what is good and what is not, and what to do about it, can be a complex and life-long process. Professional counselling or attending a self-help group can help people work through painful issues.

WHAT ARE YOUR BELIEFS?

It is not just your family background that influences your ability to have a happy sex life. The wider society plays its part as well simply because most cultures have strong beliefs about men and women and how they should relate to each other. Some religions instil feelings of guilt about sex into their followers. While you may accept that you should honour your background, you may find such teachings unacceptable and this can create a conflict.

The core beliefs you have about sex affect your views of sexual relationships. Consider these myths: men have stronger sexual desires than women; good girls don't want to have sex; as people get older they want sex less often; women should be passive in sex. On the basis of these attitudes, if a woman has stronger sexual desires than her partner, she may feel guilty because her upbringing has taught her that women should not feel like that. Such a clash can prevent you relaxing and enjoying sex.

CHANGING EXPERIENCES

Many people begin their sex lives successfully, in happiness and love, and this continues throughout their lives. Others may make an unsatisfactory start which leads them to think that sex is not all it is made out to be. Others may change the way they think about sex according to the influence of each new partner. It is also possible to feel differently about your sexuality during the course of your life. It is important that you accept these changes in yourself and know what to do about them if, or when, they happen.

A sense of your own sexuality gives you the right to say what sort of sex you want and to refuse sex if you don't want it. This should apply whether you are in a relationship or not.

Discovering your sexuality

You need to know your body well in order to have the best sex that you can with someone else. You should find out for yourself what brings you pleasure—and what doesn't. Women who rely on their partners to teach them what will bring them pleasure put the responsibility on someone else to control a sexual experience when it should be a joint endeavour—with equal pleasure for both.

When women describe their bodies, they often find fault with the way they look. But you will never be able to relax fully if you find yourself worrying about your appearance or if you are not happy with your body. Being able to concentrate on the feelings you are experiencing and what is happening to your body during sex enhances your enjoyment.

Some partners may try to impose on you standards of beauty or hygiene that conflict with your own. The pleasures of sex can be diminished if the expectations you have of each other are either unrealistic or cause you to have doubts about the other person. If you feel your physical self is not being valued as it is, your own self-respect should make you realize it is best to say "Thanks, but no thanks".

YOUR SENSUAL SELF
Your body will provide the clues to your sensuality. However, you must make time to discover what gives you pleasure. Delight in the sensuousness of touch and warmth.

LEARNING ABOUT YOUR BODY

Discovering that sex can be joyous, wonderful and pleasurable can come from a new partner or you can find it out by yourself. Getting to know your body and exploring the physical sensations that can be aroused in it can help you realize what you most appreciate and want from a loving relationship.

One way to do this is to look at your body in a full-length mirror, noting the shapes of the different parts, the folds and creases. The purpose is not to be critical, but to reveal which of these parts could be a source of pleasure. Take a warm bath, dry yourself with a fluffy towel, then slowly rub your whole body with body lotion. Use a light massage movement, stroking your arms, legs, torso and breasts, drawing your fingers and palms along the skin, teasing the nipples, moulding and pressing on muscle and tissue. Don't rush, relax into the feelings. Try different types of touch—firm or gentle, with fingertips or the whole hand—so you can feel your body responding.

MASTURBATION

In times past, it was assumed that women never masturbated. It was not considered acceptable, or possible that women could be sexually frustrated. However, masturbation is perfectly normal, an activity which many women discover by accident, usually during childhood when exploring the body is a natural process. Masturbation also helps you to know what kinds of touch you like and don't like when it comes to sex with another person.

If lack of understanding or embarrassment about your genital area prevents you from masturbating, try becoming familiar with its parts through reading a well-illustrated book about anatomy and sexual practice. When you are alone, gently touch and stroke the area to find out the response they invoke. Now imagine an unknown lover is pleasuring you; bring into your mind's eye the fantasy person you would like to have sex with. Take as much time as you want, touching and stroking your clitoris and vagina, feeling the area swelling and lubricating until you are thinking only of the pleasure.

Masturbation trains your body to react sexually, so you know your own arousal levels and

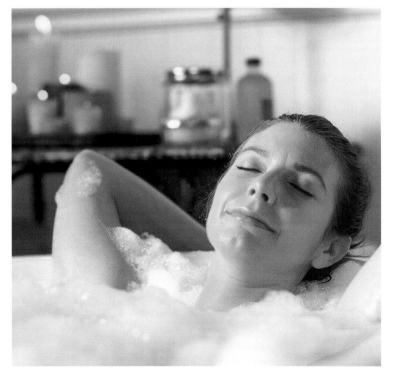

Lesbian and bisexual women

It is not unusual for girls and young women to be attracted to other women for a while, and even cuddle and kiss with these women, but still eventually find that they want a man as a sexual partner. Others realize that they are lesbian, but may have to choose their time to come out.

They may have existing family who reject anything that differs from the heterosexual "norm", or may be in a marriage they cannot leave, perhaps because of children, or illness. They may not feel psychologically able to handle the emotions that might be triggered by their revelation, and so go on denying their lesbianism to themselves.

In most cases women need to take time to come to terms with their feelings and to decide how open they want to be about their newly found identity. One of the first stages of coming out may be to contact helplines which provide understanding and advice, offer friendship and put a less antagonistic perspective on lesbian and bisexual women. You may learn, from those who have faced the problem, of ways to broach the subject with your friends and your family. You will want to talk through with them the risks of coming out.

There is in both heterosexual and lesbian society an assumption that someone is either "one of us" or not—and it is this attitude that can cause unhappiness. A woman who loves another woman can face opposition and oppression. Mothers who become lesbian may be challenged in regard to custody of their children, they may become targets of violence and at work they may be discriminated against or receive unwelcome sexual attention from men or harassment from females. Being aware that any of these might happen is preparation in itself. There is now, however, greater awareness of sexual diversity and more people accept lesbians and bisexual women as simply part of a wider society.

Being honest with yourself about your feelings is the basis of finding your true happiness. As in any partnership, each of you needs to feel equal to make it work, and any problems have to be ironed out together. A relationship that is mutually beneficial and supportive is as prized by two people of the same sex as it is by a heterosexual couple.

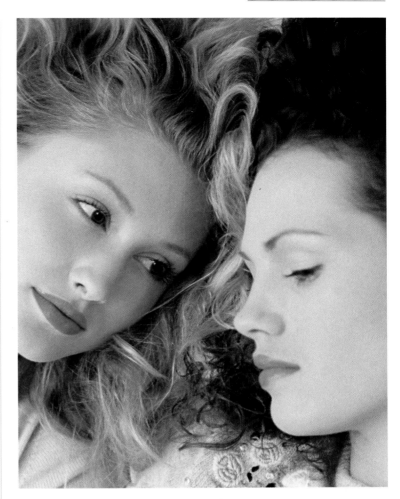

how close you are to orgasm. Women who may have trouble having an orgasm with a partner can often do so when they are alone, using their hand or a vibrator.

CELIBACY

Many women choose to spend some time in their lives without being in a sexual relationship. They choose celibacy so they can concentrate on other things, or have a period of reflection, perhaps after the ending of a long-term relationship. Others may be celibate because they cannot find a suitable partner, or for religious reasons. It may also be forced upon some by a change of circumstances, such as the death of a partner and the loss of desire.

Celibacy does not stop you having sexual feelings. You may not have the intimacy of a relationship—whether by choice or not—but you remain a sexual being. If sex is important to ensure self-esteem, masturbation and fantasy are valid options.

SEXUAL IDENTITY
Close, loving and sexual relationships between women can begin at any age. To enjoy each other you need to relate as individuals—the same is true of a heterosexual relationship.

See also:

1/BEING A WELL WOMAN
Healthy body systems p. 42
A healthy mind pp. 44–49

What a sexual relationship means

Sex within a relationship can bring a couple closer together, increase their sense of bonding with each other and give them a feeling that cannot be shared with anyone else.

There are different issues, joys and pleasures in a new relationship compared with a long-standing one. When you are first attracted to someone the mere sight of that person may be enough to make you want sex. As soon as you touch, you are excited. With the development of your relationship, you learn more about each other, mentally and physically, and a new sexual approach may replace that earlier excitement. It is not unusual for a woman to need more stimulation before she is ready for sex and her partner may indicate preferences to make penetration more enjoyable for both. Most couples find that sex improves over time, as they get to know each other's bodies and learn to trust each other implicitly. The potential for giving each other profound, deep pleasure becomes greater with time.

In a long-standing relationship, sex can be many things depending on your mood—fun, comforting or deeply, intensely loving. During the course of such a relationship, you may make love many thousands of times, but if it becomes routine you risk sexual boredom which may break the bond you have established. If you don't always do exactly the same things, in the same order, in the same place a relationship stays fresh. On the other hand, as time goes by such familiarity may be appreciated by both of you.

HOW IS YOUR RELATIONSHIP?

How sex is between the two of you often reflects how things are in the rest of your relationship. For instance, a man who is successful in his career may feel dominant over his partner who is at home with the children. At a later stage, she may be achieving in her career when he is facing a crisis in his own. Both changes are bound to have an effect on a couple's sex life—although the precise way depends on their affection for each other and their personalities.

Anger in a relationship may generate exciting sex for some. But this is not satisfactory long-term as the anger may too easily lead to physical violence. A partner who is physically stronger may hurt you even in play.

Blocked feelings or misunderstandings—particularly those that arouse resentment or jealousy—can influence your attitude to having sex. You need to find out what is upsetting you and try to work it out with your partner before it becomes a problem that divides you.

GOOD SEX, BAD SEX

Nothing is abnormal if both partners are happy with it. So if both of you only want sex in the bath or shower, always want sex in bed in the dark or want to do something that would make everyone you know burst out laughing, that's entirely up to you—providing it does not damage your relationship or hurt anyone else.

Bad sex is anything you don't want to do or find boring, uncomfortable or painful. If your partner likes certain sexual practices and you don't, you have every right not to do them. If you go along with it when you don't want to it may begin a pattern of pain and hurt. It can also too easily become physical abuse if you don't pay attention to your sense of fear. Be warned if after hurting you, your partner sends roses or makes some other "romantic" gesture and

ENJOYING SEX
For both of you to enjoy penetrative sex, you must be aroused. This is likely to happen more quickly for a male partner than for you so, if you are not ready, find a way to encourage more stimulation to arouse you fully.

promises never to hurt you again. In a relationship like this you must put your physical safety first and find a way out, bearing in mind that attempting to leave an abusive relationship is known to prompt violence. Seek help.

THE FANTASY OF SEX

The mind plays as great a part as the body in bringing about sexual enjoyment. Learning to fantasize and sharing the experience can make a relationship stronger and enhance lovemaking. The best sex is not static, it changes and grows as you discover what you like and what satisfies you. You may have fantasies that help you reach orgasm, but you may choose to share them only when you are sure of your partnership and know they won't offend.

Fantasies come in many guises, from those which take you away from reality to those that add something extra to it. The one that works for you may encompass playacting (for instance, you have never met before). It may be something that in theory you could do, but which has an element of danger (such as having someone else in bed with you). It may be an outlandish dream (such as having sex on a raft at sea). Using some form of harmless bondage may add to the fantasy as long as you both want it.

Physical and emotional abuse

Domestic violence is a significant source of women's illnesses and injuries, which they may not be willing to talk about from fear or embarrassment or pretence that it hasn't happened. Physical abuse can include anything from slapping, kicking, pinching and choking to forced sexual activity. Emotional abuse involves continuous criticism and undermining of self-worth, unpredictable responses, threats of violence, withholding of affection and manipulation through unreasonable demands. Certain factors have been identified which may indicate susceptibility to violence or battering when they are present in a relationship. Does your partner:

♀ Always want to know where you are and who you are with?
♀ Limit, control or try to stop your contact with family or friends?
♀ Throw things or hit objects when angry?
♀ Show violence toward anyone else?
♀ Abuse alcohol or drugs and is he violent when drunk or high?
♀ Put you down and belittle your opinions?
♀ Believe that he ought to be in charge?
♀ Have views about men and women that are very traditional?
♀ Imply that everything that goes wrong is your fault?
♀ Have violence or abuse in the family background?
♀ Seem to behave worse as your relationship develops?
♀ Keep weapons in the house?

If you experience any or several of these, or have been injured by your partner, you should not assume the behaviour will change. You need to remove yourself from the dangers and get help: tell your doctor, the local hospital or the police. Call a domestic abuse helpline.

LOVING MOMENTS
Affection, warmth, respect and humour bring the closeness that a sexual relationship needs to develop. Being able to express your thoughts and feelings without worrying about your partner's response is key to an emotionally and physically mature partnership.

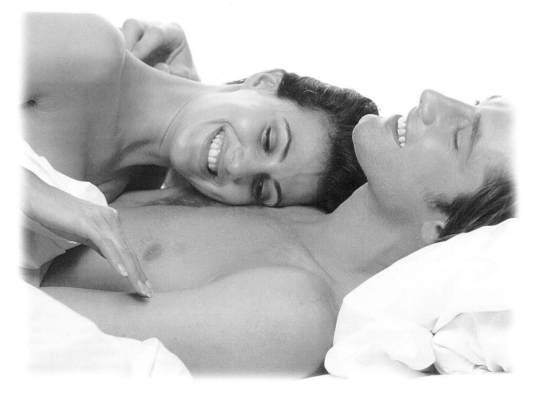

The keys to intimacy

The basis of all happy sexual relationships is intimacy. This means knowing someone as they are, rather than as they appear to be or as you would like to see them—and accepting it.

Intimacy takes time to develop and it does not happen automatically. You need to remain emotionally open to your partner and make an effort to keep getting to know him, as he needs to do with you. Wanting to find out more about your partner's responses and feelings is the best way to keep your passion healthy and thriving.

Many couples believe they are communicating because they talk to each other all the time. But talking about the practical things—such as taking the children to school, paying the bills—is only part of the communication that leads to real, deep closeness. For that, you need to be talking about yourselves and your thoughts, sharing ideas and attitudes whether they are positive or negative. Relationship counsellors find that most couples who come to them seeking their help have problems communicating on a personal level. Talking is the

first step, but you need to listen too. And you need to accept what your partner feels and thinks, even though it may be different from what you think and feel. Some subjects can be difficult to talk about honestly, but ultimately this is what leads to trust.

It is essential to spend time together as a couple, making space and taking time for yourselves as two people together. If you see each other only as parents, you may not be sexually aroused. Equally, if you are both totally involved in your individual careers, you may neglect your partnership. You need intimacy and closeness for an abiding sexual relationship.

Men do not always find it as easy to discuss or verbalize their feelings as women do. They may not have been encouraged to do this by their own families and may not see any point to it if, on the surface, everything appears to be going well. However, if his restraint affects the development of your relationship, you may need to encourage your partner to open up more. It may take time and patience. Quizzing him gently and affectionately when you are getting along well may help him turn his thoughts into words and to communicate them to you.

CHANGING PATTERNS
Inevitably the life of a couple will change when they become parents. You may not want sexual intercourse for a while after the birth, but your sexual intimacy can move to a new level through touch. Caressing and stroking can be loving and comforting at the same time, just as it is for the baby you have created together.

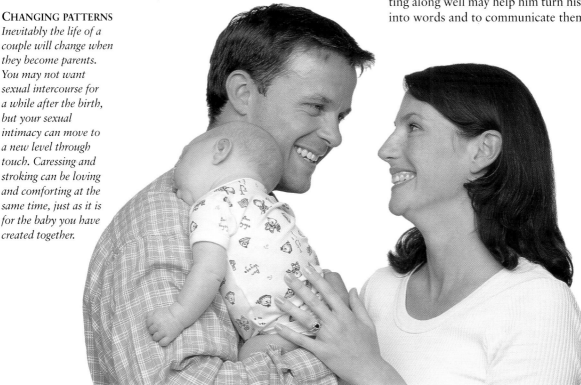

KEEPING CLOSE PHYSICALLY

The skin of the hands is extremely sensitive and the feeling of skin on skin is both sensual and comforting. Through touch you attune yourselves to each other. All sorts of touch—friendly cuddling and stroking, body massage or more intimate caressing—can relieve the stress of daily life, making you feel relaxed and close. Being touched can take you back to the warm security of childhood, while cuddling someone can make you feel nurturing and loving. Touch arouses both of you and relieves tension.

Stroking and touching, without necessarily leading to intercourse, can be helpful in bringing a couple together. Using the principles of sensate focusing (p. 71), you can take all the time you need working out what you like. By exploring your sexuality together, you will discover things about yourselves both as a couple and as individuals, helping to develop an excitement and trust that will carry you through the adverse times in your relationship.

Setting apart a time of the day when you can lie in each other's arms, being quiet and peaceful, will add to the closeness and affection that is essential to intimacy.

NEGOTIATE FOR YOUR NEEDS

Skilful negotiation is important in many parts of life and essential to your most intimate relationships. You will both have the best sex you can if you are able to ask for what you want in bed. However, the thought of talking about what you want and being honest about what does and does not work for you raises a lot of fears for both women and men. You may think, for instance, that you run the risk of rejection. Or you may find the prospect of talking about sex embarrassing. You may also fear hurting the partner you love deeply if you tell him that he is not doing what you like. At other times you may not even know what it is that you want—for instance, after the birth of a baby when tiredness and getting enough sleep become more of a concern than having sex.

The real point about relationships is that you should not expect your partner to read your mind, whether the subject is sex or the household chores. Explanation and making requests are part of a relationship between equals. You need to give some thought to what pleases you and to realize that you have a right to ask for it, as does your partner. For instance, a man may want to start penetration before the woman is ready. Asking lovingly—yet assertively—for more foreplay will add to your pleasure. Similarly, if you don't like the way he rubs your clitoris, gently redirect his hand to indicate this. You can use body language to reveal your preferences, too, to show your partner what you like by doing it to yourself. There may be other times when you have an increase in desire which your partner cannot meet—he's too tired, falls asleep or is away from home. In this case masturbation may be the best resolution.

Negotiation is part of all relationships, heterosexual and homosexual. While a woman may feel she knows instinctively what another wants, all women do not necessarily like the same thing—and if the process of finding this out is enjoyable, it makes for a better relationship. Intimacy relies on you being honest with your partner and yourself.

All relationships have troughs and peaks; by its very nature, sex can't or won't be perfect or satisfying every time. If you know this and you and your partner have learnt to be confident of each other you can laugh about it together when the unexpected happens. Such warmth and humour are as much elements of intimacy as touch, to be prized in a loving relationship.

The limits of touch

As a relationship develops it is important to take a lead from your partner as to which parts of the body it is good to touch and to convey your preferences to your partner. Although touch will be arousing in a sexual sense, it can also be worrying or alarming.

♀ With an established partner, if you do not like a particular touch, say so, even if you liked it in the past.

♀ If you are with a new partner and feel at all uncomfortable about anything, let that person know as soon as possible. If you continue to be uncomfortable and he does not change, you should leave the situation.

♀ If you are single always be clear about sexual limits right at the start of a date.

♀ If you find yourself in an abusive relationship, be aware of the risks at all times (p. 57) and take action to protect yourself from physical subjugation. Seek help from a domestic helpline or women's refuge or from the police.

CHOOSING CONTRACEPTION

The right choice of contraception can be an important part of a happy sexual relationship. The next few pages present information about the different forms of birth control to help you make the right choice for your situation.

See also:

3/GENERAL HEALTH ISSUES
Anxiety-related disorders p. 112
Blood & the circulation p. 123

4/HORMONAL HEALTH
Reproductive problems
pp. 146–149

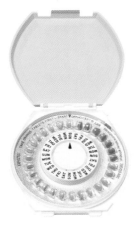

COMBINED PILL
Synthetic female hormones are used in this pill to prevent ovulation occurring.

> **! Caution**
> If you vomit within three hours of taking the pill, it may be ineffective. If you have not had your period three weeks after it was due, you may be pregnant. Make an appointment to see your doctor.

Hormone birth control methods

No method of contraception is perfect—each has advantages and disadvantages—but couples are usually able to find a type that suits them. Most types of birth control need your careful compliance. While some unplanned pregnancies are caused by the contraceptive itself not working, most result from it not being used properly—for instance, if you forget to take the pill or insert a diaphragm incorrectly. If the contraception doesn't meet the needs of you or your partner, you may feel anxious or ill or be at risk of pregnancy.

Your contraceptive needs also change during your life; what was suitable for you at the age of 20 may not be right for you at 40. Your choice may be influenced by whether you have completed your family or hope to have a child.

To find the method that's right for you, you should talk to your partner and your doctor about what you want and don't want. When you see your doctor, discuss the effectiveness of the chosen method, how easy it is to obtain and use and any possible side effects. Much will depend on whether you are in a monogamous relationship, your age and fertility history and any preferences you have.

THE CONTRACEPTIVE PILL

Since it was first made available in the 1960s, the contraceptive pill has been hailed as a revolutionary force in women's lives because during the reproductive years it allows more effective family planning and spontaneous sex with minimal risk of becoming pregnant. Modern formulations offer between 95 and 99 percent protection against pregnancy. The pill rarely causes side effects, although these may

> **Checks and balances**
> When you are taking hormonal oral contraceptives, you should reduce any potential risks by keeping your weight down, stopping smoking, having your blood pressure checked regularly and having pelvic examinations and cervical smears. If you are prescribed medicine for any reason, remember to tell your doctor you are using this birth control method.

occur in some women. A minority of women, for example, may have an increased susceptibility to blood clots. When considering your suitability for hormonal contraception, your doctor will make a thorough assessment for any risk factors, such as a family history of clotting, which you can weigh against the benefits.

COMBINED PILL

What it is The most widely prescribed pill uses synthetic forms of the female hormones oestrogen and progesterone (progestogen). Different types contain varying levels of each hormone. The lowest effective dosage is prescribed.

The "phased pill" is a combined pill with different levels of hormones for different days of the month. The pills must be taken in the right order over 21 days. Some brands have pills for 28 days, with seven containing no hormones (taking a pill daily means that you are less likely to forget to take it).

How it works Oestrogen plus progesterone prevent ovulation (the maturing and releasing of the egg), so there is no egg for the sperm to fertilize. The progesterone changes the uterine

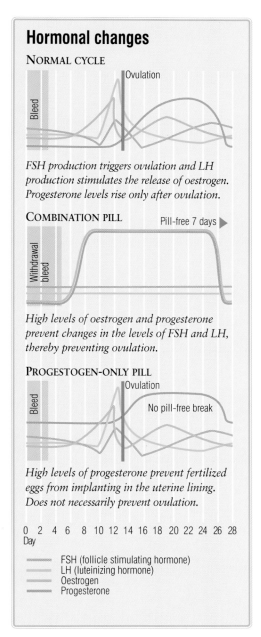

Hormonal changes

NORMAL CYCLE

Bleed

Ovulation

FSH production triggers ovulation and LH production stimulates the release of oestrogen. Progesterone levels rise only after ovulation.

COMBINATION PILL

Pill-free 7 days ▶

Withdrawal bleed

High levels of oestrogen and progesterone prevent changes in the levels of FSH and LH, thereby preventing ovulation.

PROGESTOGEN-ONLY PILL

Bleed

Ovulation

No pill-free break

High levels of progesterone prevent fertilized eggs from implanting in the uterine lining. Does not necessarily prevent ovulation.

0 2 4 6 8 10 12 14 16 18 20 22 24 26 28
Day

— FSH (follicle stimulating hormone)
— LH (luteinizing hormone)
— Oestrogen
— Progesterone

May be unsuitable if You are breastfeeding, are over 35 and smoke, have a history of phlebitis or deep vein clots, have diabetes, high blood pressure or liver diseases such as hepatitis.

May not work if You miss a pill, vomit within three hours of taking a pill or are taking certain antibiotics and other drugs such as anti-epilepsy medication. In any of these situations, use other contraception, such as a condom, in addition to the pill for seven days.

PROGESTOGEN-ONLY PILL

What it is The pill uses only one hormone, progestogen, a form of progesterone, making it suitable for women who get side effects from oestrogen or who are breast-feeding or are unable to take the combined pill for other reasons.

How it works It thickens cervical mucus and changes the uterine lining, preventing sperm reaching the Fallopian tubes. It inhibits ovulation in about 50 percent of women.

Pros Same as for the combined pill. Fertility returns to normal soon after you stop taking it.

Cons It must be taken at the same time daily, and has a slightly higher failure rate than the combined pill. Irregular vaginal bleeding and breast tenderness are possible.

May be unsuitable if You are overweight, have had unexplained bleeding or an ectopic pregnancy or have heart disease in the family.

May not work if You have vomiting or diarrhoea. If you take it more than three hours late, do so immediately and take the rest at the usual time—use another form of contraception for the rest of the cycle.

OTHER HORMONE METHODS

What they are Depo-Provera is injectable progesterone. Implanon is placed under the skin and lasts for three years.

How they work Depo-Provera is injected by a doctor during the first three days of your period, lasting 12 weeks. Implanon is inserted on the first day of your period.

Pros They are long-lasting: you can't forget them. Failure rate is low (Depo-Provera 1 percent, Implanon 0 percent). Periods are light. Fertility returns soon after Implanon is removed.

Cons With Depo-Provera fertility may not return for a year. Implanon may be visible. Both carry risk of irregular bleeding and weight gain.

May be unsuitable if You want to get pregnant in the near future.

> **! Caution**
> Stop taking the combination pill if you have migraine-type headaches for the first time, or frequent severe headaches or sudden disturbances of sight or hearing. See your doctor immediately. Stop taking the pill six weeks before having major surgery, or during prolonged immobilization.

lining and thickens the cervical mucus, making it difficult for sperm to bypass.

Pros It is convenient, reliable and allows spontaneity; you have lighter, less painful periods and reduced PMS symptoms. It can be taken for years and may protect against pelvic inflammatory disease (PID), benign breast disease, endometriosis and ovarian and uterine cancer.

Cons You may gain weight, experience mood changes, swollen breasts, reduced sex drive, migraine headaches, nausea and vaginal bleeding. You may take some months to reestablish ovulation after stopping it.

See also:

1/BEING A WELL WOMAN
Healthy body systems p. 38

2/SEX & SEXUALITY
Your sexual self pp. 52–59
Sexual infections
pp. 72–75

5/ILLNESSES & EMERGENCIES
Immune system problems
pp. 204–209

Barrier contraception

Birth control methods which prevent sperm from entering a woman's uterus are known as barrier contraception. The best known types—male and female condoms—are essential for people starting new relationships and when practising safe sex. They help prevent HIV and other sexually transmitted diseases (STDs) from being passed from one person to another. Ideally condoms should be used until you and your partner know each other's sexual history, and only abandoned if you are both in a truly monogamous relationship with each other.

MALE CONDOM

What it is A very fine latex sheath with a nipple-shaped tip, the condom is unrolled on an erect penis. Polyurethane condoms, which are thinner and provide more sensation for the man, can be used with oil-based lubricants.

How it works It covers the penis and collects the semen in the tip, so sperm are prevented from entering the reproductive tract. A new condom has to be used with every act of intercourse. It is safer if it is put on right from the start. As soon as the man has ejaculated, the penis must be withdrawn from the vagina, and care should be taken to hold the base of the condom so no sperm escape.

Pros It is very easy to obtain, protects both partners against STDs and is easily disposed of. Fertility is normal when the condom is not used. There are no side effects unless you are allergic to latex. If used properly, the failure rate can be as low as 3 percent; used with a spermicide, a condom is even more reliable. It may be used in addition to other methods of contraception for safe sex.

Cons The condom can come off or break during sexual activity, leaving you at risk of pregnancy and STDs. It should be put on before any penetration occurs (because sperm may leak out before ejaculation) and you have to stop during lovemaking to put it on. There may be reduced or altered sensation for both partners. It is wise to make sure you always have a supply.

FEMALE CONDOM

What it is A polyurethane tube fits inside the vagina, with the ring outside.

How it works Semen is contained inside the condom and doesn't enter the vagina. The

> **! Caution**
>
> Barrier methods of contraception use latex or polyurethane to protect one set of genitals from the other. Those made of latex can be delicate, however, so do not use oil or petroleum jelly (for example, Vaseline) in conjunction with these types. Do not let massage or body oil come into contact with them. You can use a water-based lubricant if additional moisture is required.

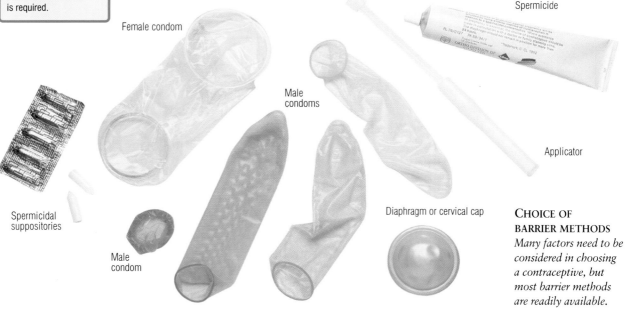

Female condom

Male condoms

Spermicide

Applicator

Spermicidal suppositories

Male condom

Diaphragm or cervical cap

CHOICE OF BARRIER METHODS
Many factors need to be considered in choosing a contraceptive, but most barrier methods are readily available.

failure rate is about 6 percent. A new condom has to be used with every act of intercourse.

Pros It is available from pharmacies and has no side effects. It is under the woman's control and protects against STDs. Unlike the male condom, it can be inserted well before sex. Fertility is normal when the condom is not used.

Cons There is reduced vaginal sensation and the ring protrudes outside the vagina. It may be difficult to insert and must be inserted correctly. It has to be obtained in advance.

May not be suitable if You find it hard to insert or you or your partner find it physically unsatisfactory.

DIAPHRAGM OR CERVICAL CAP

What it is A soft latex or plastic dome fits inside the vagina covering the cervix and is used with a spermicide. There is a range of sizes and types and hence it must be fitted to the individual by a trained professional (at your doctor's surgery or a family planning clinic). You

need to be taught the best way to insert and remove it. After removal, a diaphragm should be washed in warm water, dried and stored in its container. It should be checked regularly for signs of wear and tear; if you have long fingernails take care not to rip holes in it.

How it works It prevents semen from entering the uterus; any sperm that do bypass the cap are killed or disabled by the spermicide. To make sure that no sperm survive, the diaphragm needs to be kept in place for six to eight hours after intercourse.

Pros It works well for women who only want contraception when required—that is, infrequently rather than all the time. You have to remember to insert it but it can be put in up to two hours before intercourse. Fertility is normal when it is not used. It offers some protection against STDs and cervical cancer. Side effects are rare.

Cons It is messy. You can't be wholly spontaneous as it needs inserting before sex. You need to put in more spermicide with every act of intercourse. The diaphragm must fit over the cervix, and if you gain or lose more than 8 kg (20 lb) you should be reassessed by a healthcare professional as a new size may be needed. A diaphragm can sometimes become dislodged and some women find it difficult and messy to insert correctly. It should not be left in place for more than 24 hours because infection may result.

May not be suitable if Pregnancy would be a disaster—the failure rate is about 6 percent if fitted correctly, higher if fitted incorrectly; you are prone to bladder, vaginal or urinary tract infections—a diaphragm may increase their frequency; you have poor pelvic muscle tone or vaginal and uterine abnormalities.

USING SPERMICIDES

Various forms of spermicide are used with barrier contraception to kill any sperm that escape the condom, diaphragm or cap. There are various forms (such as cream, foam, jelly or suppository) and you may need to experiment with different types until you find the one that suits you. They are known to cause an allergic reaction in some women. It is important to remember that a spermicide used alone is not a reliable contraceptive (even at perimenopause when fertility is low) and a fresh amount must be used with each act of intercourse.

Emergency contraception

What it is Commonly called the morning-after pill, this can actually be effective if taken within 72 hours (3 days) of unprotected sex. It can prevent pregnancy after contraceptive failure (forgotten pill or diaphragm, condom accident) or if you had sex without contraception, or have been raped. This form is now available over the counter from pharmacists.

How it works One or two (depending on the sort of pill) higher-dose contraceptive pills are taken within 72 hours of unprotected sex, followed by another one or two, 12 hours later. They may prevent ovulation or change the womb lining so that a fertilized egg can't be implanted (in normal circumstances an egg can take five or six days to implant in the uterine wall). Use a barrier method of contraception until the next period.
Pros Prevents pregnancy in an emergency. The failure rate is only 2 percent.
Cons Side effects of the morning-after pill can include nausea or vomiting.

Under certain circumstances, an IUD may be fitted. It can be inserted up to 120 hours (5 days) after unprotected sex, and can be more effective than the hormonal method.

● See your doctor

If you or your partner find the presence of the diaphragm or cap physically uncomfortable or if you have recurring bladder or vaginal infections.

See also:

1/BEING A WELL WOMAN
Healthy body systems p. 38

4/HORMONAL HEALTH
Reproductive problems
pp. 146–149
Pregnancy problems pp. 174–175

Alternative contraception

The methods described here are for a woman who does not want to or cannot use the pill or barrier methods of birth control described on the previous pages.

IUD

What it is A small T-shaped plastic device coated with copper fitted through the cervix into the uterus (hence its name, intrauterine device). It has a nylon thread attached which hangs down into the vagina so the user can check it is still in place. After discussion with a family planning practitioner or doctor (and occasionally tests to check that she has no sexually transmitted disease), a woman usually has the IUD fitted in the early part of her menstrual cycle although it can be fitted up to day 19 of a 28-day cycle. It is effective immediately and can be kept in place for five years. If necessary, it can be removed after the next period.

How it works The IUD prevents implantation of the fertilized egg by disrupting the lining of the uterus. It is also possible that because it acts as a "foreign body" in the uterus, it attracts infection-fighting white blood cells which swallow invaders—in this case the sperm and the egg.

Pros It has a very low failure rate, only about 1 percent. Once it has been fitted, after each period you must check that the thread is still there.

Cons It is not first choice in women who are at risk of contracting STDs. Insertion may be uncomfortable. There is a slight risk of perforation of the uterus in the first few months of use. In rare cases, the IUD may migrate to a different part of the body and surgery may be necessary to remove it. Periods may be heavier and more painful. In other rare cases, the woman's body expels the IUD.

May be unsuitable if You or your partner are not completely monogamous, since it does not stop the transfer of STDs; you have not had children—there is a slight risk of infertility so an IUD should be the contraceptive of choice only for a woman who has completed her family or does not wish to have children; you have painful or heavy periods, pelvic inflammatory disease, anaemia or have previously had an ectopic pregnancy.

See your doctor

If you miss a period or have cramping or vaginal bleeding. If you are using an IUD and you become pregnant there is a greater chance that the fertilized egg will implant itself in the Fallopian tube and you will need urgent medical help.

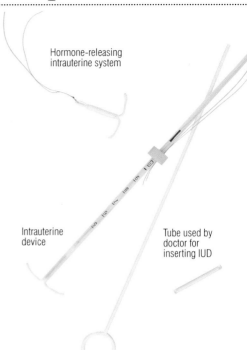

Hormone-releasing intrauterine system

Intrauterine device

Tube used by doctor for inserting IUD

IUD AND IUS
Intrauterine devices are usually made of plastic wrapped with copper. They are inserted into the woman's uterus by a medical practitioner and provide almost certain contraception. They do not, however, protect against STDs. Another method—barrier contraception—should be used for safety.

MIRENA (HORMONE-RELEASING IUD)

What it is An intrauterine system (IUS) designed to stay in the body for five years.

How it works As well as acting as an IUD, it releases low doses of the hormone levonorgestrel (in a similar way to the progestogen-only pill), thickening cervical mucus to stop sperm reaching the uterus and thinning the uterine lining to prevent egg implantation.

Pros It is especially useful as a contraceptive for perimenopausal women and is as efficient in women over 40 as the combined pill or sterilization. It is often used to remedy heavy periods, which typically become lighter and sometimes painless six months after insertion.

Cons There is a low risk of ectopic pregnancy. It may be difficult to insert in women who have not had children.

STERILIZATION

Male and female sterilization are surgical methods of contraception and should be used only by people who have completed their family or who don't want children. Sterilization should be viewed as final—although occasionally, at high cost and with difficulty, it can be reversed. It is the most popular form of family planning after the age of 35.

Tubal ligation for women
How it works The Fallopian tubes are cut or banded via laparoscopic surgery. Eggs from the ovaries cannot then reach the uterus.

Pros There is less than 1 percent chance of pregnancy. Sex can be spontaneous afterwards. Apart from the surgery, there is little risk to health. It is effective immediately.

Cons General anaesthetic is necessary. There is a slight risk of pregnancy and a 40 percent chance of it being ectopic. It does not protect against STDs.

May be unsuitable if You are not in a stable monogamous relationship. It may be difficult to adjust to it psychologically.

Vasectomy for men
How it works The two tubes (the vas deferens) that conduct the sperm from the testicles to the penis are cut and the ends are tied or heat-sealed .

Pros It is 100 percent effective. It is a short procedure, done under local anaesthetic. It does not affect the ability to have erections and ejaculate (semen without sperm).

Cons It is not effective for three months after surgery so use other contraception in this time. It does not protect against STDs. It may be a risk factor for prostate cancer. It can cause psychological problems, which can be reduced through counselling before the procedure.

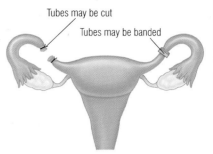

Female sterilization

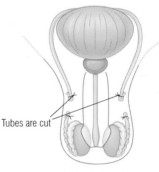

Male sterilization

NATURAL BIRTH CONTROL
What it is There are two methods. In the first method, a woman learns, with help from a natural fertility teacher, how to use a menstrual calendar (p. 183). This charts her temperature and changes in vaginal mucus in order to see which days of the month she is likely to be fertile. Most women are fertile a few days before and a day or more after ovulation.

In the second method, a small personal computer uses urine testing to check hormone levels. Over several months, it tracks your individual cycle. Then it uses a system of coloured lights to tell you whether you are fertile: green days are safe, red days (about eight a month) mean you are fertile, and on amber days you need to retest your urine.

How it works By finding out which days in the month you are fertile, you can avoid getting pregnant by not having intercourse at that time or by using barrier methods.

Pros Your fertility is not affected. Religions that do not approve of artificial birth control approve of it. There are no health risks. If natural birth control is strictly adhered to, the failure rate can be as low as 5 percent (but it is usually higher).

Cons If the method is not followed correctly all the time, failure rates can be high—nearly 35 percent for the temperature/mucus method. You need to be extremely motivated to follow it, as does your partner. It can be complicated to learn and complex to follow. Each menstrual cycle has to be plotted separately, since the day of ovulation can vary from one month to the next. Illness may alter your temperature and vaginal infections change your vaginal mucus. If you use a computer it is expensive and is recommended only for women with 23- to 35-day cycles.

May be unsuitable If you are not in an established relationship; you or your partner want to have spontaneous sexual intercourse without having to watch the calendar; it is essential that you do not become pregnant; one of you is not committed to making it work.

See your doctor
If you have been sterilized by tubal ligation and develop pelvic pain and vaginal bleeding. It may indicate an ectopic pregnancy.

See your doctor
If you miss a period. You may be pregnant and you may need to consider your options.

UNWANTED PREGNANCY

Nobody sets out to become pregnant in order to have an abortion. Yet many women, married and unmarried, find themselves in the position of having to make a choice about abortion which may affect them for many years to come. Remember that, if you are in any doubt, there is the option of giving birth to the baby and having it adopted.

See also:

1/BEING A WELL WOMAN
Healthy body systems p. 38
A healthy mind pp. 48–49

6/TREATMENTS & THERAPIES
Treatment plans pp. 262–269
Conventional treatments
pp. 282–287
Complementary therapies
pp. 292–297

Having an abortion

Many pregnancies—about one in three in unmarried women and one in four in married ones—end in abortion, which is the voluntary termination of pregnancy before the foetus can live independently. There may be many reasons for a pregnancy to be terminated. Conception may have been unintentional or the pregnancy unwanted, the woman may have a health or age problem or there may be an abnormality in the foetus or a worry about genetic inheritance.

Whatever the reason, the more thought and care that goes into the decision, the better the psychological outcome will be. Reliable advice and information should be sought on the methods used and what, if any, side effects they may have. Abortion is a legal procedure and every woman's right should she not want to go ahead with a pregnancy.

MAKING THE DECISION

Some women know immediately that they want to terminate their pregnancy and will be comfortable with their decision; others are not sure. Most will want to discuss it with people closest to them, especially with the male partner, if appropriate. Having a supportive male partner can make a great deal of difference at such a time, but for many women this may not be an option. How a woman feels about the prospect of abortion will depend on why she wants one. A woman who definitely does not want to have a child is in a different position from a woman who would ideally like one, but for financial or other reasons is unable to cope with one at present. If abortion is against the moral or reli-

gious code she was brought up with, this can cause even more conflict. If there is any uncertainty, it is important not to feel pressured into having an abortion. You may wish to consider the alternative of adoption (p. 68).

TALKING IT THROUGH

Because it is much easier physically and psychologically to have an abortion as early in a pregnancy as possible, time may be an added pressure in the decision making. To help you place the experience in perspective, you need to talk to people who know the emotional problems that may be involved and who will not be judgmental. Doctors vary considerably in their attitude to abortion—they may be supportive, condemnatory or patronizing. Counsellors at clinics where abortions are done are supportive of a woman's choice, whatever it is. Having the opportunity to talk through your decision will help you to feel more reconciled to it later.

PROBLEMS WITH THE FOETUS

Making the decision to abort a wanted baby may cause pain and trauma. You may feel it is the only option because antenatal tests show the foetus to have chromosomal or physical problems such as Down's syndrome or spina bifida. These tests (blood, ultrasound scan and amniocentesis) are offered and carried out routinely; some are done near 16 weeks and there may be a wait for the results. A counsellor or support group can help you come to terms with what may be an agonizing decision and to understand the implications for future pregnancies.

See your doctor

Your first consideration after unprotected sex should be some kind of morning-after treatment (p. 63) which can be effective in blocking pregnancy for several days after intercourse.

ABORTION PROCEDURES

Termination of a pregnancy (under 24 weeks) can be done on request by a doctor at a family planning or abortion clinic or at a hospital. The needs and welfare of the woman involved are of prime importance, particularly if there are health problems such as heart disease, blood clotting disorders or possible mental conditions.

Legalized abortion is a commonly performed surgical procedure, mostly done between seven and 12 weeks. You may have a pelvic examination or an ultrasound scan. Tests may be done to see if you are anaemic and if you have a rhesus negative blood type, and also for infection (STD). The doctor will want to know whether you have had a child or a previous abortion or miscarriage. This first appointment can be emotional and a partner or friend can be a great support.

The termination is done by vacuum aspiration or dilatation and curettage (D&C), a surgical procedure with local anaesthetic administered to the cervix. It can be painful, but the procedure is quicker than under a general anaesthetic, which is more risky. You may feel nauseated and have cramps, similar to painful periods, during the procedure which takes 10 to 15 minutes. You will probably be in the clinic for several hours and you may feel shaky. You will bleed, so take sanitary towels with you. You should ask your doctor when you can return to work (a few days' rest is usually advisable). Antibiotics are often prescribed to prevent infection.

ABORTION AFTER 12 WEEKS

At this later stage—the second trimester (12–24 weeks)—the health risks are greater and the two procedures used can be more distressing. Both induce a short labour and involve a one- or two-day hospital stay. The first, at 13 to 16 weeks, is also a D&C procedure (as above), but it is done over two days. Absorbent dilators are inserted into the cervix, where they absorb cervical fluid, thicken and gradually stretch the cervix. The next day, the dilators are removed and the foetus and other tissue are suctioned from the uterus as before.

The other method, used for later pregnancies, involves placing prostaglandin suppositories in the vagina or injecting prostaglandins into the uterus to cause contractions. Local anaesthesia or pain-relieving medicine is given. The foetus is expelled over the next 12 hours and a D&C may be done later to ensure that the uterus is clear.

The trauma of rape

Rape is one of the most traumatic things that can happen to a woman. The experience of being forced, coerced or manipulated into unwelcome sex will remain with you for life. The humiliation you feel can prevent you from trusting men, destroy any sexual relationship you might have and leave you psychologically scarred.

The number of reported rapes is increasing faster than other crimes of violence. Legally, only penetration of the vagina by the penis is rape. Anything else is known as sexual assault—even anal or oral rape or penetration by an object. Most rape is carried out by a man known to the woman; rape by a total stranger is unusual. So-called date rape, in which a woman is raped by a man with whom she has become friendly, has been a subject of controversy. However, if a woman does not want to have sex and a man makes her do so against her will, that is rape.

Contacting a Rape Crisis Centre or counsellor will provide you with emotional and physical support after this terrible event. You may wish to discuss informing the police and what this might entail. Your first reaction may be to want to take a shower, but before you wash you should have a medical check-up. This is best done by a doctor or at a hospital where there are staff experienced in examining rape victims. A complete physical examination will be done, you will be given tests for STDs and, if there is a chance you could become pregnant, emergency contraception. If this does not work, or you do not seek help after rape, you may have an unwanted pregnancy. You should make an appointment to see your doctor two weeks after the incident for follow-up care. You may need ongoing counselling to deal with your emotions.

RISKS TO BE AWARE OF

Having an abortion in the early stages of pregnancy is safe but there are a few risks. Very early abortion (before six or seven weeks) can mean that foetal matter is missed. You may remain pregnant and the abortion may need to be repeated. Sometimes tissue is retained in the uterus which may have to be removed by D&C later. You will be advised not to use tampons for three weeks after the operation because they can cause infection. Indications of infection are a high temperature, very heavy bleeding or foul-smelling discharge or severe abdominal pain; if you have these, go back to your doctor for antibiotic treatment. Have a post-abortion check-up to ensure your body has returned to normal before resuming lovemaking.

NORMAL REACTIONS

Loss and sadness are perfectly normal reactions after a termination of pregnancy, even when you are sure you have made the right decision. It is important that you show compassion to yourself at this time and avoid people who are unable to show it to you. Accept that it may take some time to recover fully, but if you feel you need help with your emotions seek a bereavement counsellor's help.

See also:

1/BEING A WELL WOMAN
Healthy body systems p. 38
A healthy mind pp. 44–49

4/HORMONAL HEALTH
Pregnancy pp. 170–177

6/TREATMENTS & THERAPIES
Treatment plans pp. 262–263
Conventional treatments
pp. 282–283

Having a baby adopted

Abortion is not necessarily the only answer for a woman with an unwanted pregnancy. She may decide to carry the baby to term and then have it adopted. In this instance it is essential that she seeks reliable information and advice on what may be involved, including help with her own physical and emotional welfare during pregnancy and after giving birth.

Once the pregnancy has been confirmed by the doctor and the normal tests done, you should ask about your options, including adoption. The doctor or member of staff should be able to provide nonjudgmental counselling—whether a family member could possibly keep the child, for example, or if there are strong feelings about who the adopter should be.

If you decide to have the baby adopted, it is generally advised that the procedure begins immediately, under the direction of a social worker in an adoption agency. A case record of the history of the child, its parents and their state of health and religious or cultural preferences will be made. It is rare for a birth mother to deal directly with the people who wish to adopt her child but an independent agency may offer support during the pregnancy for this purpose. A mother's actual consent to placing a child for adoption cannot be given before the birth though she may indicate this as her wish. The mother's consent is generally given six weeks after the birth.

If the birth mother is married, her husband automatically shares parental responsibility and his consent must be sought before the child can be adopted. If the woman is unmarried but puts the name of the father on the birth certificate (which must be registered within six weeks after the birth) he may apply for a Parental Responsibility Order so that he can be involved in the child's care. In most cases he has to agree to the adoption process.

In complicated cases, such as mental illness, ill-treatment, neglect or abandonment, an adoption agency needs the permission of only one parent to apply for a "freeing" order. The aim of proceedings to free the child for adoption is to obtain unconditional consent; once given to the court it is final. The court will give parental responsibility to the adoption agency until the adoption is completed.

CARING FOR YOURSELF

A pregnant woman who is intent on giving her child up for adoption should seek counselling to help her recover physically and emotionally from the experience. Your doctor or a local voluntary agency may have counselling facilities and may provide advice and information about the birth and the postnatal procedure. You will not be expected to provide care for your child, who will be placed with foster parents as a first step. You may decide to look after the child and share the care under the guidance of the social worker. Issues such as whether to breastfeed or not should be part of any discussion.

Finding the right person to talk freely to about the reasons for giving up the child is important. You may not agree with termination or, if conception occurred after rape or violent assault, you may not feel able to care for a child conceived in this way. Perhaps you are not prepared to be a parent at this stage. Whatever your reasons, you need to address them, to allow a time to grieve so that you recover fully. Physically you need to see your doctor for a check-up six weeks after the birth to ensure you are healing well.

A WANTED CHILD
There are prospective parents all over the country seeking to adopt a child from a background similar to their own. After a woman who chooses to have her child placed for adoption gives her consent the procedure can be done quickly so the adoptees can begin parenting without delay.

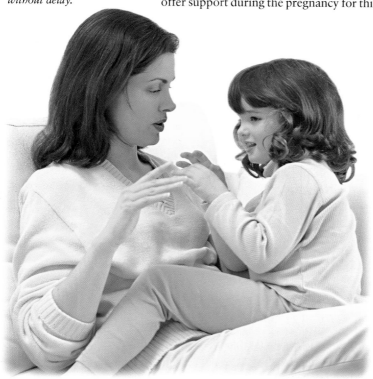

SEXUAL PROBLEMS

Not being able to make love because your body won't do what you want it to can be frightening and frustrating. It happens to men and women and can cause worry and anxiety. Medical help may be needed to investigate the problem.

When love hurts

See also:

2/SEX & SEXUALITY
Your sexual self pp. 54–55

4/HORMONAL HEALTH
Endocrine system problems p. 144
Uterine problems p. 164

5/ILLNESSES &EMERGENCIES
Acute infections pp. 244–246

Sex should be pleasurable, not painful. If something is hurting you, the first thing you should do is stop—or ask your partner to stop. Painful intercourse can be caused simply by a man thrusting too hard or too deeply. It may also happen if you have a chronic medical condition, in which case all that may be necessary is to find a more comfortable position.

If intercourse continues to be painful, there may be other reasons. Infections such as yeast vaginitis, cystitis or pelvic inflammatory disease (PID) can be the cause of discomfort. If you have an infection, you will need to see your doctor for antibiotic treatment; until the infection is gone you should not have sex. Inflammation of the vagina can also be the result of an allergy to perfume in soap and body lotion; the pain should disappear when you stop using them. If you bleed after intercourse, you should report this to your doctor who may arrange tests.

LACK OF LUBRICATION

Some women find that intercourse is uncomfortable because their vaginas are not lubricated sufficiently. This may occur because sex is infrequent or you are not yet sexually aroused, in which case more foreplay may help. Other women may not produce enough lubrication no matter how excited they are. This can apply particularly at the menopause and after, when the vaginal walls thin and shrink from lack of oestrogen. Using a lubricant can overcome the problem, as can hormone replacement therapy (HRT), which makes the tissues more like they were before menopause, or oestrogen cream.

A woman's first sexual experience may cause pain—either there is not enough lubrication or the hymen may be unbroken. Take things very slowly, make sure your vagina is moist and your partner stretches the opening with fingers first.

After childbirth the memory of physical pain can reduce desire for sex and cause anxiety. Overcoming this requires a gentle partner, much reassurance and the use of a lubricant so intercourse can be enjoyed once more.

VAGINISMUS

This is a condition where the vaginal muscles tighten so that any penetration is painful and, in serious cases, impossible (so an internal examination or cervical smear cannot be done). Vaginismus is usually caused by anxiety about sex and is not permanent. To see whether you have vaginismus, put your fingers inside your vagina to feel if the walls seem very close together. The best way of treating it is to try and establish a relaxation ritual during which, at your own speed, you find out for yourself how to relax the vagina. Then, with your partner, have lots of foreplay so your vagina is well-lubricated before any penetration.

If you have tried these suggestions and are still having pain, stop attempting penetration. Do not force yourself to have intercourse because you think you should. Your body may start associating sex with pain, affecting your desire and leading to a bigger problem. A trained sex therapist can help.

Men's problems

Some men cannot achieve an erection from time to time, and this is quite normal. Other men may ejaculate far too quickly, leaving their partners frustrated. It helps to know that some causes of erectile dysfunction and premature ejaculation are psychological and can be alleviated by simple exercises a couple can learn with the help of a therapist trained in sex therapy. Remember that if you and your partner are having penetration quickly to avoid loss of an erection, you may be compounding the problem, causing discomfort and anxiety for both of you.

When a man is unable to get an erection at all, or cannot maintain one for long, there may be a physical factor involved; encourage your partner to get medical advice.

Sex and relationships

When sex is going well, it is just one part of a loving relationship. When it goes wrong, it can feel as if it is taking over not just your relationship, but every element of your life.

The most common sexual complaints women have fall into four categories: decreased libido, difficulty with arousal, dissatisfaction with frequency of orgasm or the type of stimulation required to reach orgasm, and painful or uncomfortable sexual activity (p. 69).

Factors that can affect the first three of these include depression, anxiety, fatigue, alcohol consumption, low hormone levels and many drugs—both prescription and illegal—including antidepressants and treatment for high blood pressure and fluid retention. Your lack of sexual response should be discussed with your doctor, particularly if there is illness involved.

Both men and women can have sexual problems—and if one partner has a problem, the other is invariably affected by it. A sexual problem that has always existed is called a primary problem and may have either a physical or a deep-seated psychological cause. When problems start during a previously happy relationship, it is essential to consider the reasons rather than ignoring them.

Many couples remember a time in their relationship when sex was good. Those memories and their fondness for each other should reassure them that, whatever is causing the present upset, it can be overcome.

DECREASED LIBIDO

Between 50 and 70 percent of women report loss of desire at some time in their life. For men who complain of impotence, it may well mask a lack of desire. People can feel bewildered and upset when desire deserts them, but it is only a problem when one or both of you think it is.

It is not uncommon to find you want to have sex less frequently the longer you know each other. If you remain close and intimate, you will be satisfied by quality rather than quantity. If on the other hand you have no interest in making love, you may have relationship difficulties. This is the most common cause of decreased libido and also arousal and orgasm problems.

The reasons can be complex. What you were taught in childhood about what sexual expression should and should not be may have predisposed you to certain emotional traits that do not sit well with your current relationship—often without you realizing it.

Each new relationship brings different pleasures and problems, but people do tend to bring their sexual habits and assumptions with them. In the early days, you are likely to have a lot of fantasies about your sexual partner, because there are always new things to discover. There can be an air of secretiveness to add to the excitement. Once a relationship is established, sexual arousal can depend on different factors.

WHEN DISSATISFACTION STRIKES

The most obvious cause of many sexual problems is to be found in the pressures of day-to-day living. Work demands, little time to relax, even good events such as the birth of a child or a new job, can stop you from wanting sex. You may not be feeling well or on top of things and other parts of your life take priority.

It helps to know in any relationship that this is inevitable and will happen from time to time. However, if sex loses its importance to both of you, you will lose intimacy too. In this situation it is essential that you make time for sex and for each other. Organize it so that the two of you can be alone without other distractions. Plan a date together, doing something you enjoy, spend some time hugging, hand holding, give each other a massage or a foot rub, and see where it takes you. You may not solve all your problems but you will be closer.

RELEASING YOUR FEELINGS

Sex-related anxiety is not uncommon in both men and women and can prevent you reaching orgasm or even allowing yourself to be stimulated. If you know your love-making is likely to be interrupted, perhaps by children, it can be difficult to relax and enjoy yourselves. Or you may worry about becoming pregnant. Such concerns should be resolved before the anxiety becomes disabling to your relationship.

Changes in your lifestyle—giving up work, having a baby, changing jobs or neighbourhoods—can cause you to look anew at your sexual relationship. If you can't reach orgasm now was it always this way, or were you once able to be satisfied? Have you become stuck in certain sexual patterns or habits? Perhaps there are other reasons why you can't relax. Your desire may be inhibited by a plethora of deep feelings—other problems within the relationship can leave you with blocked anger, repressed emotions and no way of talking about them. These emotional issues can be resolved by increased communication.

If you find that you can't talk to each other or there is too much anger felt, it may be worth seeing a counsellor who is trained as a sex therapist who can facilitate communication, look at the emotions and may guide you through a series of sensual exercises to connect with your sexual self and each other.

THE PURPOSE OF SEX THERAPY

When normally loving people have problems in their sex life, a sex therapist may help them find the answers they seek. Sex therapy can be based on behaviour therapy or insight-oriented, psychodynamic psychotherapy, or preferably both. A therapist who is also trained in sex therapy will alternate between these as needed during the treatment with a couple or individual depending on the issues revealed.

A therapist can show you and your partner how to change the way you approach or have sex in order to overcome specific and solvable problems, such as premature ejaculation or insufficient arousal.

In the 1960s sex therapists Masters and Johnson developed a programme called sensate focusing, which is often used today to help couples discover more about their feelings and sensations. You are given a set of exercises to do at home in your own time. You take turns pleasuring each other through massage, touching and stroking parts of the body, but not the genitals. As you progress in your understanding of each other's reactions and have confidence in saying yes to what you like—and you both find your excitement increasing—non-intercourse related genital activity is encouraged. Finally your sex life is restored to normal, or better, so that your relationship should benefit from a return to shared values—and prosper.

FOCUS ON SENSATIONS
When a couple starts therapy for sexual problems, the first stage will encourage them to discover more about their feelings and sensations. Pleasuring each other through the gentlest massage and stroking brings new understanding of what arouses them.

SEXUAL INFECTIONS

Once called venereal diseases, sexually transmitted diseases—more commonly called STDs—are infections spread from one person to another by sexual contact. They are a worldwide problem and can have particularly serious consequences for women.

The dangers of sex

Women are at greater risk from sexually transmitted diseases than men—a woman is, for instance, more likely than a man to catch an STD from a single sexual encounter. There are about 25 different infections classified as STDs. The best known is HIV—the virus that leads to AIDS—which a woman is 17 times more likely to catch from a man than a man is from a woman. Viral STDs, such as HIV and herpes, cannot be cured; bacterial STDs can be cured if treated promptly.

If there is any chance that you have contracted a sexually transmitted disease even if you have no symptoms at present—and women often have fewer noticeable symptoms—you have a responsibility to yourself as well as to your sexual partners to be diagnosed, treated and to let any partners know the situation.

If you have caught an STD it will not clear up on its own. If left untreated some STDs, such as chlamydia and syphilis, can have long-term consequences for your health and fertility. STD infection during pregnancy can also lead to complications and illness for the baby.

HOW DO YOU CATCH THEM?

STDs are usually caught by having sex—vaginal, anal or oral—with an infected person, and exchanging body fluids such as semen, blood and vaginal fluids. Very rarely is an STD passed on though blood transfusion. STDs cannot be caught from toilet seats or swimming pools, although some, such as pubic lice, can be picked up in close, nonsexual contact. Other infections, such as cystitis and thrush, can be passed on or made worse by sex—but they can develop without sexual contact.

WHO IS AT RISK?

Almost anyone who is sexually active is at risk of catching an STD. There are only two totally risk-free choices. The first is abstinence. The

Practising safe sex

The idea of safe sex first developed out of the need to prevent HIV transmission, but anyone who is sexually active and not in a long-term monogamous relationship should take this approach to reduce the chances of catching an STD. At its most basic, a condom should be used every time you have vaginal, oral or anal intercourse so that body fluids do not pass from one person to another. But this will not remove the risk completely. You may wish to use multiple forms of latex or polyurethane protection—condoms, dental dams (covers teeth and gums) or gloves—so there is no contact with any body fluids during oral or manual sex.

Other strategies include having sex without penile penetration, restricting the number of sexual partners, discussing your partners' sexual histories with them and putting condoms on dildos and vibrators. Some men may be reluctant to use condoms as they may reduce sensation. For your own benefit, it is important to establish before you get into bed that a condom is a prerequisite for sex. The more convincing you can be about these ground rules the better. Also, do not place yourself in physical or emotional danger through getting drunk or taking drugs, which make you less capable of taking care of yourself.

second is life-long monogamy. If you and your partner have only ever had sex with each other, then you are not at risk.

Today, it is far less likely for a person to have just one sexual partner in a lifetime. You may be in a trusting and long-standing relationship but, as some STDs do not present obvious symptoms, it is possible that one of you may be infected with something caught many years previously. The more partners you have, the more you are at risk.

BREAKING THE NEWS

It may be difficult to tell your partner or partners that you may have an STD—though this can depend on the circumstances in which you contracted it. A long-standing but recently diagnosed STD, such as chlamydia, may be seen as a health condition, rather than an emotional crisis in a relationship. Professionals at the clinic you attend can inform casual partners if you don't feel able to do so yourself.

Being told that your established partner has an STD can be as hard as breaking the news yourself, although it does not necessarily mean that the infected partner has contracted the disease while in the relationship. However, you must be examined and treated as necessary if your partner is infected. Feelings of hurt, betrayal and anger—on either side—will need to be discussed and you and your partner may find counselling helpful.

> **! Caution**
>
> If it is possible that you could have an STD and you have any of the following symptoms, contact your doctor or hospital right away: unpleasant vaginal discharge, pain during intercourse, pelvic pain, pain on passing urine, swelling in the groin, sores in the genital area or flu-like symptoms. These may get worse during your period. If you are infected, you should not have sex until your treatment is complete.

SEXUALLY TRANSMITTED DISEASES

Symptoms may develop weeks, months or years after the initial exposure to the infection. A sexually active woman should ensure that she has regular pelvic examinations and cervical smears, as these may reveal problems. If you have had unprotected sex with a person who you think may have an STD, see your own doctor or one at a genito-urinary medicine clinic. There is no need to be embarrassed. Nobody knows why you are there.

Disease	Symptoms	How detected	Treatment
HIV			
The human immunodeficiency virus (HIV) is a leading cause of death of young people in many countries. After contracting HIV, people may have no symptoms for years, but over time the virus attacks the body's immune system, leaving it susceptible to acquired immune deficiency syndrome (AIDS). This is a collection of symptoms that prevents the body from fighting a range of infections and conditions.	Mild flu, which comes and goes, then vulnerability to infections such as thrush, shingles and herpes. Loss of appetite and weight.	The virus becomes apparent in blood tests, one to three months after the infection has been contracted.	Retroviral drugs (triple therapy) to reduce some viral activity, such as that of PCP pneumonia, and to prolong life. Infections treated. Change of diet and lifestyle to boost immune system.
Hepatitis B			
This liver infection is caused by a virus that is 100 times more infectious than HIV. Symptoms appear two to six weeks after infection caused by sexual contact or through infected blood or other body fluids (saliva or faecal matter). Most people recover, others become carriers and may pass it on to sexual partners as well as remaining at risk of serious liver disease later. Family and sexual partners of those with hepatitis B can be vaccinated.	Jaundice, loss of appetite, nausea, headaches.	Blood test. In rare cases, a liver biopsy.	Includes rest and restricted physical activity. For chronic hepatitis, the drug interferon.

Continued overleaf

Disease	Symptoms	How detected	Treatment
Trichomoniasis			
This is caused by a microscopic protozoan single-celled animal. It is uncommon, but is associated with other STDs such as gonorrhoea, chlamydia and genital warts. It is spread through sexual contact and may be passed on by syringes, or shared devices used anally or vaginally. Trichomoniasis does not usually produce serious disorders and only rarely reaches the upper genital tract.	Vaginal discharge is smelly, and may be green and frothy. Soreness of the vulva and pain on passing urine are common, as is discomfort on penetration.	Testing vaginal secretions.	Antibiotics: Metronidazole, Tinidazole. Pessaries: Povidone-iodine
Syphilis			
A bacterial infection, syphilis—if untreated—can develop over several years into serious illness and possible death. In modern times, syphilis is usually diagnosed and treated before it gets to the tertiary, or final, stage for which there is no treatment. Syphilis is passed on through sexual contact. If anything leads you to think that you have been exposed to the infection, you must contact a doctor immediately. Syphilis screening is carried out as part of antenatal care and for giving blood.	First stage of infection is a painless sore on the genitals, which may come and go unnoticed. Second stage, up to three months after infection, has flu-like symptoms and a body rash lasting 2 to 10 weeks.	A blood test may not be effective if infection occurred less than 10 days before. If there is a genital sore, a smear of cells is examined microscopically. A blood test is then done to confirm diagnosis.	Antibiotics, usually injected penicillin; azithromycin or doxycycline are used for those with a penicillin allergy. Partner should also be treated. This may be ongoing, depending on the results of three-monthly tests.
Gonorrhoea			
Gonorrhoea is caused by bacteria that spread around the vagina and urethra. It is highly contagious. Sufferers may have no symptoms, but if untreated it can lead to serious problems—chronic stomach pain, infertility and other STDs. It can infect a foetus in the womb via the birth canal, causing blindness. It is spread by sexual contact, including oral sex.	Unpleasant vaginal discharge, an urgent need to pass urine, pain on urination, bleeding between periods.	Testing of a sample of cervical fluid.	Often resistant to some antibiotics. Ceftriaxone, ciprofloxacin, doxycycline and cefixime can be used. Both partners must be treated.
Chlamydia			
The most common STD, caused by a bacterium, chlamydia often has no symptoms and is particularly common in young people. It has been recommended that all young women be screened annually. Left untreated in women, the infection can lead to pelvic inflammatory disease (PID), which in turn can cause infertility. Men who contract chlamydia can be made sterile. After one bout of PID, the disease tends to be recurrent.	Pain during intercourse, thin vaginal discharge, burning when passing urine.	Swab of the cervical fluid is tested.	Antibiotics of the doxycycline or tetracycline type, such as azithromycin.

Disease	Symptoms	How detected	Treatment
Genital herpes			
The most common viral STD caused by the herpes simplex virus HSV2, which is similar to the cold sore virus HSV1 and the Epstein-Barr virus of glandular fever. Genital herpes is contagious, incurable, but not fatal. The virus remains in your body, though it may not show symptoms, and can be triggered by stress and tight-fitting undergarments and clothing. It is spread by sexual contact—this can include kissing or touching infected areas. Babies born vaginally during an active herpes infection may, rarely, become infected.	A few days after infection, flu-like symptoms, pain on passing urine, burning in genital area, lower back pain. There may be vaginal discharge, swollen glands and small red bumps in or near the vagina which blister.	A doctor takes a sample of fluid from a blister and sends it away for testing. If no blisters are present, herpes can be hard to diagnose.	Antiviral drugs help healing during attacks and can be taken long term to reduce the frequency. Bathe sores in tepid salty water; use a topical painkilling cream. Wash hands after touching sores. Reduce stress.
Nonspecific urethritis			
This bacterial infection of the urethra can be caused by chlamydia, ureaplasma or trichomanas. In a man, one sign is a cloudy discharge from the penis. Early treatment prevents spread of infection into the pelvic cavity. There is no firm evidence that irritants such as perfumed soaps can cause urethritis.	Pain or burning when urinating; frequent urination.	Urine and urethral discharge testing.	Antibiotics: doxycycline, azithromycin or erythromycin.
Pubic lice and scabies			
Two types of tiny, irritating parasites that live on the skin but can't be seen. Pubic lice, often called crabs, are pinhead-sized insects that lay their eggs in hairy parts of the body, particularly the groin. Scabies is an itchy rash caused by a mite burrowing under the skin to lay its eggs. They are passed on by sexual or other close contact with an infected person.	Pubic lice: intense itching or rash in the pubic/groin area. Scabies:generalized itching.	By sight.	Your doctor or clinic will suggest relevant shampoos or creams. It is not necessary to wash clothing and bedding in very hot water, as previously assumed.
Genital warts			
These contagious warts are caused by the human papilloma virus (HPV), which can show up in cervical cells in a cervical smear. As the virus may be involved in pre-cancerous changes it is important to have regular smears. There are no obvious symptoms of infection. Warts can grow in or outside the vagina or around the anus and may be puffy and pink or hard and gray. Genital warts are passed on through sex with an infected person. Even after treatment, the virus remains in the body.	Small, painless lumps appear around genitals or anus three weeks to six months after infection. May itch. Associated with cervical dysplasia (pre-cancerous changes), caused by HPV.	By sight, during a physical examination or when a Pap smear is being done.	Visible warts can be burned off, frozen off or treated with laser surgery, but virus remains. May be self-treated with drugs such as podophylline cream at home.

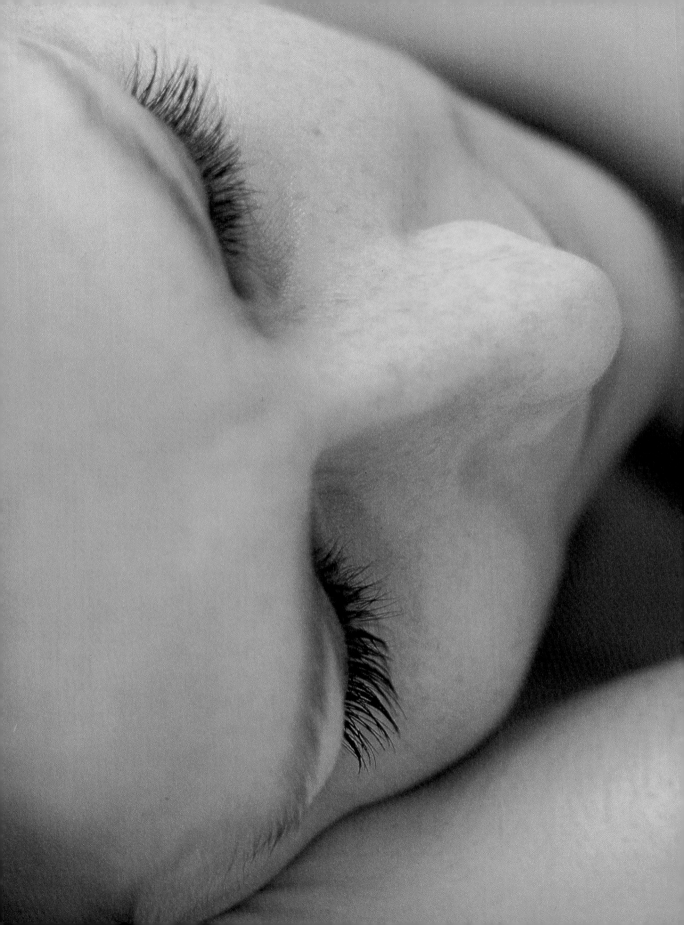

GENERAL HEALTH ISSUES

This chapter discusses illnesses and conditions that are related to a woman's lifestyle and may build up gradually over the years until a crisis point is reached and medical intervention is necessary. For themselves and the members of their families, women need to know when their health is being compromised and be aware of the telltale signs indicating that medical advice should be sought. The stresses of modern life can affect females of all ages and patterns and habits may be established that have serious, life-threatening outcomes. Knowing how to recognize these stresses and habits is the first step in formulating measures to prevent them and their associated illnesses.

SKELETAL SYSTEM PROBLEMS

Your body's frame and its network of muscles, tendons and ligaments are designed to support your weight through a range of activities. When mechanical or immune factors cause problems, they must be recognized and treated to prevent long-term impairment.

Vulnerable joints

Your body is capable of a range of movements that can occur without your conscious effort. You learnt to move as a baby, reaching out to touch, then to grasp. When your bones became stronger you were able to sit up, crawl and then walk. All of these actions are made possible by an array of joints, each one designed to meet the needs of the particular limb involved.

The brain sends out the messages and your fingers, toes, arms and legs move, enabling you to write or type, walk or climb stairs, roll your shoulders or ankles, bend to touch your toes, lift a child or shopping bags. A woman's lifestyle can put her at risk of joint pain. Too much time spent sitting at a desk or computer, without proper care and attention given to correct posture, can cause chronic problems in the back, neck, wrists and elbows. Carrying heavy loads such as a baby or toddler, suitcases or over-full briefcases can strain muscles and place undue stress on your spine, just as wearing high heels can shift your body forward and compromise the spine's alignment.

In pregnancy your body has a changing centre of gravity because of the weight of the growing baby. Your back muscles have to work harder to maintain an upright stance, and this puts more stress on the strong collagen fibres called ligaments, which have already been relaxed in preparation for the delivery. This can predispose the pregnant woman to backache.

MUSCLES AND MOVEMENT

Muscles, which make up about 23 percent of a woman's body weight, work with the largest (called load- or weight-bearing) joints to allow everyday movement. Muscles need a constant supply of oxygen to work well. If the skeletal muscles—which give the body its form and are anchored to bones—become slack through lack of stimulation and exercise, your movement suffers. Carrying extra weight can also make you prone to musculoskeletal problems.

EXERCISE AND SAFETY

Muscles work better the more they are used, which is why preventive medicine calls for regular, steady exercise. Unaccustomed effort, such as running for a bus, not warming up before an aerobics class or playing a weekend sport, can

HOW JOINTS WORK

Ball-and-socket joints in the shoulder and hip are kept mobile by synovial fluid which contains cells that remove debris and microorganisms. Hinge joints allow the elbows, fingers and knees to move. In the wrists, ankles and spine the joints glide. The head, on a pivot joint at the top of the spine, can swivel and bend.

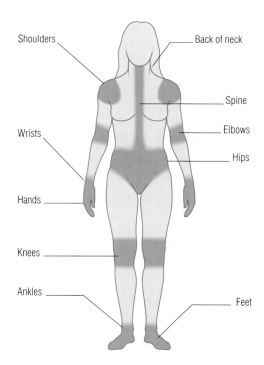

Shoulders

Back of neck

Spine

Elbows

Wrists

Hips

Hands

Knees

Ankles

Feet

cause damage such as a pulled muscle or a strained ligament.

The knee is particularly vulnerable. It has four ligaments and 13 muscles supporting it. The cartilage in the knee can wear down after a sports injury, or from wear and tear over time. Sometimes the ligaments, the supporting tissues of the knee, can tear or become damaged. In this situation, physiotherapy and perhaps surgery may be required.

PAINFUL OCCUPATIONS

Joints are guarded against friction by bursae, small fluid-filled sacs in the fibrous tissue. These can become inflamed through repeated pressure from awkward movements, a condition called bursitis. The most common symptom is pain in a knee, elbow or shoulder. Certain repetitive actions also cause joint pain. In tennis elbow, which is not restricted to tennis players, the repeated rotation of the forearm produces inflammation in the tendons of the forearm near the elbow joint. The use of a manual screwdriver over a long period of time will produce the same effect. NSAIDs (p. 81) may be prescribed and sometimes a hydrocortisone injection may be used to treat this condition.

UNUSUAL CONDITIONS

Women are susceptible to some disabling disorders that can cause joint and muscle pain. Polymyalgia rheumatica (PMR), which can appear after the age of 50, has no known cause. Symptoms include stiffness and aches in the neck, shoulders and hips, and there may be pain and swelling in the hands. In most cases of PMR, blood tests will reveal an elevation in the erythrocyte sedimentation rate (ESR), which indicates the presence of inflammation.

Treatment is by corticosteroids, generally 5–20 mg of prednisone daily. The condition may last for months or years, although most people may be weaned from treatment within two years. However, the symptoms can reappear and in some people an associated condition called giant cell arteritis may occur. The symptoms are headaches, a jaw ache and visual problems. Immediate medical attention is needed to prevent sight damage.

Women in their 20s, 50s and 60s are twice as likely as men of the same age to succumb to two autoimmune disorders affecting the joints or muscles. Dermatomyositis and polymyositis target the muscles in the arms and thighs causing inflammation and general weakness. Symptoms include difficulty reaching overhead, combing your hair or climbing stairs. Diagnosis is made by blood tests, electromyography (EMG), which records electrical activity in muscles, and muscle biopsy. Magnetic resonance imaging (MRI) may be used to pinpoint the affected area for muscle testing and biopsy. Treatment consists of high dose corticosteroids and immunosuppressive drugs such as methotrexate.

See your doctor

A ganglion is a swelling of synovial membrane in the sheath of a tendon, most usually on the back of the wrist. It may disappear by itself in time, or can be removed by surgery if the doctor thinks it necessary.

! Caution

Swollen ankles occur when fluid builds up in tissues around the joint. It happens if you sit for a long time (as on a plane journey). If it doesn't subside within 24 hours, see a doctor—it may indicate a leg vein problem or be a sign of kidney or heart disease. In a pregnant woman, swollen ankles can signify a dangerous condition called pre-eclampsia. Seek help immediately if an indentation remains after you press your finger on the swelling.

WHAT GOES WRONG?
The sleeve-like capsule of cartilage surrounding the joint prevents dislocation, and cartilage discs act as shock absorbers. Wear and tear over time causes the cartilage to break down, the bones rub together and new bone growth called osteophytes is produced by the body to try to repair the damage. In autoimmune diseases, the synovial fluid and membrane become inflamed and cartilage damage occurs.

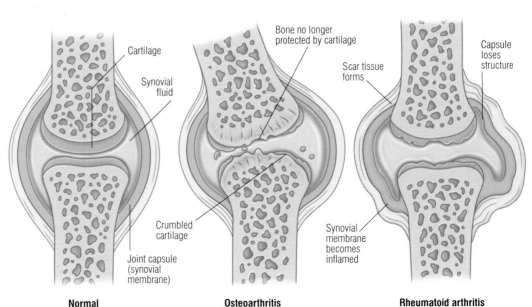

Cartilage
Synovial fluid
Joint capsule (synovial membrane)
Crumbled cartilage
Bone no longer protected by cartilage
Scar tissue forms
Capsule loses structure
Synovial membrane becomes inflamed

Normal   **Osteoarthritis**   **Rheumatoid arthritis**

Arthritis

See also

1/BEING A WELL WOMAN
Healthy body systems p. 30

5/ILLNESSES & EMERGENCIES
Digestive system problems p. 190

6/TREATMENTS & THERAPIES
Conventional treatments
pp. 272–277; p. 288
Alternative medicine
pp. 304–305

Signs and symptoms

♀ The gradual onset of pain in the joints, especially with exertion, that wears off with rest.
♀ Gradually increasing restriction of movement in the affected joint or joints.
♀ A "grating" feeling when the joint is moved.

When the tissues of a joint get disrupted, we call this a form of arthritis. There are around 100 such conditions and they afflict women of all ages.

There are several direct causes of arthritis: infection by bacteria or viruses, the degenerative changes associated with age and disorders of the metabolism or immune system. All joints of the body are vulnerable, from the hips and knees to the shoulders, hands and feet.

Some forms of arthritis can be inherited, but the genes responsible for this are not yet fully understood. Rheumatoid arthritis, for example, runs in families, and there is a strong hereditary link in both gout and psoriatic arthritis. However, if a family member has one of these forms of arthritis, it does not mean that you are destined to get it. In osteoarthritis, inactivity and overweight are factors that predispose people to the disease.

OSTEOARTHRITIS

Known as degenerative joint disease (DJD), osteoarthritis is often associated with aging, though the condition can develop at any age.

Supplements and arthritis

Recent research into tissue injury and painful joints suffered by athletes and other sportspeople has encouraged the development of dietary supplements which may aid repair and recovery of movement. Collagen, glucosamine and chondroitin are essential elements of vulnerable cartilage, tendons and ligaments; when they're under strain, the body can't provide sufficient new material to repair any tissue damage as it occurs.

Studies of patients with osteoarthritis have shown that they benefit from supplements. When the pain is eased, sufferers are less likely to remain immobilized, which is one of the major side effects of arthritis and a leading cause of other complications such as diabetes and heart disease. If you intend to try dietary supplements, discuss them with your doctor first.

The symptoms usually start to appear during middle age and are more common in women than in men. Most people over the age of 70 suffer from the condition to some degree.

Its main cause is wear and tear on a joint, when bones have lost the protective layer (cartilage) or lubricant (synovial fluid) that prevents them from rubbing against each other. A number of factors can increase the rate at which wear and tear takes its toll. These include previous damage to a joint (especially when the condition develops in a young person) or even misalignment of a joint. The two most important factors, however, are a sedentary lifestyle, and—the most common—having much too much body weight.

The progress of osteoarthritis is slow but steady. The cartilage between the bones wears away until, eventually, these bones come into direct contact with each other. At the same time, bony spurs called osteophytes develop around the edges of the joint and the capsule surrounding it becomes thicker and coarser. The cumulative effect is that the joint becomes painful and stiff and its normal movement is restricted. In extreme cases the joint may become deformed.

PAINFUL HANDS

The hands are a common site for arthritis in many older women. In the condition called erosive osteoarthritis painful bony growths form in the joints closest to the fingernails (Heberden's nodes) and middle joints (Bouchard's nodes). Pain and stiffness may be present for a few months to a few years but in general the hands can continue to function. It is not known why the bones change in this way, and there is no proven preventive measure. Degenerative arthritis can also occur at the bones at the base of the thumb.

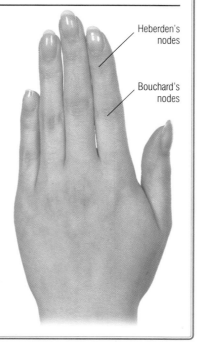

Heberden's nodes

Bouchard's nodes

APPROACHES TO TREATMENT

If osteoarthritis is in its early stages, your doctor is likely to suggest that you do exercises to keep the joints mobile and, if appropriate, lose weight—this may be all that is needed to slow down the onset of the condition.

In moderately severe cases, painkillers and a range of non-steroidal anti-inflammatory drugs (NSAIDs), such as ibuprofen, are likely to be prescribed. Losing weight becomes a priority in such cases, though be careful that any exercise taken is not too demanding, in order to avoid further wear and tear.

Physiotherapy may be suggested to ensure that appropriate exercises are used—some in water—and walking aids, such as a cane, may also be provided to take weight off affected joints. The physiotherapist may also show you how to use hot and cold compresses and other pain-relieving and anti-inflammatory techniques. Your doctor may recommend that you join an arthritis support group to learn more about ways to cope with the condition every-day. When symptoms become so severe that they interfere with an individual's ability to function, she may be referred to an orthopaedic surgeon for possible joint replacement.

GOUT AND PSEUDOGOUT

The cause of these arthritic conditions are crystals that collect in the joint and result in inflammation and pain. With gout, the crystal is monosodium urate (also found in kidney stones, p. 245); with pseudogout, it is calcium pyrophosphate. Gout is more common in men and rare before the menopause in women. Pseudogout tends to occur postmenopausally, too, sometimes with endocrine disorders such as thyroid and parathyroid disease. In gout, the usual sites are the toes, feet and knees; pseudogout commonly affects knees, wrists and feet.

The conditions are diagnosed by examining a sample of fluid from the affected joint and by checking blood levels of uric acid for gout. Possible treatments may be NSAIDs, steroid injections into the area or oral steroids.

WHEN SURGERY IS CONSIDERED

Surgery is only an option when there is severe disability and the normal range of treatments has proved ineffective. Various techniques are used, depending on the extent of degeneration and the joint in which it occurs:

Arthroplasty Part or all of an affected joint is replaced by an artificial one. Arthroplasty is usually chosen if the joint is a hip, knee, shoulder or elbow.

Arthrodesis The bones of the joint are fused. Arthrodesis is generally performed on spinal vertebrae.

Other surgical treatments These include an osteotomy, in which the bones in a joint are re-aligned to relieve pressure, and an osteoplasty, in which damaged material is removed from a joint.

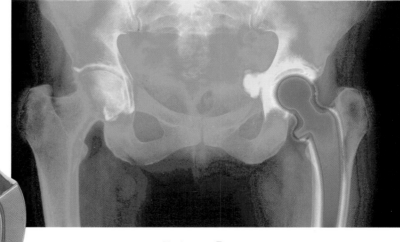

Plastic socket

Femoral hip prothesis

REPLACEMENT HIP
Standard hip replacement joints consist of a metal cup with a long spike attached to one end, and a socket made of high density polythene. During surgery, the bone ball at the top of the femur is removed and a shaft driven into the femur to take the spike. The metal cup rotates in the plastic replacement socket.

Immune-linked arthritis

See also:

3/GENERAL HEALTH ISSUES
Blood and the circulation
pp. 116–117

Several arthritic conditions are the result of an autoimmune condition and are more likely to affect women than men. The most common is rheumatoid arthritis, which occurs most frequently between the ages of 30 and 40. Women over 65 may also be at risk.

Heredity, infection and environmental factors may be the causes of this condition in which the body's cells attack themselves. The first signs appear when the delicate synovial membranes lining the joints become inflamed and start to thicken. Over time, the cartilage and then some of the bone in the joints wears away, while the sheaths of the muscle tendons around them also become thickened and inflamed. The result is pain, stiffness and swelling in the joints, and a reduction in mobility. About 10 percent of sufferers may become disabled.

Rheumatoid arthritis cannot yet be cured, though treatment can reduce its symptoms and delay its progression. It can go into remission, for example during pregnancy.

As with osteoarthritis, NSAIDs and painkillers are used, as well as physical therapy and exercise programmes. Pregnant women need medical guidance. Another treatment involves the injection of gold salts. New drugs that can halt joint destruction include infliximab. Leflunomide is also prescribed. Sulfasalazine, azathioprine, penicillamine, hydroxychloroquine, methotrexate and antibiotics can also be effective. Sometimes corticosteroid drugs are prescribed, but they must be closely monitored since they can lead to the

Diagnostic tests

After performing a physical examination, the doctor will arrange for blood tests to confirm the diagnosis. Tests will be looking for the "rheumatoid factor", common in immune-linked arthritis, and markers of inflammation and chronic disease. If there is a suspicion that joints may be damaged, X-rays will be done to look for evidence of cartilage destruction and bony erosions.

onset of Cushing's syndrome (excess of steroid hormones). Obesity, high blood pressure, diabetes and osteoporosis are other side effects of steroids. Surgery may be considered for joint deformities.

JUVENILE RHEUMATOID ARTHRITIS

This more commonly affects girls than boys and may strike between the ages of two and four or at puberty. In most cases, the arthritis will disappear after several years, although some children may be left with joint abnormalities. Juvenile rheumatoid arthritis can range from classic rheumatoid arthritis to Still's disease, in which the fever, swollen lymph nodes and skin rash last for several weeks. Pain and swelling in the joints may not appear until months later.

LUPUS ERYTHEMATOSUS

Systemic lupus erythematosus, also known as SLE, is an autoimmune disorder producing inflammation in any of the organ systems or the

Signs and symptoms

♀ Tenderness and stiffness in joints, usually the same ones on both sides of the body—the hands, wrists, elbows, shoulders, knees, ankles and feet; often occurs in the early morning and lasts several hours.
♀ Increasing pain, stiffness and swelling after periods of inactivity (sleep, a car journey, a plane flight). Stiffness lasts more than 30 minutes. There can be joint deformity.
♀ Painless nodules under the skin over joints.
♀ Tiredness, fever and weight change.

WHO IS AT RISK?

Autoimmune disorders are thought to start with a virus to which the body's immune system reacts, but then can't stop. This results in a vicious circle which may become a chronic, and progressive, disease. The challenge is to find a balance between rest and exercise without allowing the disorder to disrupt everyday life.

JUVENILE

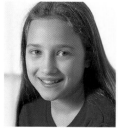

Children under five or at puberty may have fever and anaemia. Treatment may emphasize physical therapy to keep growing bodies active.

20s

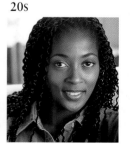

The most common age for SLE, when the symptoms may wax and wane. Care of the skin is needed because of sun photosensitivity.

30s-40s

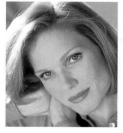

With rheumatoid arthritis the monthly cycle and fertility are not usually affected. Symptoms may go into remission in pregnancy.

tissues of the body. The skin, the face, the brain, the kidneys and the joints are especially vulnerable. It affects about eight times more women than men, and symptoms usually appear between the ages of 15 and 40. Treatment of the joint symptoms is similar to rheumatoid arthritis although there is no risk of deformity. Hydroxychloroquine, steroids, immunosuppressives and occasionally chemotherapeutic agents are used for other symptoms.

PSORIATIC ARTHRITIS

Psoriasis is primarily a skin disorder that affects women and men equally and has a strong genetic basis. In about one in 20 cases, psoriasis sufferers also develop psoriatic arthritis, but it is not known why. Psoriatic arthritis can be severe and disabling. Treatment is similar to that of rheumatoid arthritis.

REACTIVE ARTHRITIS

Although more common in men than women, this can occur in either sex after a bacterial infection. The usual sites of the infection are the genital tract (the cervix or urethra) and the intestines. The infection triggers an abnormal immune response. When it is linked with conjunctivitis and arthritis in the knee or ankle joints, it is called Reiter's disease. This syndrome is linked to people who carry the blood antigen HLA-B27. About 80 percent of those with Reiter's are HLA-B27 positive, which means it is inherited.

The first symptoms may be pain when passing urine or diarrhoea, though some sufferers have neither. Swollen, painful, red and tender joints are common. Blood and stool tests can determine the source of infection. Antibiotics may be prescribed to deal with the infection and NSAIDs for pain. The illness can last for about six months. When the genital tract is involved, practise safe sex until symptoms clear up.

> ## ! Caution
> If you find your joints are swelling and pain prevents you from pursuing everyday activities, you may need to start some exercise routine. Swimming is excellent as it is gentle on the joints but can also strengthen muscles. Also, consider consulting a physiotherapist.

Autoimmune disorders

Normally, the immune system recognizes foreign antigens that are harmful to the body and manufactures antibodies to fight them. In an autoimmune disorder, the body loses the ability to distinguish between foreign material and some of its own cells. The body then produces antibodies that act against its own tissue, which can cause inflammation and disease.

Little is known at present about the mechanism of autoimmune diseases, although genetic factors are certainly involved in some conditions. People who suffer from one autoimmune disorder may also contract others.

Research continues to identify more and more conditions as autoimmune. It is known, for example, that SLE (opposite page) is an autoimmune disorder. Antiphospholipid antibody syndrome (APS) is another. This is a disorder that can arise in conjunction with SLE and other rheumatic diseases or by itself. In APS, antibodies are directed against phospholipids, a substance found throughout the body. These antibodies promote clotting; patients may experience blood clots, heart attacks, strokes and recurrent miscarriages.

The purpose of treatment of autoimmune diseases is to suppress the immune system's response. Unfortunately, the drugs that do this, which are known as immunosuppressives, tend to reduce the activity of the whole immune system, instead of just the part of it responsible for the disorder. They often have side effects that include an increased risk of infection.

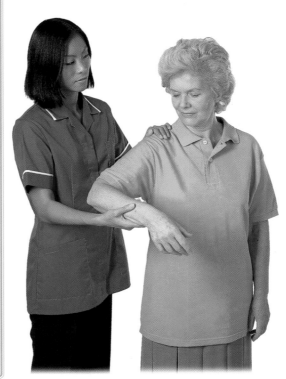

PHYSICAL THERAPY
Trained physiotherapists offer a range of treatments to remedy your particular situation. They may apply heat and electrical therapy directly to the painful area. They can also suggest different exercises to help restore movement. Exercise, combined with relaxation techniques, can alter your perception of pain, the most difficult symptom of autoimmune illnesses.

Back conditions

SPINAL CURVES
The spine has four natural curves which absorb shock and strain during movement. The curves are classified as either primary (present at birth) or secondary (developing during infancy). The convex curves of the thoracic and sacral vertebrae are primary. The concave curves of the cervical and lumbar vertebrae are secondary.

The back's intricate system of checks and balances—in the spine, joints and supporting muscles and ligaments—is vulnerable to damage. Over time, the spinal discs can get thinner and lose their ability to act as shock absorbers. Occasionally, the discs can prolapse (move out of normal position), putting painful pressure on a nerve root. The facet joints between the vertebrae can become too tight, also applying pressure to a nerve and causing pain.

There is no doubt that being overweight adversely affects the spine. Unlike muscle, which protects and supports the joints and relieves them of pressure, stored body fat merely increases the load that the joints—particularly in the lower back and hips—have to bear.

Excess weight increases general wear and tear, and can lead to osteoarthritis and to ailments such as strained ligaments and disc problems.

Overweight people who carry much of this extra fat around the stomach can weaken the stomach muscles, leaving them unable to do the important job of supporting the spine. Anyone with lower back pain will usually be encouraged to strengthen their stomach muscles through gentle exercise as a first step toward solving the problem.

LIFESTYLE HABITS

Crouching, bending, lifting and carrying places a great deal of stress on the back. In activities that tend to call for a repetitive type of work—such as digging, mowing and weeding—for several hours at a time, the level of stress is compounded if it is done in irregular spurts.

People who follow a sedentary lifestyle spend a lot of time sitting or lying down. If this is combined with lack of exercise and poor posture, a chronic back problem may result.

SPINAL CURVES

The spine has four natural curves and these allow it to absorb the shock waves experienced from the impact of walking and the stresses and strains caused by the body's weight and its movements. Everyone has a naturally

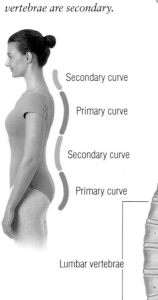

Secondary curve

Primary curve

Secondary curve

Primary curve

Lumbar vertebrae

Sacrum and coccyx

Cervical vertebrae

Thoracic vertebrae

> ## ! Caution
>
> If you experience sudden back pain, stop what you are doing immediately. If it hasn't improved in 24 hours through rest, seek medical advice. If you have a back problem, don't embark on an exercise programme without checking it out first with your doctor. Remember that high impact sports (like squash) put considerable strain on the spine. Never move anyone after an accident if you suspect that any part of the spine has been injured. Get immediate help.

ABNORMAL CURVES
Kyphosis, or hunched upper back, may result from bad posture or osteoporosis. Lordosis is excessive curve of the lumbar spine and may result from poor posture, pregnancy or obesity. Scoliosis is a lateral curve and may be caused by one leg being shorter than the other.

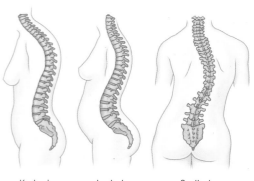

Kyphosis   Lordosis   Scoliosis

slightly different degree of curve but various conditions or postural habits can produce distorted or exaggerated curve. These then fail to absorb shock effectively and can lead to nerves not functioning properly.

WHERE THE PAIN COMES FROM

The sciatic nerve is the longest in the body—it is, in fact, six spinal nerves that leave the base of the spine and converge to form one large nerve that runs down the leg. If any part of the nerve is trapped, the effect can be felt a long distance from the back. The sciatic nerve gets "trapped" when a disc presses on it or when it is being pressed against the spine, as sometimes happens during pregnancy. The symptoms are acute, resulting in shooting and unrelenting pain in the area of the body served by the part of the trapped nerve, usually the buttock or the back of the leg.

Another cause of back pain results when a vertebra collapses on itself and causes sciatica-type pain. This is caused mostly by severe osteoporosis or bone-thinning.

Back pain is not always caused by a back problem. Pain can be "referred" to the spinal region, perhaps because two areas of the body share the same pain pathways. Medical causes of such referred pain can come from gynaecological, abdominal and chest problems.

THE SPINAL JOINTS

The 33 bones called vertebrae are stacked on top of each other with pads of cartilage known as discs between. The column is held together by strong ligaments and facet joints between the vertebrae.

Normal disc *In a healthy spine the discs are plump and resilient. They are compressed during everyday activity and return to normal during rest or sleep.*
Prolapsed disc *Under extreme pressure the centre of the disc may break out of its covering and put pressure on a nerve, a painful condition also known as a slipped disc.*
Shrunken disc *The water content of a disc may diminish with age, leading to a reduction in springiness.*

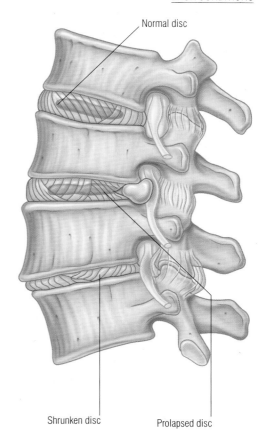

Normal disc

Shrunken disc

Prolapsed disc

WHEN BACK PAIN STRIKES …

It is extremely important to stop what you are doing and lie down on a bed or the floor. This will take the stress off your spine. Help yourself by making a positive effort to relax your mind and body.

1 *Lying flat on your back is the most effective way of reducing pressure. Bend your knees up but keep your feet flat on the floor and your arms by your side.*

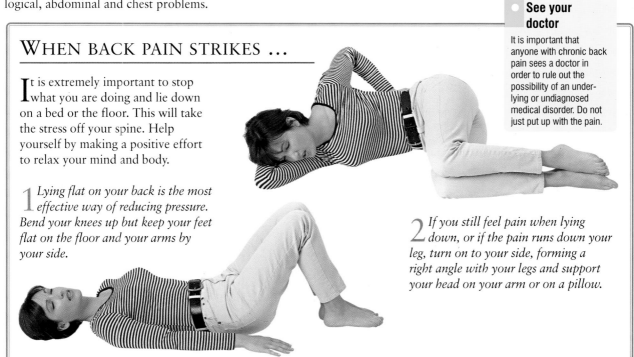

2 *If you still feel pain when lying down, or if the pain runs down your leg, turn on to your side, forming a right angle with your legs and support your head on your arm or on a pillow.*

See your doctor

It is important that anyone with chronic back pain sees a doctor in order to rule out the possibility of an underlying or undiagnosed medical disorder. Do not just put up with the pain.

Neck and shoulder pain

See also:

1/BEING A WELL WOMAN
Healthy body systems pp. 30–31

6/TREATMENTS & THERAPIES
Conventional treatments
pp. 272–277; pp. 288–291
Complementary therapies
pp. 292–297

The neck plays an important role in supporting your head, helping maintain good posture and protecting the vulnerable upper part of the spine that connects to the brain. Its wide range of movement is made possible by strong ligaments and a great number of muscles. The neck can be the site of problems which may be acute and temporary or chronic.

Muscular tension is the most common cause of chronic neck pain and results from stress or poor posture. Some muscles become taut and knotted, putting pressure on nerves in the area, while their opposing muscles become over-relaxed, making the problem worse.

Generally, acute neck pain comes from muscles that go into spasm to protect the joint and prevent movement. The neck feels "locked", there is often a deep ache and sometimes pins and needles down a limb if a nerve has been trapped. This may result from ageing, trauma or chronic muscular tension. The postural changes that occur during pregnancy can also cause neck pain. Treatment can include immobilization in a neck collar, muscle relaxants and NSAIDs. Massage therapy may help. If there is no evidence of neurological involvement, chiropractic or osteopathic manipulation and acupuncture can be used. In severe cases, the doctor may give trigger point injections or steroid injections into the joints and ligaments.

Women who have osteoarthritis may also develop cervical spondylosis, sometimes called degenerative joint disease. In this condition the discs in the cervical vertebrae wear out, causing stiffness and chronic neck pain.

SHOULDER TRAUMA

Because of its anatomical structure, the shoulder has a number of weaknesses. The socket in which the arm bone sits is small and shallow and its rim of cartilage is weak, and the three short ligaments that protect the joint are unstable. The stability of the joint depends on the short, protective rotator cuff muscles that surround it and allow it free movement.

Any damage to the rotator cuff muscles is likely to lead to inflammation of the joint capsule or tendon, a condition known as rotator cuff tendonitis, or painful arc syndrome. If the capsule thickens, called adhesive capsulitis, severe pain often shoots down the arm when movement is attempted. Because those who have the condition find that only small movements of the joint are possible, to compensate and prevent pain they tend to hunch their shoulders and use the muscles attached to the shoulder blade instead.

This condition occurs more often in people over 50. Some researchers attribute the loss of flexibility to ageing. However, the damage may be the direct result of an acute injury such as a fall or from a gradual build-up of frequent strains to the muscles—when carrying heavy items. It is also associated with various occupations—musicians, for example, are

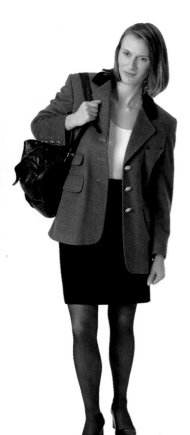

CARRYING SENSE
All too frequently women carry heavy bags and don't realize what it may be doing to their posture. If you put a bag over one shoulder your body lurches sideways to keep balanced, forcing the spine into an unnatural position (left). It is much better to carry equal weights in both hands (right), or use a back pack which rests evenly on both shoulders.

prone to this disorder. Treatment varies. In some cases, hydrocortisone injections into the shoulder may be tried along with physiotherapy, involving friction, some gentle traction and graduated stretching exercises. In severe cases, a specialist may decide it is necessary to manipulate the muscles and tendons under a general anaesthetic to increase mobility and remove any tissue adhesions. In extreme cases, it may be necessary to try and repair the cuff surgically, but this in itself may cause further problems.

Rotator cuff injuries tend to clear up over time, usually about two years, so your doctor may advise you to postpone invasive treatment. You will be encouraged to do exercises daily to gradually loosen the joint while taking painkillers and NSAIDs as needed. As the joint begins to regain some normal movement, swimming may be recommended to exercise it.

WRIST AND ARM PROBLEMS

When the hand and wrists are held in an unnatural position for long periods of time, such as during repetitive work, inflammation, tendon damage and pain can result. Typing and fine manual work are a particular risk. The condition is called overuse syndrome or repetitive strain injury (RSI).

Two of the most frequently occurring problems today are tenosynovitis and carpal tunnel syndrome. In tenosynovitis the forearm tendons or their protective sheaths become swollen and are no longer able to slide easily past each other. Carpal tunnel syndrome affects the nerves as they pass through the wrists (see box below).

The usual treatment is a combination of immobilization of the joint (in a splint for several weeks) and steroid injections followed by physiotherapy to encourage gradual movement and ensure blood flow to the area. The condition may take a long time to correct. In some severe cases, surgery may be necessary.

Repetitive strain conditions tend to recur. It is important that you recognize signs that yours may be beginning again. Make sure that your workplace environment complies with health and safety practice and take frequent breaks—five minutes or so, every hour.

> **! Caution**
>
> A stiff, painful neck may need medical investigation. If it follows a sudden jolt to the head (as in a car accident), a whiplash injury may be indicated—ligaments may be stretched or torn, or one of the tiny neck vertebrae may be fractured. With either, long-term support from a surgical collar may be necessary.
>
> If there has been no jolt, an acute stiff neck may be a sign of meningitis, especially if there is a headache, fever, dislike of bright lights, feelings of nausea or drowsiness (p. 250). You should seek medical attention as soon as possible.

CARPAL TUNNEL SYNDROME

The carpal tunnel is formed by the first row of carpal bones in the wrist and a ligament (the flexor retinaculum) that runs across and over them. A branch of the median nerve, which supplies the thumb, first two fingers and the thumb side of the third finger, passes through this tunnel, with various muscle tendons. In carpal tunnel syndrome, the median nerve becomes compressed, causing a numbing pain in the hand (often at night or on waking), clumsiness when using the hand (holding a needle or pen is difficult), pins and needles or tingling in all the fingers except the little one. Sometimes there is pain in the arm and when pushing the thumb and little finger together. You may get some relief by massaging or shaking the hand.

Carpal tunnel syndrome (CTS) often has no identifiable cause, although it may be associated with trauma of the wrist and chronic inflammation of the tendon sheaths as a result of RSI (above). CTS is seen during pregnancy and in people with an inflammatory autoimmune disorder such as rheumatoid arthritis. It is also associated with diabetes and hypothyroidism.

Treatment may involve a wrist splint, exercises to stretch the wrist muscles and steroid injections. The last resort is surgery to release the trapped nerve. Before this is tried, a nerve conduction test may be performed to check the nerve fibres.

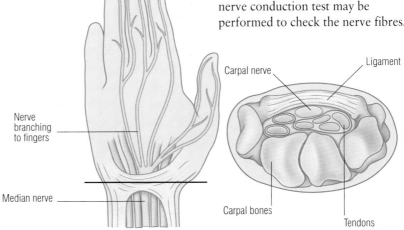

Nerve branching to fingers

Median nerve

Carpal nerve

Ligament

Carpal bones

Tendons

Muscle and tendon problems

Pain in the muscles or the tendons (the sinews that attach muscles to the bones on which they act when they contract) is a common problem.

CRAMP

The cause of a cramp in the leg is not completely understood. It is thought that a chemical imbalance within the muscle may be responsible, causing excessive contraction. Other possibilities are a loss of salt, potassium and magnesium, which can occur

> **! Caution**
> Batheing in extremely cold water can give you cramps, which can be highly dangerous if you are in deep water. When you are swimming, get used to the water temperature gradually.

through excessive exercise, a bout of diarrhoea or alcohol or drug use. During pregnancy muscle cramps are more common.

In the feet cramp is usually the result of over-stretching your foot; in your calf muscles it may be over-exertion; in your hands and wrists it may stem from a constant repetitive movement. The problem may be avoided by warming up your muscles before exercise and cooling down afterwards, by taking a salt tablet or drinking slightly salted water.

Once a cramp strikes, massage the muscles until the pain subsides, usually in a few minutes. Regular night cramps may be treated by a prescribed drug containing quinine or an over-the-counter remedy. Recurrent cramps in the legs, especially after walking, should be investigated by a doctor. They may also be a sign of restless leg syndrome, a sleep disorder in which the legs move irresistibly and wake you up.

PULLED MUSCLES OR TENDONS

The usual cause of a "pull" in a muscle or a tendon—often called a strain—is an excessive demand on the tissues as a result of unusual movement, often after periods of inactivity.

The degree of damage caused varies from a simple overstretching of the fibres to a tear in them. In response, the muscle contracts or even goes into spasm to protect the damaged tissues. This disrupts the blood supply and alters the muscle's internal chemistry, causing pain.

Immediate treatment is by RICE (see box opposite). If muscles and tendons are damaged, physical therapy, involving massage, friction techniques and ultrasound, may be necessary. When exercising, gentle warm-up and cool-down routines before and after help prevent the problem, as does correct posture and a conscious effort to make movements flow.

SPRAINED LIGAMENTS

Ligaments are bands of fibrous tissue that support and stabilize joints by binding together the bones that meet in them. In the ankle, where the fibula (the outer bone of the leg) meets the talus (an inner bone of the foot), there are three ligaments. Many common accidents in which

PRESSURES ON YOUR FEET

Many foot problems are the direct result of the feet being subjected to pressures for which they were not designed.

The foot contains 26 bones, linked in a series of joints and supported by numerous ligaments. The whole weight of the body must be carried by these bones and by the arches that they form in the instep. Being overweight and wearing unsuitable footwear can contribute to pain.

High-heeled shoes, from a medical standpoint, are always unsuitable as they put strain on the muscles of the lower leg. High heels shift body weight forward, straining the tissues of the arches. And tight shoes of any type increase the risk of bunions, corns and nail or toe deformities.

Pain in the feet can also occur in pregnancy. Choose shoes with low heels, in natural materials such as leather or canvas to allow your feet to breathe. You may need a wider fitting shoe or a different size

in the later stages of pregnancy. Wearing correct footwear will help with your posture and may prevent backache during these months.

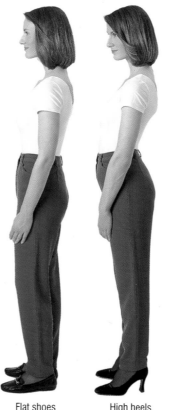

Flat shoes   High heels

THE WORDS DOCTORS USE

There are many ways in which your muscles and the associated tissues can cause pain or characterize long-term disorders. Here are some of the terms that describe the symptoms of muscular and skeletal problems and which your doctor may use in diagnosing or explaining your problem.

Disease	Description
Fibromyalgia	A modern term for what used to be called "muscular rheumatism", fibromyalgia has no known cause, although it has been suggested that it is connected with stress. It mostly affects middle-aged people and may disturb sleep. Symptoms include pain and tenderness in muscles all over the body. There are specific "trigger points" within the muscles that set off sharp, shooting pains—hence the condition's other name "trigger point syndrome". It may also be referred to as fibrositis. Fibromyalgia is treated by deep massage and stretching exercises. Antidepressants and muscle relaxant drugs are sometimes prescribed.
Fibrositis	Another name for fibromyalgia.
Myalgia	Any pain in a muscle.
Paresthesia	The medical term meaning "pins and needles", paresthesia usually occurs in a limb that has been in the same position for a long time. The tingling numbness indicates temporary disruption to the nerve or blood supply. It can also be a symptom of disc protrusion on a nerve in the lumbar or cervical spine or disorders such as Raynaud's phenomenon (p. 124), carpal tunnel syndrome (p. 87), diabetes (p. 136) and hypothyroidism (p. 138).
Rheumatism	This is not a word ordinarily used by doctors, but rheumatism is a common description by non-medical people for general pain and stiffness in muscles and joints. So-called rheumatic pain may derive from osteoarthritis, rheumatoid arthritis or polymyalgia.
Sciatica	Sciatica is caused by pressure on the sciatic nerve as it leaves the spine. It is the result of inflammation of the facet joints of the vertebrae between which the nerve emerges, or may be due to a disc protrusion between these vertebrae caused by poor posture, lifting heavy objects or unaccustomed activity. Irritation of the nerve by the bony pelvis can occur during menstruation and pregnancy. The nerve compression gives severe pain along its length from the lower back to the foot, often with pins and needles and numbness. Treatment is by anti-inflammatory injection, painkillers, rest, manipulation and exercises.

you trip or miss a step can cause the joint to lose its stability and twist inward, resulting in a sprained ankle. The torn fibres bleed and become inflamed, and the muscles in the area go into spasm to prevent any further damage. With serious sprains treatment involves ice application, support from elastic bandages and ultrasound. Ligaments that have been badly torn may require surgical repair.

MYASTHENIA GRAVIS
Women are particularly affected by this autoimmune disorder, which involves the muscles used in chewing, swallowing and speaking, and causes weakness in the limbs. It may become apparent in early adulthood with signs of weakness of the eyelid and double vision. The condition is usually progressive, with some periods of remission.

Treatment involves drugs to restore nerve transmission to the muscles, immunosuppressive drugs and steroids. Surgery to remove the thymus gland may also be considered in young women.

First aid for strains
R—Rest.
I—Apply an ice-pack to injured area.
C—Compress the ice with a bandage.
E—Elevate the injured area for 20 minutes. Then wrap injured part in an elastic bandage.
Repeat RICE twice a day.

Osteoporosis

See also:

1/BEING A WELL WOMAN
Essentials of good health
pp. 16–29
Healthy body systems pp. 30–43

A hormone-related disorder, osteoporosis, which literally means porous bones, generally afflicts the whole skeleton of postmenopausal women. Bone thinning leads to increased risk of fracture—often it is only after a fracture occurs that osteoporosis is diagnosed.

The condition comes about gradually, causing the thinning of the honeycombed inner layer, rather than the compact outer layer, of the ends of the long bones of the lower arms, the hip ends of the thigh bones and the spinal vertebrae. These bones become extremely susceptible to breaks and the fractures are likely to take longer than normal to heal, increasing the risk of infection and deformity, both of which may lead to disability or death. It is estimated that about 20 percent of women who fracture a hip die from complications and half of those who survive are disabled.

With osteoporosis, the gradual collapse of the spinal vertebrae, as a result of the loss of bone density and the load that they bear, causes a reduction in height and a forward bend and hunching of the upper spine. Medically termed a thoracic kyphosis (p. 84), this is traditionally known as a "dowager's hump".

WHO IS AT RISK?

Osteoporosis is a particular hazard for postmenopausal women, women who have had a premature menopause, a hysterectomy with removal of both ovaries or reduced oestrogen levels for a prolonged length of time. There are a number of other factors that may increase their vulnerability. These include:

Inadequate bone mass formation This is the most important risk factor. If there is insufficient bone mass before it starts to decrease, the effects of osteoporosis become apparent much earlier. Reasons for the inadequacy may involve any of the other risk factors.

Family history Osteoporosis is a condition that tends to run in families. It is more prevalent among white and Asian women than African and Caribbean women.

Hormonal deficiencies Any condition that lowers oestrogen levels (for instance, anorexia nervosa or exercise-indued amenorrhea) accelerates loss of bone mass.

Inadequate diet and exercise A lack of calcium or vitamin D through poor nutrition means that less bone is renewed and more calcium leaches out of bone into the blood to make up for the deficiency. Regular weight-bearing, repetitive exercise promotes an increase in bone mass. Without it, bone loss continues.

WOMEN AND BONES

Everyone's skeleton starts out as cartilage and soon after conception begins to be strengthened by calcium, supplied by the pregnant woman's diet. In this ongoing process, more cartilage is laid down as the bones—and the foetus—grow. Bone, like any other living tissue, is broken down and replaced throughout life, an activity in women which is influenced by the hormones oestrogen and progesterone. Bone strength is established in young adulthood through a healthy lifestyle, a diet made up of a wide variety of foods rich in calcium and vitamin D (which helps the calcium to be absorbed) and regular weight-bearing exercise which stimulates bone growth.

Bones reach their peak mass between the ages of 20 and 30

and your bone mass level will depend on the efficiency of your hormones, how healthy you are, your genes and if you drink and smoke. Many women with osteoporosis never reached their optimal mass, for reasons mostly related to lack of oestrogen and calcium. This essential mineral is used by the heart, nerves and muscles as well, and if those vital parts do not have not enough of it the bones release it into the bloodstream so affecting the bone-building process.

Bone mineral starts to be lost from the skeleton from the age of about 35 and is part of natural ageing. The greatest loss occurs in the first year after the menopause. Later the rate of bone mass loss may be as much as five percent a year.

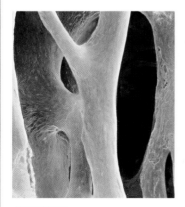

Normal bone

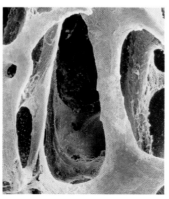

Osteoporotic bone

HELP YOUR BONE STRENGTH

If you are at risk of developing osteoporosis, your doctor may suggest ways in which you can increase bone mass and reduce the effect of mineral loss. If you have been diagnosed with osteoporosis, the following strategies also play an important part in the medical treatment of the condition.

Treatment	Action
More calcium	Increase your intake of calcium-rich foods, such as milk, eggs, cheese, bread, leafy green vegetables, canned fish with bones (sardines, salmon), almonds and peanuts.
More vitamin D	Found in red meat, liver, oily fish, full-fat or semi-skimmed milk, margarine, butter and egg yolks and is also made in the body through the action of sunlight on the skin.
Increase weight-bearing exercise	Regular physical activity of a kind that allows the bones to bear the body's weight and is repetitive helps the bone-making process. A brisk 20 to 30 minute walk, two or three times a week, may be enough. In some cases vigorous exercise may not be appropriate.
Stop smoking and reduce alcohol consumption	Smokers and heavy drinkers are at greater risk of developing osteoporosis as well as many other diseases.
HRT	Discuss the pros and cons of HRT with your doctor if you had a premature menopause, are approaching the menopause or are postmenopausal.

Small build Slight women have less bone mass to start with, so the effects of loss of bone mass may become evident more quickly. They are more likely to have a history of fracture.

Smoking Tobacco increases the risk. Most smokers have menopausal symptoms up to two years earlier than non-smokers.

High alcohol consumption Consuming more than two drinks every day is associated with a higher risk of osteoporosis, because alcohol attacks the cells that form bone and inhibits the absorption of calcium.

Excessive caffeine Consistently drinking more than three cups of caffeine-containing drinks, such as coffee, tea and cola, can increase the risk of developing osteoporosis. Drinking more milk can counteract this.

Prescription drugs Long-term use of a number of drugs can cause osteoporosis. They include anticonvulsants, thyroid hormone, antacids that contain aluminium, methotrexate (used to treat cancer, immune disorders and arthritis), heparin (used to prevent blood clotting), cholestyramine (used to reduce levels of cholesterol in the blood) and some glucocorticoids, such as cortisone and prednisone given

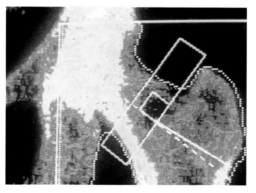

FRACTURE POINT
The hip is possibly the most vulnerable area of the skeletal system in anyone susceptible to osteoporosis. It is one of the bones scanned by dual-energy X-ray absorptiometry (DEXA, p. 92).

to treat osteoarthritis, rheumatoid arthritis, asthma, allergic reactions, multiple sclerosis and chronic skin disorders.

Certain medical conditions Bone loss may be caused by two conditions: Cushing's syndrome, in which the adrenal glands are overactive and produce excess glucocorticoids; and hyperparathyroidism, an overactivity of the parathyroid glands. The hormone from these glands controls blood calcium levels and if there is not enough it removes calcium from bone tissue. Thyroid disease and malabsorption (from digestive disorders) may also affect bone mass. ▸

> **! Caution**
> The signs and symptoms of osteoporosis are few and become apparent over the long term. It is possible for osteoporosis to be so advanced that you might fracture a bone without knowing that you have the condition. Preventive measures such as dietary changes and exercise are the best approach to take.

> **! Caution**
> You should not stop taking any medication because you suspect it may put you at risk for osteoporosis. Instead, discuss the matter with your doctor.

DIAGNOSING OSTEOPOROSIS

Bone mineral density (BMD) can be measured by dual-energy X-ray absorptiometry (DEXA). In this test you lie fully dressed on a table for approximately 15 minutes while a low-powered X-ray scanner is moved above your spine, hips and wrists. A bone densitometer calculates the density of the bone by analysing how much X-ray is absorbed by it and how much passes through. The information is sent to a nearby computer where it can be processed.

The results are graded according to a World Health Organization classification, comparing your BMD with the average bone mass of a young female adult. Under this system, "mild" osteoporosis (osteopenia), has a BMD between minus 1 and minus 2.5 and "moderate" to "severe" has a BMD of less than minus 2.5. The measurements are particularly relevant for menopausal women because of oestrogen loss associated with the menopause.

DEXA is recommended for women over 65 and before that age in women with risk factors. A scan can be arranged privately if you prefer.

A DEXA BONE SCAN
The density of your bones can be measured by this type of X-ray scanner. The scan takes only a few minutes and the results are recorded on a computer for analysis by the doctor.

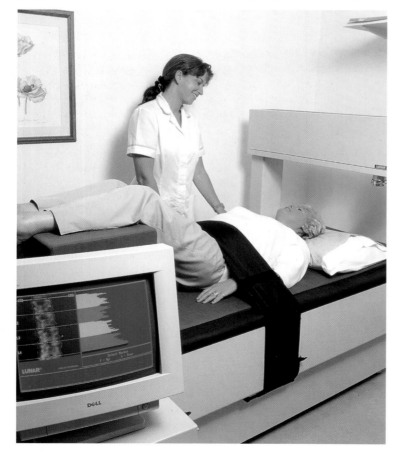

HOW OSTEOPOROSIS IS TREATED

Calcium and vitamin D supplementation does not increase bone mass, but it may be prescribed to prevent bone loss. The typical daily requirements for a postmenopausal woman not using hormone replacement therapy (HRT) are 1,200 mg of calcium (carbonate or citrate), with 400–800 IU (international units) of vitamin D. Women on HRT and premenopausal women should take 1,000 mg per day. The calcium should be taken at bedtime. An excess of vitamin D—more than 2,000 IU a day—can be dangerous and lead to kidney damage and the formation of calcium deposits in the skin.

Oestrogen therapy for those at risk can delay the onset of osteoporosis while you are taking it, if given early enough. Many doctors suggest it should be taken from the start of menopausal symptoms, when hormone levels begin to fluctuate (measured by blood testing). It can halt bone loss in those who have osteoporosis.

Progestogen is also given to reduce the risk of developing uterine cancer that exists when oestrogen is given on its own. This, however, is not necessary in a woman who does not have a uterus. Various HRT regimes are available, depending on individual circumstances and preferences (pp. 144–145). Whether or not to choose HRT is a decision for a woman to make with her doctor after careful study of the facts and discussion of the risks and benefits. Unless there is a health reason for not taking it (such as existing heart problems), it is generally accepted that it is beneficial in the case of women susceptible to osteoporosis.

There are two alternatives to HRT, but neither is suitable for premenopausal women. They can be used as first-line therapies or when there is a contraindication to HRT—in conditions such as liver disease, breast cancer, blood clotting disorders and unexplained vaginal bleeding—or when a woman chooses not to have HRT. They are the bisphosphonates and selective oestrogen receptor modulators (SERMs), the most prescribed one being raloxifene. Bisphosphonates affect bone by inhibiting its breakdown; raloxifene mimics the effect of oestrogen on bones, but does not appear to reduce the risk of hip fractures.

Calcitonin may sometimes be prescribed as a nasal spray to prevent bone loss. It may be administered by injection in cases of painful spine fractures.

OSTEOMALACIA

The adult form of rickets, osteomalacia, is a condition in which a deficiency of vitamin D leads to insufficient calcium being laid down in bone. The bones become soft, weak and prone to fracture. In severe cases, the leg bones may bow under the body's weight and they ache.

Lack of sunlight, which helps the body make vitamin D, is the main cause in women who are housebound or rarely go out of doors. The lack of dairy products such as milk in the traditional Asian diet may be a factor too. The condition has also been diagnosed in people who diet excessively and who have eating disorders such as anorexia nervosa (p. 102).

Vitamin D and calcium deficiency can sometimes be attributable to a failure of the intestines to absorb them properly or to kidney disorders. Osteomalacia responds quickly to treatment with vitamin D supplements and a diet rich in calcium. Milk (not fat free) is a main source of vitamin D and should be consumed daily.

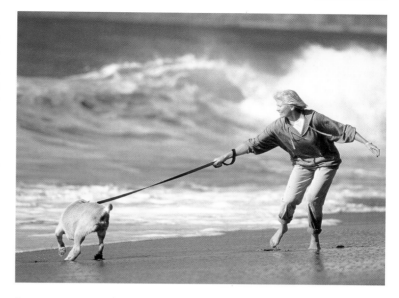

SEE THE LIGHT
The strength of bones depends on the way the mineral calcium works with vitamin D. The vitamin may be obtained from sunlight on skin, from certain foods or taken daily as a supplement.

COLLES FRACTURE

Because it is instinctive to put a hand out to break a fall, the bones of the wrist are susceptible to damage. In a young woman, such a fracture may often be the first sign of a disease that has weakened the bones and made them brittle. The most common fracture, known as a Colles fracture, affects the wrist, which suffers from the impact when the palm hits the ground. The scaphoid bone at the base of the thumb may be fractured too. The radius and ulna in the forearm are forced out of position, which in turn forces the wrist into an unnatural upward position.

The bones may need to be realigned under a general anaesthetic, and then the whole joint immobilized in plaster for about six weeks. There is a danger of the joint remaining stiff after this and physiotherapy may be required to restore the full range of movement. Anyone who has had a Colles fracture would be advised to discuss the implications with her doctor. An older woman may not be able to put out her hand quickly enough and it is more likely that she will fall on her hip and fracture it.

WRIST DAMAGE
The many bones that make up the wrist can be damaged by a fall and take time to repair themselves. The situation is made worse if the break is a symptom of bone disease or another medical condition.

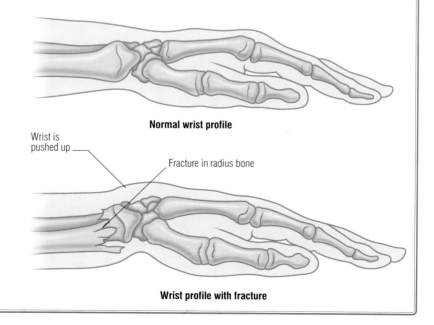

Normal wrist profile

Wrist is pushed up

Fracture in radius bone

Wrist profile with fracture

PROBLEMS OF THE MIND

Habits may not be recognized as destructive for a long time. They begin in your mind and, once they have taken over your body, they are hard to stop. Addictions to alcohol, smoking and drugs or a lack of control over eating habits have a direct impact on a woman's life, including her relationships, and increase her risk of developing illnesses.

See also:

4/HORMONAL HEALTH
Endocrine problems pp. 136–137
Conception problems pp. 182–183

5/ILLNESSES & EMERGENCIES
Digestive system problems
    p. 193; pp. 202–203
Respiratory problems
    pp. 213–221
Problems of the senses
    pp. 236–237

Addiction

An addiction is an unnatural craving for a particular feeling or sensation and for the food, drink, drugs or behaviour pattern that satisfies it and results in temporary euphoria, excitement, well-being or relief from pain.

THE CAUSES OF ADDICTION

Almost all addictions have harmful, sometimes fatal, physical consequences and can profoundly disrupt the lives of the addict and the people around him or her. Early recognition of growing dependency is the best way to avoid addiction. Once a person is addicted, cures are difficult, often painful and expensive.

Why is it that one person who experiments with, or indulges in, occasional substance abuse will become addicted, while another person, from an apparently similar background, does not? Four major factors of addiction have been studied. It is unlikely that only one of them is responsible for the tendency to addiction. More likely, all four factors are involved, with the relative importance of each one varying from one person to another.

Physiology Some experts believe that something akin to an allergic reaction takes place in those people who are predisposed to addiction. This in turn creates the craving for more of the addictive substance.

Genetics There is evidence that addiction—particularly alcoholism—runs in families. However, no specific genetic markers have yet been identified. The role of gender is uncertain. Women seem more likely to abuse prescription drugs such as pain medication and tranquillizers, whereas men are more likely to abuse hard drugs and alcohol.

Environment Lifestyle, socioeconomic status, peer pressure and family background have been shown to have an important influence on the development of addiction. Women who have alcohol problems or dependence on other substances may have been physically or sexually abused as children, have a partner who drinks heavily or may be socially isolated. Some professions and ethnic groups are more prone to heavy drinking than others.

Psychological disturbance Addiction may be a response to an inability to cope with different elements of the outside world, including relationships and employment or with some aspect of the addict's life history. Low self-esteem, aggression and a refusal to recognize and confront problems are common features of addictive behaviour. Underlying psychiatric disorders like depression and anxiety commonly need to be treated in addicts.

The most common addictions

♀ Alcohol, whether binge drinking, steady and heavy daily intake or combinations of both types of behaviour.
♀ Nicotine.
♀ Hard or illicit drugs, including heroin and cocaine, and laboratory-produced drugs such as LSD and E (ecstasy or MDMA).
♀ Prescription drugs used in the treatment of medical conditions, for example codeine painkillers, amphetamines and some antidepressants and tranquillizers.
♀ Cannabis or marijuana.
♀ Solvents (glue sniffing).
♀ Food.
♀ Abnormal behaviour patterns, such as gambling and shopping—both of which involve spending money regardless of income—or compulsive sexual activity (called nymphomania in women).

Alcohol

Alcohol abuse is a major problem in most Western countries today. While moderate alcohol consumption may be a pleasant and harmless aspect of social life, excessive intake of alcohol is much more dangerous.

Alcohol abuse is estimated to affect at least one in 10 people and to be directly responsible for long-term liver damage, heart disease and some cancers. It is implicated in about a third of accidents in the home and nearly the same proportion of murders and drownings. It is a factor in nearly half of all violent crime, including incidents of domestic violence and is a major cause of death and injury on the roads.

Women are more susceptible than men to alcohol because one of the digestive enzymes that metabolizes alcohol doesn't work as efficiently in them. Alcohol enters their bloodstream faster, making the risk of liver damage for them greater. Women also on average weigh less than men and have more fatty tissue, which contains a lower proportion of water to dilute alcohol. This susceptibility appears to increase during menstruation.

Young women between the ages of 18 and 29 need to be especially conscious of the effect alcohol can have on their lives. Women in this age group are prone to abuse or dependence and to bouts of binge or social drinking during which the risk of violence, sexual assault or having unsafe sex increases.

You have a drinking problem if:

♀ You cannot fulfil obligations at work, at school or at home.
♀ You have blackouts after which you can't remember how you got home or what you said or did the night before.
♀ You continue to use alcohol despite possible legal problems (for example, driving under the influence of alcohol) and disruptive effects drinking has on your personal relationships.
♀ You need a drink first thing in the morning to steady your nerves or get rid of a hangover.

WHEN TO AVOID ALCOHOL

It is recommended that a woman who is trying to conceive or is pregnant or breastfeeding should stop drinking altogether.

If you have liver disease or damage such as hepatitis or cirrhosis, a digestive disorder such as gastritis, or epilepsy, you should not drink.

Certain medications, for example, metronidazole (used to treat some dental and vaginal infections) and some sleeping pills, pain medications, tranquillizers and antihistamines react badly with alcohol—or alcohol may negate the effect of the drug. Seek your doctor's advice about alcohol consumption when you are taking prescribed drugs and planning to drink. ▸

See also:

4/HORMONAL HEALTH
Endocrine problems pp. 136–137
Conception problems pp. 180–183

5/ILLNESSES & EMERGENCIES
Digestive problems
p. 193; pp. 202–203
Immune system problems
pp. 204–207
Respiratory problems
pp. 213–221

! Caution

Drinking alcohol in social situations is obviously acceptable but, for women, particularly if they are on their own, it is worth being extra vigilant when among strangers. Certain drugs or even a clear spirit can be added to a drink and not be noticed. However, the effect can be dramatic, causing blackout and memory loss.

WHAT IS SAFE DRINKING?

The recommended limit is 14–21 units for women a week. One unit is:
♀ 300 ml (½ pint) beer or cider or
♀ 50 ml (1½ fl oz) of fortified wine (port, sherry, marsala and Madeira) or
♀ 25 ml (¾ fl oz) of spirits such as gin.
♀ A standard glass of wine (125 ml/ 4¼ fl oz) is 1½ units.

Moderate drinking, within these limits, may help protect against heart disease. However, this only applies to post-menopausal women and to men over the age of 40. For women, even moderate drinking increases the risk of breast cancer.

COMPARING DRINKS

The alcohol content of different drinks varies. A small amount of any spirit is stronger than a glass of wine or beer.

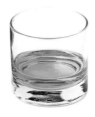

Spirit

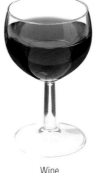

Wine

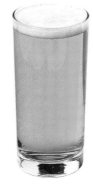

Beer

SEEKING HELP

It is difficult for alcoholics to give up drinking without assistance, but there are various kinds of treatment, depending on the degree of dependency and the extent of physical and mental damage. Medical intervention may be required to counteract withdrawal symptoms. Delirium tremens (DTs), hallucinations and seizures require the administration of tranquillizers called benzodiazepines such as Diazepam, possibly by intravenous drip. Vitamin supplements, in particular vitamin B_6 and thiamine, may be given to repair liver and nerve damage caused by poor nutrition.

Aversion therapy, in the form of drugs such as Acamprosate, which produces a severe and unpleasant physical reaction to alcohol, may be prescribed. Antidepressants and anti-anxiety medications may be prescribed if there is an underlying psychiatric illness.

Maintaining long-term sobriety can depend on the degree of support available. Alcohol addiction is hard on the drinker's family, and outside support, perhaps psychotherapy or counselling, is vital. Voluntary support groups, notably Alcoholics Anonymous (AA) and its related organizations Alanon (for the families of alcoholics) and Alateen (for young drinkers), provide emotional and practical support for recovering alcoholics on a long-term basis.

Heavy drinkers or alcoholics tend to be secretive; they hide alcohol supplies and go to great lengths to disguise their consumption. Being in an environment, such as a support group, where the problem is publicly acknowledged is a big step toward dealing with it.

GIRLS' NIGHT OUT
A drink at the end of the day with friends or colleagues can be relaxing and pleasant, but you should be sure you want to take part. If the outings become a daily occurrence, you may feel pressured into participating and drink far more than you want to. You need to be able to limit the number of nights out per week and when you do go out to set yourself a limit of how much you drink and keep to it.

Short-term effects of heavy drinking

The first effects are loss of inhibitions—the drinker may become lively, talkative, confident and relaxed. At the same time, however, judgment and coordination are affected. After a period of time, which differs from one person to another, the deleterious effects may dominate. The drinker may become aggressive or full of maudlin self-pity; speech may become slurred and he or she may fall down, bump into things or knock things over.

A bout of heavy drinking may result in a hangover due to dehydration and toxins building up in the blood. Symptoms can include acute headache, shakiness, nausea, listlessness and an inability to remember the activities of the night before (known as alcoholic amnesia). In severe cases, there may be nausea, vomiting, mental confusion, visual disturbance, delirium tremens and possibly coma. Death from acute alcohol poisoning, or from the inhalation of vomit while in a coma, could also result.

Long-term effects

Major medical conditions associated with alcoholism include:
♀ Cancer of the mouth, throat, stomach, colon, liver and breast.
♀ Heart and circulatory disorders such as stroke and congestive heart failure.
♀ Brain and nerve damage, often causing pain in the arms and legs and sometimes leading to permanent intellectual impairment and severe memory loss.
♀ Organ damage, most notably to the liver (causing cirrhosis and hepatitis), but also to the stomach and pancreas.
♀ Gastrointestinal disorders such as gastritis, ulcers, pancreatitis, intestinal bleeding, diarrhoea and nausea.
♀ Malnutrition due to avoidance of food and regular meals in favour of alcohol. This leads to physical weakness and muscle wasting and a variety of disorders related to a deficiency of nutrients.
♀ Sexual problems, possibly infertility or impotence.
♀ Foetal alcohol syndrome.

ONE DAY AT A TIME

One of the most important things to remember when trying to overcome alcoholism is to take each day at a time and view each alcohol-free day as a triumph. There will be good days and bad days but, if you have a lapse, try to put it behind you immediately and start again. A reward system may work for you, in which the money saved that you might have spent on drink or some other motivating factor can help to steer you past temptation.

Most alcoholics find that it is better not to drink at all than to try to limit themselves to one drink, because once alcohol is in the blood it can trigger the craving for more. You have to be honest with other people and yourself and avoid the places, people and occasions that you associate with alcohol.

MONITOR YOUR DRINKING

If your ticks on this questionnaire fall mainly on the right-hand side, you have an addictive drink problem that needs addressing. If you cannot reduce your alcohol consumption, cut it out totally. Talk to your doctor and/or join a support group.

How often do you drink alcohol?

☐ Never
☐ Monthly or less
☐ 2–4 times a month

☐ 1–2 times a week
☐ 2–3 times a week
☐ 4 or more times a week

How many drinks do you have a day when you do drink?

☐ I don't drink
☐ 1–2 drinks
☐ 3–4 drinks

☐ 5–6 drinks
☐ 7 or more drinks

How often in the last year have you had four or more drinks on one occasion?

☐ Never
☐ Less than monthly
☐ Monthly

☐ Weekly
☐ Daily/almost daily

How many drinks does it take before you begin to feel the effects of alcohol?

☐ 1 drink or less
☐ 2 drinks
☐ 3 drinks

☐ 4 drinks
☐ 5 drinks
☐ 6 drinks or more

Have you had any legal difficulties because of alcohol?

☐ No

☐ Yes

Do you currently use any illicit drugs (marijuana, cocaine, heroin, pills)?

☐ No

☐ Yes

Have you used illicit drugs in the past?

☐ No

☐ Yes

The effects of smoking

Tobacco is the most common of all addictive substances and is one of the most important single causes of premature death. Women who smoke subject themselves to a wide variety of health problems.

As a group, young women represent the biggest increase among users of tobacco. Despite the recognition that nicotine, the active ingredient of tobacco, is physically addictive and carcinogenic (it causes cancer), warnings on the packs and elsewhere have not been successful in deterring tobacco use by this vulnerable group.

Reasons given for this include the stresses of modern living and an increase in the number of women spending evenings in bars, which were once a predominantly male environment. Worries about body shape lead young women to smoke as a way of losing weight because it suppresses the appetite.

Women may be more at risk from smoking than men because they have a different chemical response to nicotine. This increases their susceptibility to cervical, lung, bladder and other cancers, and also the risk of starting the menopause earlier by up to two years.

SMOKING AND YOUR BODY

There are about 3,600 chemicals in cigarette smoke, many of which are carcinogenic. Once inhaled into the lungs, toxic substances cross into the bloodstream and then to the liver. In the liver, enzymes detoxify substances considered dangerous to the body, breaking them down so they leave in the urine or faeces or through the skin as perspiration.

Tobacco smoking can certainly be connected with various sorts of cancer—most notably lung cancer, pharyngeal cancer and cancer of the tongue, lips and mouth. Evidence connecting smoking with breast cancer remains subject to debate but, for some women at least, a link between smoking and the likelihood of developing breast cancer can be drawn. In women who have a gene called NAT2 the detoxifying enzymes work slowly, giving the carcinogens more time to travel through the body reaching every organ. The same research also suggests that postmenopausal women with the slow-acting gene NAT2 who smoke may be more likely to develop breast cancer. Percentages of women who have this gene vary according to ethnic group.

GIVING IT UP

The withdrawal symptoms from tobacco are less severe than those from other drugs. But quitting is far from easy since the physical craving for tobacco may persist for months or years. Common complaints include irritability, jitteriness, anxiety and a tendency to gain weight (because eating is used as a replacement for the oral gratification derived from smoking). Techniques that involve mind and body, so that you understand the physical changes and reinforce your strength of purpose, appear to give the longest-lasting results. There are many methods to choose from.

Nicotine skin patches, nasal sprays and gum provide small amounts of nicotine, but take care not to become addicted to these instead. All replacement therapies present this problem.

Hypnosis, acupuncture and similar techniques work on your subconscious desires to encourage your body to reject smoking and to begin the healing process. Both group therapy and individual counselling are based on behavioural techniques and aim to strengthen your resolve.

The drug Bupaopion, available only through a doctor, is useful when part of a quit programme.

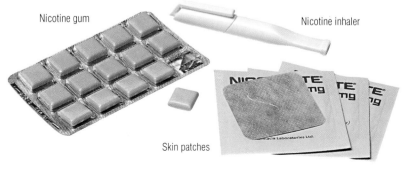

Nicotine gum

Nicotine inhaler

Skin patches

Smoking is also related to increased blood pressure (hypertension), and this in turn increases the risk of stroke, heart failure or coronary artery disease and possibly kidney damage. Cigarettes cause vascular disease (heart disease, stroke and leg gangrene) by increasing the stickiness of platelets in the blood and increasing thrombus formation, leading to narrowing of the arteries.

SMOKING AND CHILDBEARING

There exists a great deal of medical evidence about the dangers of smoking before conception and during pregnancy.

It is known that women who smoke find it more difficult to conceive naturally. Miscarriages, stillbirths and infant deaths are more common when the mother smokes.

Babies are twice as likely to be born prematurely and the newborn is usually smaller and lighter than average. The risk of congenital abnormalities, such as cleft palate and limb deformities, is increased.

The overall physical and mental development of the child may be adversely affected. Furthermore, children who become passive smokers because of their parents' habits or are taken into smoky environments are more likely to suffer from pneumonia and ear problems.

Where smoking hurts most

Smokers compared with non-smokers are at risk of:

♀ An increased incidence of cancer, notably of the lungs, but also of the pancreas, bladder, mouth, tongue, larynx and oesophagus.

♀ Chronic bronchitis, emphysema and susceptibility to lung infections including tuberculosis. The transportation of oxygen by the blood is impaired, resulting in shortness of breath even in the absence of physical activity.

♀ Heart and circulatory diseases. Smoking leads to an increase in coronary artery disease (angina and coronary thrombosis or heart attack) and to poor peripheral circulation particularly in the legs.

♀ An increase in dental and gum disorders.

♀ A perforated ulcer, since the presence of nicotine in smoke prevents ulcers in the stomach and duodenum from healing themselves.

WHEN YOU QUIT SMOKING

When you give up smoking, the returns in the context of improvements in your health are almost immediate. If you can focus on these benefits, it will help you stop successfully.

20 minutes after

Your blood pressure and pulse rate will fall. The temperature of your hands and feet return to normal.

8 hours after

Carbon monoxide in the blood drops to normal. The oxygen level increases to normal.

24 to 48 hours after

Your chance of heart attack decreases. Your ability to taste and smell is enhanced.

2 weeks to 3 months after

Your circulation improves. Walking becomes easier. Your lung function increases as much as 30 percent.

9 months to 1 year after

Coughing, sinus congestion, fatigue and shortness of breath decrease. Lungs are clearer and more resistant to infection. The risk of coronary heart disease is reduced to half that of a person still smoking.

3 years after

Risk of coronary heart disease and stroke decreases to that of people who have never smoked.

5 years after

The lung cancer rate for the average, former 20-per-day smoker decreases by almost half. Risk of cancer of the mouth, throat and oesophagus is half that of a smoker.

10 years after

The lung cancer death rate is similar to that of non-smokers. Precancerous cells are replaced. Risk of cancer of the mouth, throat, oesophagus, bladder, kidney and pancreas decreases.

See also:

1/BEING A WELL WOMAN
A healthy mind pp. 44–47

5/ILLNESSES & EMERGENCIES
Anxiety-related disorders
pp. 104–115
Nervous system problems
pp. 210–212

Drug addiction

Substance abuse, in its numerous forms, is a major problem in modern society. Illegal drugs are one of the biggest threats to law and order in all cities, and the cycle of deprivation, addiction, sickness and despair that comes from drug abuse is well documented in the media. But abuse of prescription drugs is even more common, especially among women, and harder to detect. Some drugs are physically and psychologically addictive; other drugs are only psychologically addictive or habit-forming.

Women suffer both from being addicted themselves and from concern for their families. Young and vulnerable children have been lured into drug use by dealers or even by their peers. Drugs may provide the adolescent with a means of escape or of rebelling against parental and other authority. Being aware of telltale signs may help prevent a tragedy.

If drug use is suspected, parents should confront the child and also seek help from the family doctor or a mental health professional who can advise and guide them. The social and personal consequences of drug addiction are as bad as those of alcoholism and the legal implications may be worse.

DRUGS AND ADULTS

It is not just children or young people who become addicted to drugs. Adults too can be in danger in certain situations. An adult may begin to take a prescription drug to relieve pain and become addicted. Drugs used to treat chronic or long-term illness range from painkillers like codeine to more addictive narcotics. Stress or the pressure of work may lead you to try illegal drugs; adults also can be susceptible to peer pressure, if people in their social circle are experimenting with drugs.

ILLEGAL SUBSTANCES

So-called recreational drugs usually have less serious long-term physical effects than either alcohol or tobacco. The chief risks for drug users are overdose, which is often fatal, or infec-

tion with hepatitis B or HIV (the AIDS virus) through the sharing of dirty needles.

Narcotics Opium and opiates—including heroin ("smack" and "scag") and morphine ("morph")—are among the most addictive, physically and psychologically, of all abused drugs. They act on the body's nerve transmitters and withdrawal symptoms can be severe. Narcotics may be injected, with the attendant risk of HIV infection, taken orally or by smoke inhalation ("chasing the dragon").

Cocaine Cocaine is most familiar as a white powder ("snow", "Peruvian marching powder", "nose candy" and "coke"), which is inhaled ("snorted") through the nose. It releases a neurotransmitter that distorts the signals in the brain and produces a rush of pleasurable sensations and an increase in alertness. Cocaine is both harmful and highly addictive (particularly in the purified form called "crack'). In the long term, it causes irritability, weight loss, depression, personality change and paranoia.

Hallucinogens Some hallucinogenic drugs (psychedelics) occur naturally, for example in peyote, mescaline and psilocybin ("magic mushrooms"). However, most are synthetic, including LSD ("acid") and PCP (phencyclidine and "angel dust"). Hallucinogens cause sensory, especially visual, distortion, and users experience intense emotions. The pupils dilate and breathing becomes erratic. Hallucinogens may also cause intense feelings of paranoia, confusion and depression, with potential consequences for psychological health. They are habit-forming rather than addictive.

Amphetamines In night-time club culture, ecstasy ("E", "adam" and MDMA), ketamine ("K") and other drugs easily made in backstreet laboratories are popular. Some of these can be altered so that they remain outside the category of proscribed substances. Amphetamines are referred to as "uppers" because they stimulate the nervous system, causing alertness, wakefulness and euphoria. They sometimes produce hallucinations. They are psychologically rather than physically addictive. Long-term abuse leads to irritability, personality changes and paranoia.

Cannabis Also known as marijuana, hash or hashish, pot and grass, cannabis is one of the least addictive and most widespread of illegal

Children and drugs

The warning signs are:
♀ Associating with known drug users.
♀ Unexplained truancy or consistent and unexplained late arrival at school or returning home after school or social activities.
♀ Deterioration in the quality of schoolwork and homework.
♀ Secrecy, unsociability and unaccustomed aggression.
♀ Neglect of personal appearance.
♀ Covering up of the arms to hide needle marks.
♀ Disappearance of money, from a purse, for example, since an addicted child may steal to pay for drugs.

drugs. It is usually smoked, in herbal form or as a resin, and produces feelings of relaxation, euphoria, disorientation and sometimes hallucinations. It can cause sudden food cravings (the "munchies"), sleepiness and, occasionally, paranoia. It is dangerous mainly because it may act as an introduction to drug culture.

Solvent abuse Solvent abuse, or glue sniffing, is most common among young teenagers, particularly boys. The most frequently used solvents are glues containing toluene or acetone, nail polish remover, butane lighter fuels and some aerosols. Fumes are generally inhaled from a plastic bag held over the face. Symptoms are similar to those of alcohol. A visible rash may also develop around the mouth and nose. High doses may cause hallucinations and coma and can, in severe cases, lead to permanent loss of coordination or death. Solvents are not addictive; most abusers grow out of the habit.

ADDICTIVE PRESCRIPTION DRUGS

Drugs that your doctor may prescribe for you can be addictive. These are usually prescribed for acute or chronic pain and for anxiety or depression. You should be aware of this risk when you are prescribed any painkiller or mood-altering medication and ask your doctor about its effects. When you are taking any of these drugs, you should monitor your responses closely to check for dependence.

Narcotic drugs include opium derivatives—morphine, codeine and methadone and other drugs such as percodan—and are often prescribed for the relief of severe pain. People with terminal cancer or other illness or cancer do not become addicted.

Amphetamines ("pep pills") are sometimes prescribed for chronic fatigue, depression and, because they suppress the appetite, obesity.

Benzodiazepines and barbiturates (otherwise known as sedatives) are used medically to treat insomnia, anxiety and depression. This group contains some of the best known of the prescription drugs that have been abused including Librium, Valium, temazepam, Seconal and phenobarbitone. They are known as "downers" from their tranquillizing and sedative effects, producing a pleasant feeling of relaxation, mood-enhancement, occasionally euphoria and, in rare cases, hallucinations. Large doses can cause confusion, coma and death. PCP (phencyclidine or "angel dust") produces

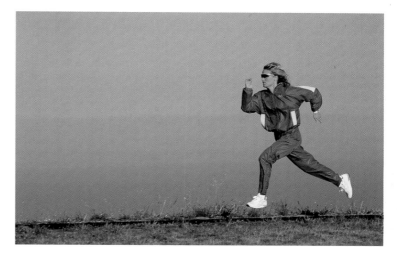

hallucinations and other extreme physical and psychological effects.

Probably the most common mood-altering drugs prescribed for women are antidepressants. Some are selective serotonin reuptake inhibitors (SSRIs) like Prozac. While not addictive to the extent of hard drugs, withdrawal symptoms include confusion and depression.

Cannabis has been prescribed to control nausea in cancer patients undergoing chemotherapy and in the management of chronic pain, muscle spasm (as in multiple sclerosis) and anxiety (Parkinson's disease). Many health professionals support its use as a prescription drug and clinical trials are being conducted to assess its effects and safety for medical use.

DANGERS FOR ATHLETES
The use of drugs in sports has caused controversy worldwide. Anabolic steroids are synthetic hormones taken to increase energy, build muscle bulk and to prolong stamina. Apart from giving the user a physical advantage over the non-user, they may have lasting, adverse effects on the body such as damage to the liver.

Treating drug addiction

There are two stages in the treatment of a person who is addicted—withdrawal and rehabilitation.

The withdrawal symptoms caused by some types of drugs—notably narcotics and tranquillizers—can be severe. They include sweating, diarrhoea, nausea, vomiting, abdominal cramps, goose pimples, running eyes and nose, yawning, irritability, sleeplessness, confusion, anxiety and depression. Symptoms can last for a week or more, and medical supervision is often necessary. Sometimes a less addictive substitute, such as methadone in the case of withdrawal from narcotics, may be given in decreasing doses to ease the severity of the symptoms.

Rehabilitation and the prevention of relapse require a programme of long-term maintenance. This generally involves counselling or psychotherapy. It is virtually impossible without the active help of family members or a support group and without strong motivation on the part of the former addict. Some form of behaviour therapy, such as aversion therapy, may be effective, so that the addict begins to associate the substance with nausea or disgust. There are many self-help groups, including Narcotics Anonymous.

? Did you know?
Anorexics do not, in fact, lose their appetite until the late stages of the illness, but their interest in food may be diverted into food-related activities such as cooking for others, hiding food, collecting recipes or obsessive calorie counting.

Eating disorders

Overeating and excessive dieting both increase a woman's health risks, but the problem becomes even greater when these pre-occupations become obsessive. Women are especially vulnerable to eating disorders which involve their weight, self-esteem and the image they have of themselves.

ANOREXIA NERVOSA

Although usually associated with adolescent girls, anorexia nervosa—which means "nervous loss of appetite"—can occur at any age and in either sex. However, it is about 10 times more common in women than in men.

There may be a genetic component to the disease, since it tends to run in families. It is associated, too, with a family history of serious depression—nearly half of all anorexics are clinically depressed. Almost as many show symptoms of obsessive-compulsive disorder, which often afflicts other members of the family. The condition is particularly common in women whose ideal of female beauty is linked to an image of thinness.

Anorexics frequently come from families in which the parents are extremely strict or over-protective. They often claim that dieting gives them greater control over their lives, especially during the teen years or young adulthood when it may feel as if other aspects of life are uncontrollable. They may be perfectionists and less sociable than their peers. Dieting to excess may be a form of rebellion, a way to reject their

Signs of anorexia nervosa

Anorexics usually deny that there is anything wrong with them. The following are all strong indications that someone is suffering from anorexia nervosa:

♀ Loss of weight to a level below 85 percent of normal for the individual's age and height. Most anorexics are usually 25 percent or more below normal weight.

♀ Excessive concern over gaining weight or becoming fat. Anorexics have no ability to perceive their own body weight and shape correctly—they see normal weight as fat. Even when they are painfully thin, they insist that they are fat.

♀ Physical debility due to starvation, including tiredness, anaemia, constipation, low blood pressure, brittle bones (osteoporosis), swollen joints, yellowing of the skin and sensitivity to cold. Anorexics often wear layers of baggy clothes to disguise their thinness and to keep warm. Fine body hair called lanugo appears, possibly to retain the body's heat.

♀ Menstruation may not begin or will cease if body weight is below about 80 percent of normal. Missing three or more periods in a row is a strong indication of anorexia.

♀ Anorexics may take laxatives and emetics (which prevent proper absorption of food). They often avoid eating in public and may also exercise obsessively, often at night and in private, where nobody can see them.

WHO IS AT RISK?

Eating disorders are most often encountered in young women who are going through emotional upheavals associated with adolescence or lifestyle pressures in their early 20s. A family history of parental control or emotional starvation can be factors. Often there may be, in fact, a family history of eating problems.

PUBERTY

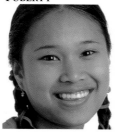

Anorexia nervosa is very common in teenagers and affects more than one in every 100 school and university students aged 15 to 25.

20s

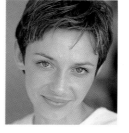

In this age group women may tend to either anorexia or bulimia. Obsession with food can be a substitute for a satisfying emotional life.

30s-40s

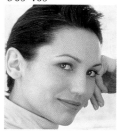

Women in this age group are more rarely affected by anorexia but may be driven by depression to bulimia or compulsive overeating.

parents' care and a means of asserting their own individuality. Because anorexia suppresses menstruation and often begins around the age of puberty, it may also be a way of avoiding the cares and responsibilities of growing up by remaining in a state of childhood innocence. What is clear is that anorexia is a sign of an underlying psychological disorder, often triggered by some stressful life event.

HOW ANOREXIA IS TREATED

If the condition is life-threatening—the anorexic has a pulse rate of less than 40—she may have to be treated in a hospital. Intravenous feeding is often needed and this requires the cooperation of the patient.

SSRI antidepressants may be prescribed to raise levels of serotonin. Serotonin is a chemical transmitter in the brain that regulates mood. SSRIs can alleviate depression and anxiety.

Long-term counselling or psychotherapy will be necessary, often over many months or years. Therapy may consist of private sessions or include the family, followed by group sessions so that problems can be expressed and shared. The purpose of therapy is to help the anorexic feel deserving of love, enhance her self-esteem and lessen her need to be in control. She can also learn strategies to assist her through difficult times, such as family meals, parties and other social situations.

The outlook for recovery is not good. Only about half of all patients will have recovered completely after four years and about a quarter will remain severely underweight. In this group, the risk of suicide, heart attack or starving to death is high.

BINGE EATING AND BULIMIA

More women than men, particularly young women, suffer from these related disorders. First an excess of food is eaten, then it is purged from the body. Binge eaters are seized by an uncontrollable craving for food, which they consume—usually in secret—in vast quantities at a single sitting. As well as inducing vomiting, bingers may use laxatives, enemas, diuretics and excessive physical exercise to control weight. Between binges, most will diet strictly. Unlike anorexics, binge eaters have a realistic perception of their weight and are generally motivated by a desire to lose excess fat. Most binge eaters have a history of dieting. Recurrent

episodes of bingeing (two or three a week) over an extended period (three months or more) can be defined as bulimia. The common characteristics of "bulimics" include the experience of some stressful event that acts as a trigger, some other form of mental problem—for example, depression or a personality disorder—or drug or alcohol problems. There may have been sexual abuse in the past.

A family history of depression may be a factor in both anorexia and bulimia. Some physical signs specific to bulimia include grazed knuckles (from sticking the fingers in the throat to induce vomiting), infection of the salivary glands, pitting of the teeth (due to acid in the vomit) and stomach bleeding. Mineral imbalances caused by constant vomiting may have serious side effects, such as an irregular heart beat. However, bulimia rarely causes death.

Bulimics are less secretive and less inclined to deny the problem than anorexics and so are more easily treated by long-term counselling or behavioural or cognitive therapy. SSRIs can also be useful. Psychoanalysis may be recommended if earlier sexual abuse is an underlying cause.

COMPULSIVE OVEREATING

Like bulimia, compulsive overeating involves eating binges, but they are not usually followed by purging. Compulsive overeaters are normally overweight. The condition is associated with feelings of guilt, shame, stress, low self-esteem and a preoccupation with body shape. It may result from fear of having to compete with other women.

When obesity could be life-threatening—such as when blood pressure is seriously elevated—drastic measures may be necessary, including surgically reducing the size of the stomach.

Treatment of compulsive eating generally requires therapy or counselling. Cognitive and behavioural therapies are usually the most successful. Many people also find that self-help groups such as Weight Watchers, where problems are discussed with those who are similarly affected, can help enormously in restoring and maintaining healthy eating habits.

> ### Signs of compulsive overeating
>
> ♀ An urge to eat when not hungry—for example, eating to relieve feelings of depression, boredom or unhappiness.
>
> ♀ A constant preoccupation with food.
>
> ♀ An abnormal interest in dietary information in books and magazines.
>
> ♀ Alternate episodes of dieting and overeating.
>
> ♀ Feelings of guilt at being unable to control the craving for food.
>
> ♀ Being ashamed of your weight and body shape.

ANXIETY-RELATED PROBLEMS

Various nervous states can commonly occur with many women and make their daily life difficult. The events causing the problems can be forgotten while the anxiety or fear remains. But these states of mind can be helped by relaxation exercises or therapy.

See also:

1/BEING A WELL WOMAN
A healthy mind pp. 44–47

6/TREATMENTS & THERAPIES
Conventional treatments
pp. 272–277; pp. 282–289
Complementary therapies
pp. 292–297.

Fears and worries

Everyone is familiar with those sensations, such as a dry mouth, pounding heart, rapid breathing and sweating, that occur when you are in a threatening or unpleasant situation.

Dizziness and light-headedness

Sweating, pale skin tone and blushing

Constant dryness of the mouth, nausea, belching and flatulence, and sometimes diarrhoea and vomiting

Fast, throbbing heartbeat

Lightness in the chest, accompanied by stabbing pains, breathlessness and hyperventilation or a choking sensation

Frequent urge to empty the bladder and bowels

Muscle tension, leading to headaches, back pain, shakiness, aching muscles and an inability to relax

PHYSICAL EFFECTS
Anxiety-related mental illness can have physical symptoms ranging from the visible, such as sweating or blushing, to the internal, such as a racing heart and headaches.

Anxiety is the normal reaction to stress; in fact, its presence is what defines a situation or event as stressful. Anxiety may be harmless or even useful. A reasonable degree of anxiety before an exam or interview is likely to help you perform better. However, if it becomes so severe that it interferes with everyday life, it becomes an illness that requires treatment.

WHO IS AT RISK?
Anxiety appears to affect women more than men and there may be an inherited disposition. It may also stem from early experiences of deprivation—loss of or separation from parents, for example, or a perceived lack of parental attention. This is particularly the case when current events in an older person's life seem to mirror an earlier traumatic experience.

Personality may be a factor. Some people are born worriers. Those with rigid and perfectionist personalities or excessively meek and submissive personalities are most vulnerable.

Physiologically, anxiety is thought to be related to an excess of the hormone noradrenaline—a transmitter of nerve impulses—in the brain. There are also some physical conditions, such as disorders of the thyroid gland and oestrogen deficiency at and after menopause, that can cause or mimic the effects of anxiety.

WARNING SIGNS
Throughout life you have to deal with stressful events that cause some degree of anxiety, for example, if someone you love is ill or a relationship breaks down, if you lose your job or move. Most people are able to get through the bad time and eventually the anxiety dwindles

and ceases. But in susceptible individuals, the symptoms may reach disabling proportions known as adjustment disorders and become persistent. This is genuine mental illness.

There are common symptoms which should be watched for. Prominent is a feeling of foreboding, sometimes amounting to unfounded dread or terror. There may be nervousness, irritability and jumpiness. The person appears to worry constantly, has regular insomnia and subsequent feelings of exhaustion. She shows a fear of physical illness, reinforced by the physical symptoms of anxiety. These may lead to periods of feeling detached from the outside world (depersonalization) or of feeling that the outside world is unreal (derealization).

OBSESSIONS AND COMPULSIONS

People with obsessions are unable to prevent certain thoughts or ideas from recurring constantly and persistently. Common forms of obsession involve cleanliness, tidiness and doubts about whether particular tasks have been performed. The obsession leads to the performance of ritualized, repetitive actions—compulsions—for example, constant washing of the hands or endlessly checking that all doors and windows are locked. Obsessives are aware that their behaviour is irrational and time-wasting, but are unable to control it.

Obsessions are a learned response to anxiety. They also appear to be linked with disorders of brain chemistry, specifically with the serotonin system. Serotonin is implicated in depression and some antidepressant drugs have proved useful in the management of inherited obsessive-compulsive disorders.

PHOBIAS

Irrational fears of objects or situations are phobias. People may be phobic about particular animals, such as cats, spiders or birds, or about specific situations, such as heights, enclosed spaces (for example, lifts) or flying. Most phobias are inconvenient rather than severely disruptive. Some, however, such as agoraphobia (fear of open spaces) and social phobia (fear of being observed by other people), are symptoms of more generalized anxiety and can affect all aspects of life.

Phobias are learned responses to a stimulus. They may result from an unpleasant or traumatizing experience in childhood, being ▶

COPING WITH A PANIC ATTACK

One of the most frightening manifestations of anxiety is a panic attack. In this, the anxiety caused by the initial situation is compounded by the fear caused by the symptoms themselves. The increased anxiety further increases the fear, in a vicious circle that rapidly spirals out of control and the person becomes convinced she is having a heart attack or stroke or that she is going insane.

Panic attacks, however, can be arrested before they reach this stage. Once you recognize the signs, you can take corrective measures.

Mentally, you need to find something to distract your attention from the anxiety you feel—if you're on a street focus on an advertising board, read every word on it and think of its meaning. Or concentrate on an activity or conversation going on around you. If you're alone, think of the birthday of every member of your family.

Physically, you need to take action to slow the rate of breathing to combat hyperventilation (overbreathing). Try deep breathing (see below). Alternatively, breathe in and out of a paper bag held over the mouth and nose for several minutes. This will reduce the intake of oxygen and increase the intake of carbon dioxide. Soon your normal breathing will be restored and your heart will stop racing.

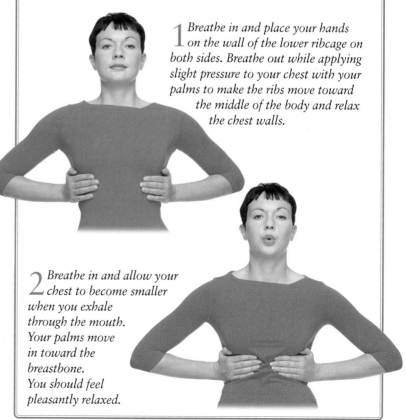

1 Breathe in and place your hands on the wall of the lower ribcage on both sides. Breathe out while applying slight pressure to your chest with your palms to make the ribs move toward the middle of the body and relax the chest walls.

2 Breathe in and allow your chest to become smaller when you exhale through the mouth. Your palms move in toward the breastbone. You should feel pleasantly relaxed.

TRIGGERS OF FEAR
Anything, even a fluffy affectionate cat, can be the cause of a phobia in susceptible people whose fear may stem from a childhood experience. The best way to learn to cope with such triggers is through desensitization in cognitive behavioural therapy.

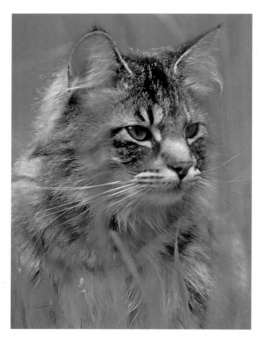

> **! Caution**
> It is important to remember that someone whose symptoms are mainly in the mind suffers as much pain and discomfort as she would if there were a genuine physical cause. Both the physical discomfort and the underlying cause need to be treated.

See your doctor
There may be a physical cause of some of the symptoms that appear to come from a stressful reaction. It may be a medical problem or the result of conflicting medication. In either case investigation is needed.

bitten by a dog, for example, or sometimes they may be learnt from parents or other adults. Mere anticipation of a situation is enough to arouse fear and then failure to confront and deal with it intensifies the anxiety. In the worst cases, the only way the person sees to control the fear is to avoid the situation ever arising. This can give rise to complete withdrawal and can reach the stage of being life-threatening.

OTHER DISORDERS

A number of factors can both cause anxiety and be a symptom of it. Physical health is one of the most important of these. Some disorders, for example, overactivity of the thyroid gland, cause anxiety as a direct symptom of the disease. Anxiety is also a fairly common reaction to serious illness.

Difficulties with personal and work relationships and sexual problems are also both a symptom and a cause of anxiety. Conversely, several mental conditions manifest themselves as physical symptoms.

Hypochondriasis This is a condition in which people obsessively worry about their health and may display symptoms that appear to have a psychological rather than a physical cause. They interpret minor ailments as symptoms of more serious disease and constantly seek medical advice and help.

Somatization In some cases, anxiety is experienced and expressed in terms of physical symptoms. Generally, these take the form of vague, unidentifiable illness. Somatization is thought to be the result of an inability to deal mentally with stress and anxiety.

Dissociative disorder Sometimes called conversion reaction, this used to be known as hysteria. Physical symptoms—often unusual ones, such as temporary blindness or the loss of use of a limb—have no apparent cause. However, the inability to find a physical cause does not necessarily mean that there isn't one.

POST-TRAUMATIC STRESS

Survivors and witnesses of terrible, violent or shocking events—train or plane crashes, earthquakes, random shootings, terrorism, assault—can suffer from a form of anxiety known as post-traumatic stress. The condition is characterized by recurrent memories and images of the event, the development of phobias about things associated with the event, disturbed sleep and other psychological symptoms of anxiety. There may be feelings of guilt, about having survived when others did not, and depression, which may become severe. The symptoms may develop soon after the event or they may not appear until months or years later.

Treatment may involve various approaches including psychotherapy, cognitive behavioural techniques, desensitization and psychopharmacological medications. Eventually the person comes to terms with the event and is able to remember it without distressing symptoms.

TREATING ANXIETY DISORDERS

One cause of anxiety is stress and an important aspect of treatment is learning to cope with it. Effective stress management can help to reduce anxiety in many situations, but if this does not work treatment may be needed. There are two main types of treatment: counselling or psychotherapy, and drugs. The general aim of therapy is to unlearn the inappropriate response.

Behavioural therapy Phobias and obsessions may be treated using a specialized form of behaviour therapy which involves gradual desensitization through increasing exposure to the feared object or situation. An alternative technique sometimes used is flooding: the person is made to confront the situation head-on, with a trained therapist always present to deal with the acute anxiety that may result.

Drug assistance Behavioural therapy may also be used in conjunction with a course of drugs. Three types of drug are in common use.

Beta-blockers counteract the physical effects of anxiety. They reduce the activity of the autonomic nervous system, so slowing down breathing and heart rate and reducing tension.

Antidepressant and anti-anxiety medications are the mainstays of drug treatment and can be beneficial both for acute situations and chronic cases. The combination of psychotherapy and medication is often the most successful.

Treatment of anxiety disorders has a good success rate. Many cases are completely cured or substantially improved, and most show some degree of improvement.

RELAXATION TRAINING

Many people find that some form of relaxation training can help with anxiety-related disorders, including physical disorders such as asthma as well as mental stress.

Trained hypnotherapists induce a state of deep relaxation and then encourage the patient to feel relaxed and stress-free. Patients can also be trained in self-hypnosis. In biofeedback, sensors on the body measure various functions such as brain waves, heart rate and muscle tension. The patient can learn to produce changes in these functions first through watching the meters and then gradually without the meters.

Autogenic training

A form of self-suggestion or self-hypnosis that can be practised at home or at work or whenever you are threatened by stress or anxiety, autogenic training (AT) can help stress-related conditions such as migraine and irritable bowel syndrome. It can also be used to combat addictions such as smoking.

You have to receive training in AT by attending 8 to 10 sessions with a trained practitioner, who teaches you some exercises to switch off stress in the body. In each of these exercises, you suggest to yourself the physical state you want to induce and gradually let it develop.

The exercises are geared to general relaxation as well as your specific need. So, with phobias, you would concentrate on calming the breathing and heart rate and then suggest to yourself that the object of fear was not too frightening, after all.

Some suggestions of phrases you can repeat to yourself for several minutes to encourage relaxation include:
♀ My heartbeat is strong and slow.
♀ My stomach is warm.
♀ My forehead is cool.
♀ My breathing is slow and calm.
♀ My muscles are limp and relaxed.
♀ My limbs are heavy and warm.
♀ I'm getting more and more relaxed.

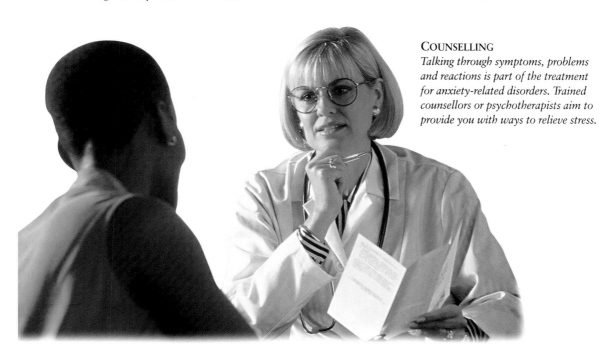

COUNSELLING
Talking through symptoms, problems and reactions is part of the treatment for anxiety-related disorders. Trained counsellors or psychotherapists aim to provide you with ways to relieve stress.

The effects of stress

See also:

1/BEING A WELL WOMAN
Essentials of good health
pp. 22–27
A healthy mind pp. 44–49

Stress acts as a stimulus to performance and makes you more alert and aware. However, there is a point, and it is different for each person, at which the beneficial effects are outweighed by symptoms of anxiety. At this stage the body is stressed by events and this can have physical repercussions.

HOW THE BODY REACTS TO STRESS

Within minutes of the immediate release of fight or flight hormones by the adrenal glands other reactions to the situation follow. The hippocampus in the brain activates memory and learning, so that you can remember and deal with the situation if it recurs.

In the immune system, activity shuts down, so that energy can be used for fight or flight.

The liver quickly converts stored fat to fuel that can be used by the body and the adrenal glands continue to release hormones.

The problem is that the effects can become chronic and affect health. Ongoing production of the hormone cortisol by the kidneys can be damaging to the brain, the immune system, the intestines and the circulatory system. Infections are not fought, memory and emotions are adversely affected, digestion is upset and blood pressure rises (which can damage the heart and blood vessels).

MEASURING STRESS

Many life happenings can cause stress—and not all of them need be unpleasant. Even propitious events, such as going on holiday or getting married, can cause stress. And stress is cumulative. The stress caused by losing your job is not displaced by the stress of loss of income, it adds to it. Since stress is closely related to anxiety and susceptibility to physical illness, it helps to be aware of situations that contribute to changes in the way your body functions.

In the 1960s, two American researchers Thomas H. Holmes and Richard H. Rahe devised a now frequently used scale to measure the impact of stress. They ranked common stress-inducing life events in order of their effects on the body and gave each a score on a scale of one to 100—the higher the figure the greater the stress. The theory is that the total score in any one 12-month period accurately predicts the likelihood of future illness.

Apparently straightforward events can turn out to be surprisingly stressful when all factors involved are taken into account. Getting married, for example, may mean moving home, changing financial circumstances, gaining new members of the family which, with other events, result in a high level of cumulative risk.

WOMEN AND STRESS

Some stressful life events or more long-term problems are specific to women. Infertility or even the lack of children as a result of a conscious decision can cause anxiety and feelings of low self-esteem. Tests have shown that infertility may have as great an effect on a woman's psyche as a life-threatening illness. On the other

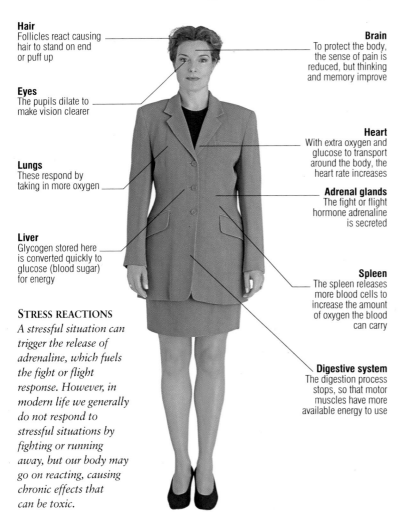

Hair
Follicles react causing hair to stand on end or puff up

Eyes
The pupils dilate to make vision clearer

Lungs
These respond by taking in more oxygen

Liver
Glycogen stored here is converted quickly to glucose (blood sugar) for energy

Brain
To protect the body, the sense of pain is reduced, but thinking and memory improve

Heart
With extra oxygen and glucose to transport around the body, the heart rate increases

Adrenal glands
The fight or flight hormone adrenaline is secreted

Spleen
The spleen releases more blood cells to increase the amount of oxygen the blood can carry

Digestive system
The digestion process stops, so that motor muscles have more available energy to use

STRESS REACTIONS
A stressful situation can trigger the release of adrenaline, which fuels the fight or flight response. However, in modern life we generally do not respond to stressful situations by fighting or running away, but our body may go on reacting, causing chronic effects that can be toxic.

hand, stress can lead to infertility, probably because the adrenal hormones released by stress affect the reproductive hormones.

Bringing up a family is also a potentially stressful job. When children are very young, if the mother does not have adequate support, she may feel trapped by the situation. She needs to be able to get out of the house, to have the child-care taken off her hands every so often and possibly to have the support and company of other mothers. Another time of crisis is when her children are teenagers and she may be worrying about their future or feel that they no longer respond to her care or control.

Girls or women commonly suffer from sexually or physically abusive situations. This may happen when the child is too young to be able to act for herself and will have repercussions throughout her life. When she is older, a woman may enter an abusive relationship, often because of low self-esteem. These events may cause severe stress or depression (pp. 110–112), which in turn produce physical symptoms, and may need long-term therapy to overcome.

THE HOLMES AND RAHE LIFE CHANGE INDEX

To assess your stress level and the risk of illness developing, check off the events that have happened to you in the previous 12 months and then add up your total score. Each successive event will add to your stress level. You may have to accept some things but be able to alter others.

Rank	Event	Points	Rank	Event	Points
1	Death of spouse or partner	100	21	Child leaves home	29
2	Divorce	73	22	Trouble with in-laws	29
3	Marital separation	65	23	Outstanding personal achievement	28
4	Prison term	63	24	Spouse or partner begins or ends work	26
5	Death of family member	63	25	Begin or finish school	26
6	Personal injury	53	26	Change in living conditions	25
7	Marriage	50	27	Change in personal habits	24
8	Loss of job	47	28	Trouble with employer	23
9	Marital reconciliation	45	29	Change in working hours or conditions	20
10	Retirement	45	30	Moving house	20
11	Change in health of family member	44	31	Moving school	20
12	Pregnancy	40	32	Change in recreation	19
13	Sexual problems	39	33	Change in religious activity	19
14	Gain new family member	39	34	Change in social activity	18
15	Changes at work or in business	39	35	Having a small mortgage	17
16	Change in financial circumstances	39	36	Change in sleeping habits	16
17	Death of close friend	37	37	Change in number of family get-togethers	15
18	Change to new line of work	36	38	Change in eating habits	15
19	Change in frequency of arguments with spouse or partner	35	39	Going on holiday	13
20	Having a large mortgage	33	40	Christmas	12
			41	Minor law violation	11

0 to 100 points
Low stress levels seldom cause problems. At around 100 points, there is a small increase to the risk that an illness will develop over the next two years.

100 to 200 points
Moderate levels of stress carry a 10 to 35 percent increase to the risk of an illness occurring over the next two years.

200 to 300 points
High stress levels carry a 35 to 50 percent increase to the risk that an illness will develop over the next two years.

300 plus points
With extremely high stress levels, there is a strong probability—80 to 90 percent—of illness developing over the next two years.

Understanding depression

See also:

1/BEING A WELL WOMAN
Essentials of good health
pp. 22–27
A healthy mind pp. 44–49

2/SEX & SEXUALITY
Your sexual self pp. 56–57

4/HORMONAL HEALTH
Endocrine system problems
pp. 140–141

Women are especially vulnerable to depression. For many people, depression may be transient and mild—a feeling of dissatisfaction, self-doubt, a loss of energy and enthusiasm and a sense of the pointlessness of life.

Many people suffer deeper symptoms for a while, for example, after bereavement or divorce. However, there are times when these feelings escalate into something more serious—overwhelming feelings of loss, sadness, guilt and despair. There may be physical symptoms, such as loss of weight and appetite, lethargy and fatigue, which become real obstacles to leading a normal life. At this stage, depression becomes a serious psychological disorder.

WOMEN AND DEPRESSION

Depression occurs in all age groups, but it is more common from young adulthood up to middle age. In the age group over 65, it begins to diminish. It is twice as common in women as in men and between 2 and 25 percent of

women will at some time in their lives suffer from it. The gender difference is found in severe depression/depressive disorder and in various other types of depression such as dysthymia (mild depression), seasonal affective disorder (SAD) and rapid-cycling bipolar disorder (rapid mood swings).

The difference in incidence of depression between women and men begins after puberty and is probably linked to hormonal changes. Women are also more susceptible to depression in the premenstrual phase and after giving birth—times linked with hormonal activity. Depression at the menopause may be more linked to social factors such as retirement from work or children leaving home, although investigation continues.

The part hormones play in depression is not wholly clear. Oestrogen and progesterone affect the levels of two of the neurotransmitters called serotonin and noradrenaline in the central nervous system. Bouts of depression appear to be associated with low levels of these transmitters. The same hormones regulate the body's cycle of metabolism throughout the day and this may be the reason why some women appear to be more susceptible than men to SAD—their metabolic rate slows in the hours of darkness.

Women's self-esteem tends to be based on relationships with others rather than having firm foundations in their own personalities. This is also associated with women being less esteemed in society and, especially in more traditional cultures, being given a restricted role to play. Women and men also appear to respond differently to drug treatment with antidepressants, presumably again because of hormonal differences, and women are likely to have recurring depressive episodes.

WHAT CAUSES DEPRESSION?

Depression can be triggered by various factors separately or a combination of factors. The two main causes are traumatic events and inherent predisposition. The genetic linkage to a tendency to depression has been well demonstrated in studies with twins. Traumatic life events may include events in the past, such as loss of a parent in childhood or, even more powerfully, recent events, such as a breakdown

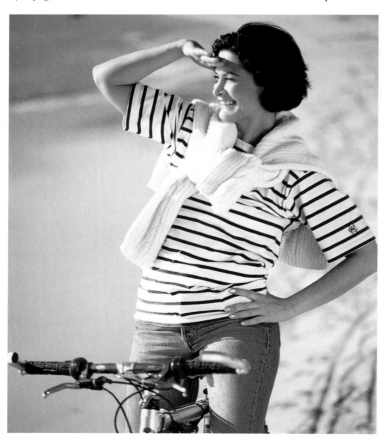

SPORT CAN HELP
Physical exercise outdoors can stimulate the circulation and digestion and combat the depression that may arise from lack of daylight.

of a relationship or the death of a family member. Physical illness can often cause depression, especially if it is long-term or life-threatening, such as multiple sclerosis or cancer. But depression can follow a viral illness, such as flu. It is also a feature of chronic fatigue syndrome (myalgic encephalomyelitis, also known as ME or post-viral syndrome) and may be linked with another psychological condition such as a panic disorder.

Surgery and medication can both have depression as a side effect. Drugs, including oral contraceptives, some tranquillizers and surgical anaesthetics, can cause depression. Alcohol and drug abuse can be symptoms or causes of depression and, in the extreme, lead to suicide. Anxiety and depression are also common symptoms of withdrawal from drugs or alcohol.

Events in a woman's life can give rise to depressive phases or sometimes a more long-term disorder. Childbirth triggers depression in more than half of all new mothers. Menstruation and menopause are times when women may feel emotionally low as well as physically uncomfortable. More traumatic events, such as an abortion or a hysterectomy, may be followed by depression. Infertility, or the inability to have children, can also produce severe depression, which may become chronic.

Generally, older people are less prone to depression, although bereavement or loneliness are common causes of sadness in the elderly.

Lack of daylight can cause SAD ("winter blues"), a form of depression that occurs during prolonged periods of daylight deprivation such as winter. SAD can be treated by antidepressant medication or regular exposure to natural light. There are lights available that simulate natural daylight.

RISK FACTORS

There are several reasons why some people are more likely to develop depression than others.

Genetics Depression appears to have a strong inherited component. With identical twins, if one is depressed there's a 60 percent chance that their twin will also be. In a family with a history of severe depression, about one in eight of family members are likely to develop the condition. The greater susceptibility of women may be linked to female sex genes.

Abnormal brain chemistry Two substances in particular are known to be involved in

Signs to watch out for

There are a number of observable symptoms which indicate depression.
♀ Lethargy and listlessness—sufferers are sometimes unable to summon the energy to go out or to get out of bed.
♀ Change in appetite and weight, which demonstrates a lack of interest in food, compounded by constipation, or an increased dependence on "comfort" eating, especially carbohydrates.
♀ Loss of interest in sex.
♀ Disturbed sleep and insomnia. Sleep is intermittent and interrupted by constant worrying.
♀ Depression tends to be worse in the morning, (except with sufferers of SAD) with an elevation of mood toward the end of the day.
♀ Inability to concentrate.
♀ Anxiety, with possible trembling or panic attacks.
♀ Low self-esteem, perhaps coupled with irrational guilt.
♀ Slowing of mental and physical activity. Speech may become soft, halting and monotone, without emphasis or inflection, often tailing off into silence. Movement may be reluctant and requires effort, often with a slow, shuffling gait.
♀ Mental confusion including forgetfulness, irrational thinking and disorientation occurs particularly in older people. The symptoms may be mistaken for dementia.
♀ Thoughts of death and suicide.
♀ Delusions and hallucinations are symptoms of serious psychotic depression.

See your doctor

Depression can affect anyone. More serious depression affects twice as many women as men, yet only about 30 percent seek professional help. It is important to remember that depression is not a weakness, but an illness that can be treated. The type of treatment will depend on the person, for everyone is a unique mix of physiology and experience. A good specialist will try to find out what's gone wrong with your own normality and choose the therapy and drugs accordingly.

depression: the neurotransmitters serotonin and noradrenaline. During intervals of depression, the levels of both chemicals are low and this is thought to lead to the transmission of faulty messages, which is responsible for some of the symptoms of depressive illness. Drugs that increase the levels of serotonin and noradrenaline in the brain have been used successfully in treating the illness.

Social and environmental factors Social deprivation, poor living conditions and alcohol or drug addiction all contribute to depression. Unemployed single mothers without adequate emotional or physical support from family or friends often become depressed, for example. ▶

TREATMENTS FOR DEPRESSION

Many people get through a period of depression simply by talking to friends and relatives, joining a self-help group or reading books and following the advice they offer. People who need more help should make an appointment to see their doctor. Depending on the severity of the symptoms and the type of depression, the doctor is then likely to recommend one or more of three types of treatment.

Drugs There are various types of antidepressant, including SSRIs (selective serotonin reuptake inhibitors) such as Prozac. SSRIs help to maintain the levels of serotonin in the brain and are relatively free of side effects. Drugs are important in relieving mood and physical symptoms but they do not tackle underlying emotional or psychological problems.

Therapy or counselling The long-term treatment for depression normally involves identifying and dealing with the problems that caused it in the first place. The most effective form of therapy is usually cognitive. This is a form of behaviour therapy in which treatment corrects habits of thought rather than patterns of behaviour. Cognitive therapy can replace negative perceptions with more positive accurate ones, so reversing the destructive spiral caused by constant depressive thinking. Psychotherapy or psychoanalysis seek deeper hidden causes of depression, often going back to childhood memories. It is a long process and may not work for everyone.

Electroconvulsive therapy This consists of the administration of electric currents to the brain through electrodes attached to either side of the head. It is only used in severe depression when other forms of treatment have failed, or when there is an immediate danger to the patient's health, for example from suicide. It is successful in many cases. Treatment is generally only given after full hospital evaluation and there will need to be support facilities available at home or in the community.

THE "BABY BLUES"

Half or more of all mothers experience mild depression, called post-natal depression, after the birth of their baby. They feel generally low, tired and listless. They may cry for no particular reason and they may feel worried and tense. They may also experience unexplained pains and feel generally unwell.

Hormonal changes following childbirth may play a part in producing the blues, but other factors are probably equally important. Many mothers are unprepared for the exhaustion that follows childbirth and may not have fully appreciated the impact that a baby, particularly their first, will have on their lives. Any uncertainty about the child's health or problems before or after the birth will be magnified greatly. Psychological and physical support are needed so that the mother gets both sympathy and rest. In most cases the symptoms pass in a few days.

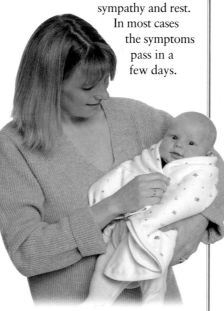

POST-NATAL DEPRESSION

About 10 percent of new mothers develop serious post-natal depression, which usually arises several weeks after giving birth. The symptoms are similar to other forms of depression and may include delusional beliefs—that the mother has the wrong baby or has not had a baby at all—and hallucinations. If there is any danger that the mother may hurt her baby or contemplate suicide, she should seek help immediately. A family member who recognizes the symptoms should not ignore the situation. Tact and sympathy should be used to encourage the mother to see her doctor. At this time, practical and uncritical emotional support from friends and family is essential.

The doctor may prescribe antidepressants or tranquillizers to deal with the more debilitating symptoms. SSRIs may also be prescribed for six to 12 months. They have few side effects and can prevent future episodes. Sleep is important to therapy and help from the family or medication may both be necessary to ensure the mother gets enough rest. The doctor will also probably recommend counselling to deal with deep-seated or long-lasting effects. In severe cases of post-natal depression, in-patient treatment under psychiatric care may be required for the mother and her baby, especially where safety issues are involved.

Headaches

Many women experience recurrent headaches which may be a response to various problems such as tiredness, hunger, dehydration, menstrual problems or a medical condition. Treatment is often more successful than finding the cause. In medical terms, there are three main types: tension (muscle-contraction) headaches, migraine (vascular) headaches and combination (tension and migraine) headaches.

In some cases, the symptoms may be due to a disease or disorder, in which case they are known as secondary headaches. Sinusitis, for example, often produces a throbbing headache. It helps to identify which one afflicts you so you can take the appropriate action.

COMMON CAUSES

Tension is one of the main causes of headaches in 90 percent of people. It affects women three times more often than men. Mental strain produces muscular tension and results in low-level aches, often on both sides of the head, forehead and the back of the neck. They usually last for no more than a few hours, but can continue for as long as a week. Pain is usually moderate.

Hormonal factors may trigger tension headaches from adolescence on. They can appear either before or during menstruation and some women may develop them at and during the menopause. Oestrogen is a known cause for headache sufferers taking the oral contraceptive pill and using some types of hormone replacement therapy (HRT). A gynaecological problem, such as ovarian cysts, may be a cause.

A bacterial or viral infection or parasitic infestation can often have headache as a symptom, particularly where there is fever. Examples include influenza, pyelonephritis and generalized infections, such as measles, ear, nose and throat infections, dental problems and shingles. Headaches may also signal rare but potentially life-threatening conditions (p. 115).

Infection or inflammation of the lining of the sinuses—the air-filled cavities on either side of the nose—causes a dull pain in the upper

> **? Did you know?**
> Women rarely get cluster headaches—most sufferers are men, and smokers in particular. Cluster headaches get their name from the fact that they tend to occur in clusters of one to four attacks over a period of several weeks. Each attack lasts for between 30 to 90 minutes and is centred on one eye, with sharp and stabbing pain felt on one side of the head and face. The headache is accompanied by watering of the affected eye and a stuffy nostril on that side of the head.

cheeks, around the eyes or across the forehead. Sinus headaches are generally accompanied by fever and a congested nose. They are made worse by bending over and can intensify when barometric pressure and temperature rise.

Cervical degenerative disease (affecting the upper spine) and neck pain can cause spasm in muscles in the base of the skull and going forward to the forehead. These muscle spasms can cause headaches.

Jaw malfunction can affect different areas of the head—the temples, cheeks, ears and the back of the neck. Known as temporomandibular joint syndrome (TMJ), the disorder involves the joint on both sides of the head which connects the jaw bone to the skull. Women between 25 and 40 are most prone to TMJ, which usually results from clenching the jaw or grinding the teeth, often while asleep; malocclusion (when the upper and lower teeth fail to meet properly), and other orthodontic problems; or dislocation of the jaw. Among the symptoms are tinnitus (ringing or other sounds in the head), earache, dizziness, a clicking noise when you chew and pain which gets worse after eating or yawning. People under stress and sufferers of osteoarthritis and rheumatoid arthritis may develop TMJ. It can be treated with muscle relaxants, analgesics or NSAIDs. A mouthpiece can be worn to prevent grinding the teeth during sleep.

Alcohol, drugs or fumes from chemicals can all produce headaches, as can spending too long in a polluted environment, such as lack of ventilation when decorating with paint. ▸

See also:

3/GENERAL HEALTH ISSUES
Skeletal problems pp. 86–87
Problems of the mind pp. 94–99

4/HORMONAL HEALTH
Endocrine system problems pp. 140–143

5/ILLNESSES & EMERGENCIES
Digestive problems pp. 196–199
Problems of the senses pp. 236–239

6/TREATMENTS & THERAPIES
Conventional treatments pp. 286–291

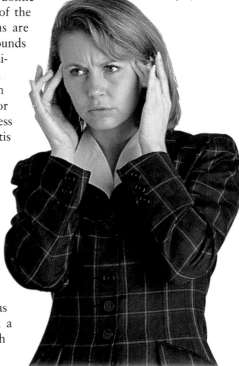

FEEL THE PAIN
There are many causes of a headache, but when one occurs all you want to do is get rid of it. Pain can be felt in different areas of the head—at the temples, on the forehead, above or below the eyes—and is generally relieved by paracetamol or ibuprofen.

LIFESTYLE CAUSES OF HEADACHE

In social terms, headaches can be caused by alcohol (when drunk in sufficient quantities to produce a hangover), tobacco smoke, caffeine (both in excess and when withdrawn) and toxic fumes from industrial chemicals.

Lack of food or fluids (especially plain water), eating ice cream or other cold foods, a sudden change in the weather (impending rain particularly), eyestrain, intense physical exercise, poor air conditioning in the workplace ("sick building syndrome"), fatigue, exposure to intense bright light, continuous loud noise, strong odours and motion sickness can all trigger headaches. Stress, anxiety, depression, anger and lack of sleep may also be causes, as can some prescription drugs, such as nitrates, prescribed for angina, and calcium channel blockers for angina and hypertension.

SIMPLE SOLUTIONS

The best way to deal with a headache is to prevent it. If the headache is due to posture—for example, working at a desk or computer for long periods of time in such a way that your muscles are tense or strained—change your ways. Alter the way you sit, have frequent breaks and do simple stretching exercises from time to time to release tension.

If a headache does develop, it is best to try to deal with it immediately as the over-the-counter painkillers, such as aspirin, paracetamol or ibuprofen, work best in the early stages. (Note that aspirin should not be given to children under the age of 12 as it may cause Reye's syndrome.)

Find a quiet, dimly lit corner or darkened room where you can rest for a while with your eyes closed. Cover your eyes with a cold, damp cloth. If you know any relaxation techniques, put them into

POSSIBLE TRIGGERS
Some people become sensitive to certain foods. The body's response is a headache, a sign of difficulty in digestion. Among the most common triggers are alcohol, some types of cheese and chocolate.

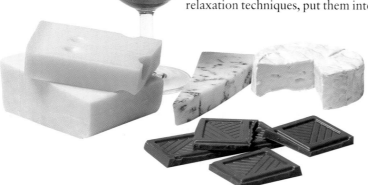

practice. Otherwise, simply breathe slowly and regularly, close your eyes and think pleasant thoughts. Gently massage your temples and the base of the skull, starting beneath the ears and gradually working round to the back of the neck. Or press your fingers on your forehead above the eyebrows, pressing and moving them gradually up to the hairline (these are acupuncture pressure points). If it is possible, take a warm, relaxing bath.

If a headache responds to over-the-counter remedies and other simple self-help techniques, or if it occurs only infrequently, there is no need to see a doctor.

MIGRAINE HEADACHES

Many people who suffer from migraines believe that they are merely experiencing severe headaches, but this is not the case. Migraine headaches are a disorder of the nervous system. They affect vision as well as the other senses, and the gastrointestinal system as well. They tend to run in families, although the genetic mechanism involved is not known.

Migraines are three times more common in women than in men. They cause a painful throbbing, usually behind the eye and often on only one side of the head. In severe cases the pain can be intense and completely disabling. Movement of the head tends to make the pain worse as can light, and relief only comes by lying down in the dark until the attack passes—generally in hours, but in some cases it can last for two or three days. Migraines may occur as isolated or infrequent attacks, or strike on a regular basis, as often as once a week.

There are two main types of migraine headache, common and classical, and a third category, menstrual migraine headache, is also identified by some doctors.

With common migraines people have nausea and sometimes vomiting as well as the severe head pain. Some people also experience painful sensitivity to light, noise and/or strong odours. There may be dizziness, confusion, visual and speech disturbance and weakness on the affected side of the body.

Classical migraines are comparatively rare, accounting for about 15 percent of attacks. Sufferers sense an imminent attack through a visual "aura", in which a gradually expanding area of blindness is surrounded by a sparkling halo. It usually disappears after about 20 to 30 minutes. In other respects, the symptoms are the same as in common migraines.

Other migraines are related to hormonal changes. Menstrual migraines occur at the start of menstruation and are thought to affect as many as two out of three women at some stage in their lives. Oral contraceptives, pregnancy and HRT may all trigger migraine headaches in some women. Auras are very rare and symptoms are almost always of the common type. The trigger is likely to be increased production of the female hormone oestrogen, which is thought to be responsible for the greater susceptibility of women to both tension and migraine headaches.

Certain foods are known to cause migraine headaches. These include: chocolate (although recent research suggests that chocolate may be no more guilty than many other foods); some dairy products, particularly matured cheeses; citrus fruits; cured meats (hot dogs, ham); nuts; onions; pickled foods; the food additive monosodium glutamate; and artificial sweeteners containing aspartame.

It is important when diagnosing to distinguish between a migraine and a headache caused by a potentially serious condition. Brain

scans (X-rays, CAT or MRI) or blood tests may be required if diagnosis is uncertain.

Inside the skull, your brain cells are fed by a vast number of arteries which are vulnerable to hardening and narrowing (atherosclerosis). Migraine and combination headaches are associated with a widening of the blood vessels in the head, as well as the tightening of the muscles that surround the head, as can happen during periods of emotional stress or when reading in dim light. Both seem to arise from the brain chemical serotonin which controls the narrowing and widening of blood vessels. It is likely that a wave of electrical activity, stimulated by a trigger factor, crosses the brain and sets off a sequence of events that alters the blood vessels for better blood flow. In the process, the brain is deprived of serotonin which irritates the nerves and produces the headache.

MANAGING MIGRAINES

There is no cure but much can be done to alleviate the symptoms of an attack, and to help in long-term management and prevention. Treatment reduces pain, or prevents it from developing after the initial onset. It usually involves one or more of the following:

Over-the-counter (OTC) painkillers Paracetamol, ibuprofen or aspirin may be tried.

Drug treatments If the OTC painkillers are ineffective, more specific drugs that counteract the swelling of the blood vessels in the brain may be prescribed (ergotamine or sumatriptan). An antiemetic, such as metoclopramide, taken before a painkiller, may be recommended for vomiting. Prophylactic drugs such as beta blockers may be prescribed if you have more than one attack a week.

Help yourself As soon as possible after the onset of symptoms, rest in a quiet, darkened room. If you can identify the triggers, you can learn to avoid them. Keeping a migraine diary (see right) is an important aspect of this. Get in touch with one of the organizations set up for migraine sufferers (addresses pp. 312–315). Contact a local self-help group, or reach other sufferers on the Internet. Find out about exercise routines that generate a relaxation response, relieve stress and depression.

When to seek medical help

Headaches may be a symptom of other medical conditions such as meningitis or malaria. You should seek medical advice if your headaches:

♀ Are frequent and very severe.
♀ Become worse over hours or days.
♀ Start suddenly and without warning.
♀ Are present when you wake in the morning.
♀ Come on after a head injury, particularly if there is any degree of mental confusion.
♀ Are accompanied by other distinct symptoms such as high fever, nausea and vomiting, visual disturbance, dislike of bright light, pain and tenderness around one eye, dizziness or signs of mental confusion.

Pain in the back of the head, particularly on waking and which lessens during the day, may indicate hypertension and should be checked out by your doctor. High blood pressure that is not treated can lead to heart attacks and strokes.

See your doctor

Migraine sufferers who have a severe headache which does not correspond to the normal common or classic pattern should seek help. This is especially true of a pregnant woman in the last trimester who may have high blood pressure, swelling of the face, hands and feet and rapid weight gain. These are symptoms which may indicate pre-eclampsia and need immediate medical treatment.

A MIGRAINE DIARY
A pattern may emerge if you keep a daily diary in which you record everything you eat and drink, how you feel (mentally and physically), what you did: for example, drove a car (fumes may be a trigger), went swimming (suspect presence of chlorine in the water). Note the symptoms of any attack, its severity and how long it lasted and the treatment you used. After several weeks, you and your doctor can assess the record to try and find the common triggers in the attacks.

BLOOD AND THE CIRCULATION

Every cell in the body depends on a constant supply of blood for nourishment and protection. In the average woman, blood takes around 60 seconds to complete one circuit. Certain disorders of the heart, the blood and the blood vessels can seriously affect your health.

See also:

1/BEING A WELL WOMAN
Essentials of good health pp. 16–19
Healthy body systems p. 34

4/HORMONAL HEALTH
Pregnancy and motherhood
pp. 172–175

Anaemia

People with anaemia either have too few red blood cells or the cells are not able to carry enough oxygen for the body's needs. A blood test to measure the level of haemoglobin—the protein that transports oxygen—will determine if you have the condition and whether further investigation is needed, since there are several reasons why it may develop in women.

The symptoms of anaemia include tiredness and breathlessness, especially after any kind of physical effort, very pale skin, a general feeling of weakness and being unusually cold.

The most common cause of anaemia is that your food intake does not include one of the components needed to manufacture the red cells in blood. Iron is particularly important as

it is essential to make haemoglobin—the recommended daily amount (RDA) is 14.8 mg. Vitamin B_{12} activates the making of red cells in bone marrow—the RDA is 1.5 mcg. Folic acid, a B vitamin, helps cells divide—the RDA is 200 mcg (400 mcg in pregnancy).

WHO IS AT RISK?

Iron and vitamin B_{12} (which are usually obtained from animal sources) may be missing from the diet of vegetarians who do not have

COMPONENTS OF BLOOD

Blood, composed predominantly of red cells, is normally bluish in the veins and turns red when it is exposed to the outside air as a result of a cut or other injury. White blood cells are part of the immune system and defend against infection and disease, reacting to the presence of alien substances such as bacteria or viruses by destroying or neutralizing them. Other cells called platelets are part of the mechanism that enables blood to clot to seal a wound.

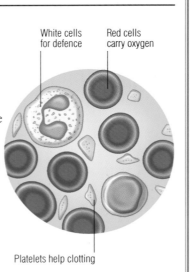

White cells for defence

Red cells carry oxygen

Platelets help clotting

Blood types

You inherit your blood type or group from your parents. There are four types: A, B, AB and O. In the UK, the most common is A followed by O. The compatibility of blood types is crucially important in blood transfusions, since people cannot receive blood from incompatible types:

    A can receive A or O;
    B can receive B or O;
    AB can receive any type;
    O can only receive O.

Another element of blood is the rhesus (Rh) factor. The Rh system classifies blood according to the absence or presence of certain red blood cell protein molecules (antigens). About 85 percent of people have the antigens and are Rh positive; the rest are Rh negative. Special care must be taken to match Rh negative blood in transfusions. Problems may arise in pregnancy if the woman is Rh negative and the father is Rh positive; the baby may in turn be Rh positive and the mother's antibodies may attack the baby, causing haemolytic disease.

a well-balanced food intake. People who have pernicious anaemia lack the substance that enables B₁₂ to be absorbed from the intestines into the blood and will usually need monthly injections of the vitamin. A number of diseases cause red blood cells to be destroyed, among them sickle cell disease and thalassaemia, in which the red blood cells are abnormal.

Loss of blood can also result in anaemia, which is why it sometimes affects those with peptic (digestive) ulcers. Women who experience heavy menstrual loss over a long time may become anaemic. It can occur in pregnancy when the baby draws on the mother's iron for its developing blood supply, or if the mother was deficient in iron before pregnancy began. This deficiency can continue postnatally. Taking aspirin and NSAIDs over a long time can cause microscopic blood loss.

DIFFERENT TREATMENTS

If you suspect you are anaemic, consult your doctor rather than trying to treat the condition yourself since some symptoms may have causes other than anaemia. A blood test will determine your haemoglobin level—normal is about 12g per 100g of blood—and haematocrit (the ratio of blood cells to total volume of blood). If the level is low, your doctor will aim to establish the reason before deciding on treatment.

Any underlying problem such as a stomach ulcer or unusually heavy menstruation will need to be treated. A blood transfusion may be necessary if the anaemia is severe. Iron may also be prescribed—as pills or, in some cases, injections—if you are not getting enough in your diet or are not absorbing it properly. Do not take iron supplements without your doctor advising you to do so.

DIETARY IRON

Adding iron to your diet means eating plenty of fresh green vegetables (such as broccoli, watercress and cabbage), either raw or lightly cooked; consuming protein from sources such as almonds, eggs, offal (liver and kidney) and shellfish; and eating pulses such as beans and lentils. Vitamin C helps iron to be absorbed, so eat plenty of fresh citrus and kiwi fruit, green and red peppers, tomatoes and potatoes (with the skin on). Avoid too many drinks containing caffeine—such as tea, coffee, or cola—which can prevent iron being properly absorbed by the body.

When you're pregnant

During the middle months of pregnancy, the amount of blood in your body increases by more than a third. You need a constant supply of iron for the extra red blood cells that make up a part of this new volume of blood. The ratio of haemoglobin to blood volume may be slightly lower than normal because of this increase in total volume, but this doesn't necessarily mean that you are iron deficient.

Anaemia usually develops, if at all, in the last trimester of pregnancy, although it may occur earlier if you are carrying more than one baby. You will have regular blood tests as part of your antenatal monitoring and if you are found to be anaemic you will be given advice on boosting your iron intake. Your doctor may also prescribe supplements.

IRON-RICH FOODS
The mineral iron is essential for the health of your blood, throughout your lifetime. To ensure that you have a regular daily supply, choose from a variety of green vegetables and protein-rich foods. Keep up your intake of fresh foods containing vitamin C, so that the body can absorb the iron.

Atherosclerosis

See also:

1/BEING A WELL WOMAN
Essentials of good health pp. 16–23

3/GENERAL HEALTH ISSUES
Women and heart disease
    pp. 132–133

4/HORMONAL HEALTH
Endocrine problems pp. 136–137

5/ILLNESSES & EMERGENCIES
Digestive problems pp. 190–191

6/TREATMENTS & THERAPIES
Treatment plans pp. 262–265
Conventional treatments
    pp. 272–277

Commonly known as hardening of the arteries, atherosclerosis reduces the blood flow and increases the risk of angina, heart attack, stroke and gangrene.

As part of the process of ageing, small deposits of fat begin to build up on the insides of your arteries causing the walls to become less flexible and more rigid. If this natural deterioration is exacerbated by conditions such as hypertension, diabetes, obesity, high blood cholesterol or other personal factors, such as smoking, a high-fat diet and lack of exercise, the inner surface becomes lumpy, making an even narrower space for blood to flow through.

If the walls develop small cracks as well, they are sealed by patches called plaques, made up largely of blood fats such as cholesterol, dead cells and calcium. These plaques can eventually block the artery or they may break off and be carried around in the bloodstream until they end up blocking the blood flow completely. The consequences depend on whether the blockage is complete or partial and the artery affected.

WHO IS LIKELY TO GET IT?

A number of interrelated factors determine whether a particular individual will develop atherosclerosis. Some you can do nothing about while others can be reduced by a definite change in lifestyle. A minority of people may have an

Five steps to prevention

♀ **Stop smoking** This is the most important step you can take to reduce your risk. Smoking is an important risk factor in itself, and also multiplies the effect of any others, such as raised cholesterol levels.

♀ **Reduce blood pressure** Elevated blood pressure may be an indication of arterial damage, so regular monitoring is needed. All women should have their blood pressure checked and recorded yearly. If diabetic, it should be done more frequently.

♀ **Change your diet** Try to have at least five portions of fruit and vegetables each day, reduce your overall fat intake, choosing polyunsaturated or monounsaturated varieties rather than those from animal sources (saturated fat) and keep sugar and salt to a minimum.

♀ **Exercise more** Aim for 30 minutes a day of brisk walking, cycling or swimming, or three 20–30 minute sessions of more vigorous aerobic exercise every week.

♀ **Maintain a healthy weight** Try to stay within the normal weight range for your height. Obesity is a risk factor in itself and may also increase your chances of developing type 2 diabetes (adult onset) and hypertension, which makes you more susceptible to arterial disease.

BLOOD VESSELS AND WHY THEY NARROW
In normal arteries the walls are muscular and elastic and with the help of the heart push the oxygen-rich blood around the body to all the cells. For a variety of reasons the walls lose this elasticity and as fatty deposits, called atheroma or plaques, build up on them, the space through which the blood flows becomes narrower. The heart has to work harder to circulate the blood.

Mild sclerosis

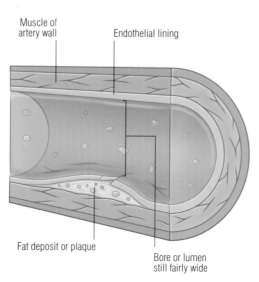

Muscle of artery wall

Endothelial lining

Fat deposit or plaque

Bore or lumen still fairly wide

Severe sclerosis

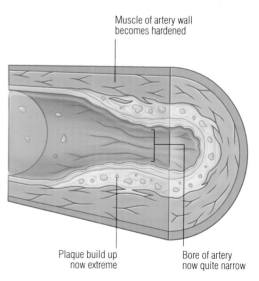

Muscle of artery wall becomes hardened

Plaque build up now extreme

Bore of artery now quite narrow

THE RISKS AT DIFFERENT AGES

While some women may be genetically predisposed and may need monitoring closely, for most other women the cause may be in their diet or lifestyle. If they eat foods high in saturated fats, cholesterol may collect in their arteries. If they have little exercise, their weight and blood pressure may suffer. If they smoke, toxic gases from the cigarettes can damage the artery lining.

TEENS

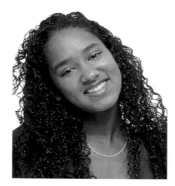

Eating high-fat "junk" foods during childhood and teenage years can be the start of the fatty deposit build-up, though without symptoms at that stage.

30S

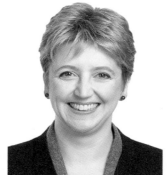

Women have protective oestrogen working for them, but this may start to diminish from mid 30s. Oestrogen keeps the level of good cholesterol high until menopause.

OVER 50

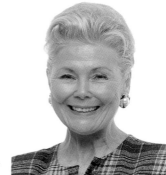

After menopause, without oestrogen, a woman's risk of developing atherosclerosis approaches that of men (in whom the condition is more common).

---

inherited disposition to develop fatty deposits because they produce abnormally high amounts of a type of cholesterol known as LDL (low-density lipoprotein). People in this category usually have one or more close relatives who have experienced coronary heart disease (CHD) or strokes at a relatively early age (under 50). Atherosclerosis is one of the causes of cerebrovascular disease, in which the arteries of the brain are narrowed.

Women develop atherosclerosis later in life than men mainly due to the female sex hormone oestrogen, which appears to provide some protection in premenopausal women. The hormone promotes high-density lipoproteins (HDLs) which protect against the development of CHD. After the menopause, in women who are not using oestrogen replacement, HDLs tend to fall and LDLs to rise. Other factors which increase the risk include premature menopause (including removal of the ovaries, and without HRT), hypertension, smoking, diabetes and obesity, and everyone becomes more susceptible in older age. Regular monitoring of cholesterol levels and blood pressure is important for all women, but essential for those at high risk. Another blood test, of homocysteine levels, may be done because high levels are associated with increased risk of CHD, strokes and peripheral vascular disease.

Atherosclerosis is a common and increasing problem in most Western countries, particularly in northern Europe.

DIFFERENT TREATMENTS

As well as the five steps outlined (box, left), which should be followed even if you have already developed atherosclerosis, your doctor may suggest other treatments, including drugs. Aspirin can help to dissolve blood clots, statins reduce cholesterol levels and a range of other types are designed to improve blood flow. Angioplasty (p. 130) can be used to open up the arteries or surgery can remove or replace blocked sections of arteries, though this may not be appropriate for all with the condition.

ULTRASOUND

Doppler ultrasound is a non-invasive test used to diagnose atherosclerosis. It assesses the state of the blood vessels by measuring the rate of blood flow in the arteries and the heart.

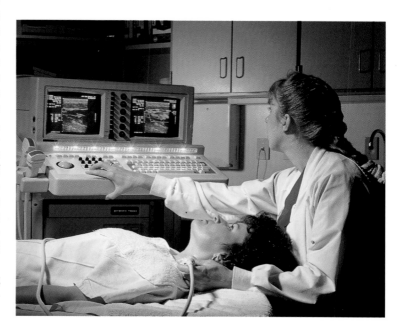

Stroke

Sometimes referred to as cerebrovascular accident, strokes are more common in men than women and in older people. A stroke affects the blood supply to the brain, and its consequences will vary depending on the degree of damage and on which part of the brain has been affected.

The most usual cause is a blood clot blocking an artery in the brain, known as an infarct or ischaemic stroke. Until investigations are done, it will not be certain whether the clot was formed elsewhere in the circulatory system and was carried in the bloodstream to the brain (embolism), or whether it formed in the brain artery itself (thrombosis). In most sufferers the artery has narrowed because of atherosclerosis (p. 118) and a blockage occurs when a piece of plaque breaks off.

A stroke may also be caused by bleeding into the brain, after a weak part of an arterial wall (aneurysm) has given way, called a cerebral haemorrhage. Often the only symptom may be a severe headache. Brain cells and the surrounding tissue die when their blood supply is cut off.

If the damage is only minor, the person may recover completely, may have problems with speech or vision or a part of the body may have been weakened or become paralysed. There may be longer-lasting paralysis or loss of sensation down one side of the body or the face, difficulties with comprehension, slurred speech, incontinence and loss of balance. The most dangerous type is bleeding into the brainstem which directly affects breathing and heartbeat.

New treatments, if given early, can prevent permanent damage. Intensive treatment from specialists in rehabilitation can minimize the after effects of brain damage and can often enable the person to regain some movement in paralysed parts and recover the ability to speak.

REDUCING YOUR RISKS

Regular blood pressure checks are essential—untreated hypertension is a major risk factor. If you are on medication to reduce your blood pressure you must continue to take it, even if you have no symptoms. High cholesterol is also linked with stroke and blood cholesterol levels should be regularly tested.

As well as following the advice given for preventing atherosclerosis, you should limit alcohol intake to what is considered the safe maximum a week for women (p. 95) and avoid binge drinking or drinking without eating food.

Taking less salt in your diet is important as this can help to bring down elevated blood pressure—a contributory factor in many strokes. If you have diabetes or

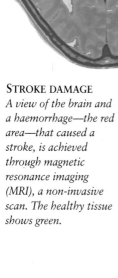

STROKE DAMAGE
A view of the brain and a haemorrhage—the red area—that caused a stroke, is achieved through magnetic resonance imaging (MRI), a non-invasive scan. The healthy tissue shows green.

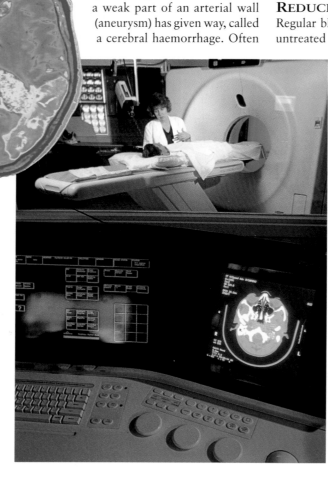

SCANNING THE BRAIN
For an MRI scan, the body is placed in a unit with an intense magnetic field. The radio waves emitted by the body's atoms are detected by the unit and built up into a picture for specialist analysis.

are extremely overweight or obese, you run a higher risk of stroke. Smokers fall into the same category. In some migraine headaches, symptoms such as numbness or tingling in the arms or legs may indicate that there are changes in your cerebral blood flow and should be drawn to your doctor's attention.

MINI STROKES

Transient ischaemic attacks, also known as TIAs and sometimes referred to as little or mini strokes, are caused when the blood supply to the brain is interrupted briefly and temporarily, usually by a tiny clot which then disperses. Symptoms last for less than 24 hours and include dizziness, weakness or numbness in one arm or leg, loss of vision and/or difficulty in speaking. The condition is more common in older people and needs to be investigated so that treatment to prevent further clots can be given if necessary to avoid a full stroke.

Stroke and the salt connection

Salt—chemical name sodium chloride, or NaCl—plays an important role in maintaining the body's fluid balance and blood pressure. One of the key conclusions of nutritionists is that everyone in Western countries eats too much of it. The average consumption is 7.5 ml (1½ teaspoons) a day, yet as little as 2.5 ml (½ teaspoon) can lead to high blood pressure in susceptible people, and this can lead to stroke. Cutting down to between the two is recommended.

Most foods—including fruit, vegetables and grains—contain some salt, but over 75 percent of what we eat is hidden in prepared foods, added both for taste and preservation. Always read labels on bought, preprepared or packaged food. If you see salt or sodium or Na among the first few ingredients listed, the amount of salt in the food is high. If last on the list the amount included may be low. If sodium bicarbonate (baking soda) is included on the list, that food should be avoided by anyone with heart or kidney problems.

It is worthwhile knowing that if you don't buy prepared foods, don't add salt when cooking and use only coarse sea salt in a grinder at the table (rather than from a shaker which allows more out), you will still provide the body with sufficient salt for fluid balance and health.

PERIPHERAL VASCULAR DISEASE

Peripheral vascular disease is the name given to blocked arteries or other conditions of arteries such as aortic aneurysm. Symptoms include painful cramps in the feet, calves, thighs or hips when walking or exercising but which stop with rest. Smoking is the most common cause.

Phlebitis is a general term meaning inflammation of a vein. Thrombophlebitis describes clotting at the site of the inflammation usually in the superficial leg veins. The skin over the affected areas is tender and feels hard when touched. Although unpleasant, it is not a risk to a woman's general health. The symptoms can be eased with rest, warm compresses, painkillers or NSAIDs, by propping your feet up to help blood flow or by gentle use of an over-the-counter remedy such as zinc oxide. Wearing support tights or stockings can help.

A blood clot that affects a deep vein—called deep venous thrombosis—is potentially serious. It can be fatal if the clot breaks away and travels through the bloodstream to block an artery in the lungs, called a pulmonary embolism. Thromboembolic disease is treated with blood-thinning drugs such as aspirin, heparin and warfarin, which dissolve the clot and prevent any more forming. People with varicose veins rarely face an increased risk of this disease.

A woman considering the oral contraceptive pill or HRT should tell her doctor of any personal or family history of thrombosis, as oestrogen medications—even in low doses—may increase the risk of clotting.

Deep venous thrombosis
Blood clot forms in a deep vein, breaks free and may travel to the lungs

Thrombophlebitis
Blood clot lodges in a surface vein, causing tenderness and pain

See also:

2/SEX & SEXUALITY
Choosing contraception pp. 60–65

5/ILLNESSES & EMERGENCIES
Digestive system problems p. 190

VEINS UNDER PRESSURE
The leg veins are the most hard-working in the body. They need to be strong to go against gravity to return deoxygenated blood to the lungs for cleansing, oxygenation and redistribution.

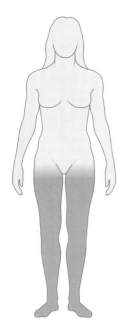

Varicose veins

From a medical point of view, varicose veins are rarely considered to be a serious problem. But their appearance can cause concern and they may be an indicator of a more serious circulatory disorder such as thrombosis.

Varicose veins occur mainly in the legs and may be disfiguring; they are usually hard, lumpy and blue because the walls of the veins become enlarged or twisted. They may also cause symptoms such as aching, heaviness, skin damage, ulcers and swollen ankles. As these can also be symptoms of other medical conditions, you should discuss them with your doctor.

Women and men are probably equally susceptible to varicose veins. The condition tends to run in families, which implies an inherited weakness in the blood vessels. They also seem to be more common in people whose job involves standing for long periods of time. Varicose veins can occur during pregnancy and can be the result of it. They are also found in people who are overweight or obese.

WHICH VEINS ARE AFFECTED?
The veins most likely to have problems are those closest to the skin—the superficial veins. In particular, the long saphenous vein, which runs up the inside of the leg from ankle to groin,

Treatment methods
Since healthy, deep veins are capable of keeping the blood flowing, superficial veins that are badly affected can be stripped out under a general anaesthetic or epidural block anaesthesia. Before this is done, your veins are assessed using a Doppler ultrasound technique (p. 119), which measures blood flow and enables the surgeon to identify and mark the veins that are varicosed. After the operation there will be some bruising which will fade and some pain and discomfort. For a few days you will need to wear compression stockings which help blood flow.

Injection treatment, known as sclerotherapy, can work well for small veins, especially those below the knee. It involves injecting the affected veins with a substance which, in effect, causes the walls to become glued together so that blood cannot flow through. The vessel collapses and the blood then reroutes itself to nearby veins.

Tiny spider veins are not considered a medical problem, but they can be sealed with laser surgery or sclerotherapy.

HOW VEINS BECOME VARICOSED
In a healthy body, veins have valves that work like locks on a canal. They automatically open to let a certain amount of blood through, then shut while the next amount accumulates. If the valves aren't working well or the walls of the vein stretch, blood collects in one area and distorts the system. The medical term for this distortion is "varicosed".

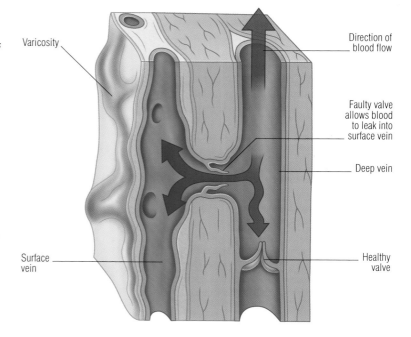

Varicosity

Direction of blood flow

Faulty valve allows blood to leak into surface vein

Deep vein

Surface vein

Healthy valve

and the short saphenous vein, which is visible on the outside of the leg from the ankle to around knee level, are usually involved.

Most of the blood that flows through veins has to travel upward. Not being pumped in the same way as blood in the arteries, it would flow back under the influence of gravity without the valves that allow only so much blood through before shutting, then reopening. It is thought that varicose veins are caused when these valves stop working properly, possibly because the vein walls become weak and distended. The blood collects and distorts the vein, slowing the flow from one valve to the next.

WHEN TREATMENT IS NEEDED

Most people want their varicose veins dealt with for cosmetic reasons, but some seek help when skin changes occur—commonly eczema and/or skin darkening or discoloration, which may eventually result in ulcers. If you experience bleeding from varicose veins, which is relatively unusual, this is a sign that they need to be treated, as is a sudden feeling of heaviness in the legs and swelling. See your doctor.

VARICOSE ECZEMA

The supply of blood to any area affected by varicose veins is reduced and the skin therefore receives less nutrient-enriched blood. It is here that eczema may develop. The scaly patches and blisters that form may be treated with corticosteroid ointments and you may be advised to wear support (compression) tights or stockings to help reduce the swelling.

VARICOSE VEINS IN PREGNANCY

One of the common complaints of middle to late pregnancy is varicose veins. The head of the foetus presses down on the pelvic veins, causing blood to pool in the legs and placing pressure on the walls of the veins. You will be advised to avoid gaining too much weight and not to be on your feet for long periods . Sleeping with your legs raised will help and daily exercise will improve circulation. The tendency to develop varicose veins increases with each successive preganancy you have.

Haemorrhoids (commonly known as piles) can also be a problem for pregnant women who are susceptible to constipation. Haemorrhoids are varicose veins of the anal canal, a direct result of straining to pass faeces. When you

HELP YOURSELF

Take short walks whenever possible and repeatedly lift your heels off the ground for a few minutes at a time. This activates the "muscle pump", which helps to keep the blood moving. Exercise that stimulates blood circulation is beneficial for women at any age and during pregnancy.

Excessive weight is thought to be a contributory factor in varicose veins. You may be less likely to develop them if you keep your weight within the normal range for your height.

You can relieve heaviness and aching by raising your legs so that they are supported at a level with or above the rest of your body. Remember that sitting immobile in a chair for long periods will make the symptoms worse.

Wearing special support stockings or tights during the day helps to compress the veins and eases discomfort. It is not advisable to wear them at night.

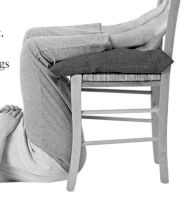

strain, the blood bears down on the lowest vessels, causing them to stretch. Unlike other veins, the blood vessels in the anal canal have no valves to regulate the flow of blood and the pooled blood becomes a haemorrhoid. It can be internal or, if it extends from the anus, prolapsed. Consult your doctor before using any ointments and suppositories from a pharmacy. A high-fibre diet and drinking plenty of still water may help to ease the constipation.

If haemorrhoids continue to be a problem after your baby is born, they can either be injected with a chemical to shrink them or tied with an elastic band to halt circulation to the area. In serious cases—that is, when the haemorrhoids are large and don't respond to treatment or bleed—anaemia can result.

Pregnant or not, it is important to report all instances of bleeding from the anus or blood in the stools to your doctor. It may need further investigation with a proctoscope or colonoscope to examine the anus, rectum or colon.

Scleroderma

See also:

1/BEING A WELL WOMAN
Healthy body systems pp. 42–43

3/GENERAL HEALTH ISSUES
Skeletal system problems
    pp. 78–83

6/TREATMENTS & THERAPIES
Treatment plans pp. 262–269

A relatively rare disorder which mostly affects women, scleroderma changes the look and feel of skin on the face, arms, hands and feet, and it can also involve some internal organs.

Scleroderma is part of a family of disorders characterized by skin thickening, due to disturbance of connective tissue called collagen, and a drastic reduction in the number of blood capillaries that feed the skin. This tissue, which normally gives skin its elasticity and bounce, becomes hardened and has fewer sweat glands and hair follicles. The skin thickens and appears shiny and smooth to the touch. The underlying subcutaneous fatty tissue and muscle may also be affected. If the skin tightens, it can limit the range of motion of joints and limbs.

It is not known what actually causes the collagen to overproduce. Scleroderma tends to be regarded as an autoimmune disorder in which the body produces antibodies against its own tissues. If the sclerosis is progressive, the kidneys, lungs and heart may be affected.

Scleroderma is a multi-system disease which may be managed by a medical team comprising a rheumatologist, a nephrologist, a chest physician, a gastroenterologist, a dermatologist and a cardiologist. It is a chronic disease that needs to be carefully monitored so any physical changes can receive prompt attention. There is no cure and drug treatment includes corticosteroids, anti-hypertensives, antacids, painkillers and sometimes chemotherapy. In severe cases calcium channel blockers may be used.

How scleroderma is diagnosed

Diagnosis of the condition is based on a physical examination and occasionally a skin biopsy may be done. The doctor will look for what is known as CREST syndrome:

C—calcinosis (calcific deposits under the skin),

R—Raynaud's phenomenon (see box),

E—Oesophageal dismotility (thickening of the oesophagus which prevents simple digestion),

S—Sclerodactyly (thickening skin on the fingers affecting shape and movement) and

T—Telangiectasias (collection of tiny blood vessels on the skin's surface, most usually the face).

WHO IS AT RISK?
The disorder can occur at any age, but is most likely to be found in Afro-Caribbean women in their 20s, and in white women between 20 and 40. Thought to be an autoimmune condition, scleroderma can be limited (affecting only the hands and face) or diffuse (skin over the entire body is involved). The condition is rarely life-threatening, but it can be disabling and affect quality of life.

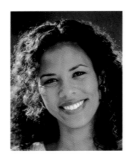

between 20 and 30

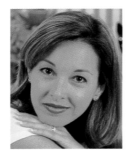

early 20s to late 30s

RAYNAUD'S PHENOMENON

This circulatory disorder, which mostly affects women under 40, has no known cause. It can be triggered by emotion and appears when the temperature drops. Sufferers are hypersensitive to cold because the small arteries close to the surface of the skin go into spasm, restricting blood flow.

During an attack, usually lasting only a few minutes, the fingers and toes (and sometimes the nose and/or the earlobes) turn white, then blue and feel numb. They may then turn red and you experience a tingling or burning sensation.

Prevention is the first line of defence. Dressing in warm layers when going out in cold weather and remembering to protect the head (most heat is lost from the body here) and hands and feet will help. Stopping smoking is crucial. You have to be alert to changes such as ulcers, sores or skin discoloration on fingers or toes. If they occur, report them to your doctor as they may indicate lack of blood to these vulnerable parts.

Self-help tips

During an attack, have a warm (not hot) bath if possible.

Keep a hot drink in a flask by your bed if you are prone to attacks at night.

Regular, vigorous exercise may help by improving your circulation and toning your muscles. Be careful not to get chilled—in a swimming pool, or in the changing room afterwards, for example.

Blood and lymph cancers

There is a close relationship between blood and lymph, which run in parallel. Both reach all parts of the body and may be involved in the spread of cancerous cells. Women are at relatively low risk rate for these cancers.

LEUKAEMIA

There are several different types of leukaemia (cancer of the blood) and some are more dangerous than others. All involve excess production of various types of white blood cells and tumours may form in bone marrow, spleen and lymph nodes.

The symptoms differ according to the particular type of leukaemia, but may include tiredness and a general feeling of being unwell, susceptibility to infections, aching bones, night sweats and a raised temperature. Diagnosis is based on a blood test and bone marrow sampling. Sometimes leukaemia that causes few or no symptoms may only be diagnosed when a blood test is done for some other reason. Chronic types mostly affect people over 50.

Leukaemia classified as "acute" and chronic myeloid or lymphocytic leukaemia are treated with powerful chemotherapy and, in some cases, with a bone marrow transplant. For some chronic forms, a milder form of chemotherapy with fewer side effects may be adequate.

MULTIPLE MYELOMA

This rare condition, which involves uncontrolled growth of plasma cells in bone marrow, generally appears in middle to old age. It occurs when something causes the B lymphocyte cells to overproduce one type of immunoglobulin so that the body is then not protected against infection. Diagnosis is by blood test and bone marrow biopsy; treatment includes anticancer drugs used in chemotherapy.

HODGKIN'S DISEASE

At the earliest stage of this not very common cancer, the only symptom may be enlarged lymph nodes in the neck or under the arm which are painless. However, as malignant cells develop in the lymphatic system fever, loss of appetite and weight and night sweats add to a general feeling of being unwell. The cause of the disease is not known, but it is more likely to affect women between the ages of 20 and 30, and over 55. Gradually, as the lymphoid tissue spreads, it impairs the immune system, leaving the body vulnerable to infections that would not worry anyone who was healthy.

The progress of the disease is assessed by tissue biopsy (from a lymph node, affected organ or bone marrow), chest X-ray and CAT or MRI scans. If diagnosed in its early stages, Hodgkin's disease can be cured. Chemotherapy is the most likely treatment, in some cases combined with radiotherapy. In other cases, relatively low-dose radiotherapy on its own is likely to be effective.

NON–HODGKIN'S LYMPHOMA

A malignancy of the lymph system that is not Hodgkin's disease, non-Hodgkin's lymphoma mostly affects people over 50. It may begin with swelling of lymph nodes in the neck or groin, but the spread of cells can speedily overwhelm the immune system. There are several types of the disease: one is caused by the Epstein-Barr virus (which also triggers glandular fever).

Treatment is decided after biopsy. Radiotherapy may be given if the cells are contained in a group of lymph nodes. If the disease is affecting the spleen, liver or other organs treatment is anticancer drugs possibly combined with radiotherapy. A bone marrow transplant may be the only option in serious cases.

See also:

1/BEING A WELL WOMAN
Healthy body systems p. 34;
pp. 40–41

6/TREATMENTS & THERAPIES
Treatment plans pp. 262–269
Conventional treatments
pp. 272–287
Complementary therapies p. 292

! Caution
Brain tumours can cause major problems, depending on their location and size. A cancerous growth may arise directly from brain tissue (called primary cancer) or be spread via the blood from tumours in another part of the body (called metastases or secondary cancer). One benign growth, meningioma, is more common in women than men; symptoms include seizures, severe headaches, double vision and difficulty in controlling a part of the body. Always check unusual symptoms with a doctor.

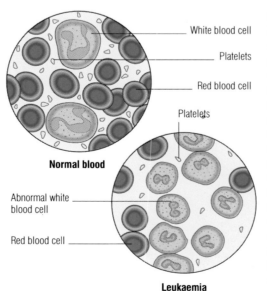

White blood cell

Platelets

Red blood cell

Platelets

Normal blood

Abnormal white blood cell

Red blood cell

Leukaemia

CELL CHANGES

Healthy white blood cells are carried in blood and lymph fluid to fend off disease. When something causes certain white cells to grow uncontrolled, the healthy ones are crowded out. As all blood cells are made in bone marrow, a bone marrow transplant may be viewed as the best way of treating blood cancer. The development of drugs that work on affected cells may change this.

WOMEN AND HEART DISEASE

The heart is the perfect pump, sending blood to all parts of the body every second you are alive. It is a complex organ with four chambers separated by valves and operated by powerful muscle. Cardiac disease affects the whole of your body and your life.

See also:

1/BEING A WELL WOMAN
Essentials of good health
pp. 16–29
Healthy body systems pp. 34–35

3/GENERAL HEALTH ISSUES
Problems of the mind pp. 94–99

4/HORMONAL HEALTH
Endocrine system problems
pp. 136–145

6/TREATMENTS & THERAPIES
Conventional treatments pp. 272–277
Complementary therapies
pp. 292–293

Reducing the risk factors

Before the menopause, women are much less likely to develop coronary heart disease (CHD) than men. After the menopause, they become more vulnerable and by their 70s are nearly on a par with men. Protection is thought to be provided by the female hormone oestrogen which is secreted by the ovaries during the fertile years. Studies strongly suggest that hormones in replacement therapy may offer women without known coronary heart disease some protection from developing the condition in later life. You may not be able to change pre-existing or inherited conditions but heart disease is less likely if you adopt a healthy lifestyle.

Do not smoke There is no doubt that smoking is the most important risk factor for heart disease. Smokers are at least twice as likely to die of it as non-smokers; even women who smoke very little have significantly higher risk of heart disease. Among other things, the chemicals in cigarette smoke can cause temporary narrowing of the blood vessels and an increase in the stickiness of blood platelets, which makes clotting more likely. Chemicals also contribute to plaque build-up on the inner walls of arteries which can result in angina and heart attacks.

Eat far less fat Reduce intake of saturated fat and trans fatty acids (in foods from animal sources) and substitute polyunsaturated or monounsaturated fats. This raises the levels of protective HDL cholesterol. Eat more fresh fruit and vegetables, pulses and whole grain foods—wholemeal bread, brown rice and oats.

Hormones and cardiac disease

When considering hormone replacement therapy (HRT) you will want to weigh the pros and cons. Among the factors to be discussed are the menopausal symptoms you are experiencing and the protection HRT may offer some women against the later development of heart disease and the bone-thinning disease osteoporosis.

If you do decide to choose HRT, you may find it takes a certain amount of trial and error to find the type of treatment and dose which suits you best; there are different combinations of hormones and ways of using them and the first one or two you try may not suit you.

For postmenopausal women who do not want to use conventional HRT, a relatively new type of treatment called selective oestrogen receptor modulators (SERMs) offers protection against osteoporosis without any associated increased risk of breast or endometrial (womb lining) cancer. Side effects may include hot flushes and thrombophlebitis.

HOW THE HEART BEATS

Your heart rate alters according to what you are doing. When the body is at rest, the nutrients in the blood are carried to the cells for repair. Activities such as eating and walking need more energy, so the rate increases. When the body is in action, when playing tennis for example, the lungs take in more oxygen and the heart beats faster to produce the energy needed for the movements of the game.

Exercise Your heart will become stronger and fitter with regular exercise. To give your heart a reasonable workout aim to leave yourself feeling slightly breathless but still able to talk.

Weight If you have accumulated excess fat it's especially important to bring your weight down to the normal range for your height.

Diabetes Diabetics should not smoke and blood glucose, blood pressure and cholesterol levels should be closely monitored.

Check-ups You should have your blood pressure checked regularly and also your cholesterol levels measured. Elevated blood pressure and hyperlipidaemia (high blood fats) are considered important contributing factors to CHD and myocardial infarction (heart attack).

THE BLOOD FLOW IN THE HEART

A woman's heart weighs around 250 g (9 oz), about 50 g (2 oz) less than that of the average man. Protected by the breastbone and the ribs on the left side of the chest, the heart beats about 70 times a minute, the rate increasing when demand for blood goes up—during exercise or at times of stress, for example, when the body systems prepare for "fight or flight".

The heart has four chambers, two on each side, separated by a membrane called the septum, which stops oxygen-rich blood from mixing with blood depleted of oxygen. Valves between the upper and lower chambers on both sides open and close to ensure that blood flows in one direction only (p. 34).

The coronary arteries carry blood containing oxygen and nutrients to the myocardium (heart muscle). It contracts under stimulation from a series of electrical impulses controlled by nerves—this is the heart's natural pacemaker. These impulses regulating the heartbeat are measured during an electrocardiograph (ECG).

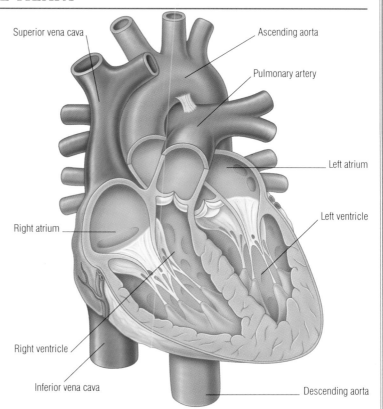

Superior vena cava

Ascending aorta

Pulmonary artery

Left atrium

Left ventricle

Right atrium

Right ventricle

Inferior vena cava

Descending aorta

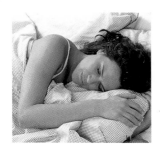

Sleeping 60 beats per minute

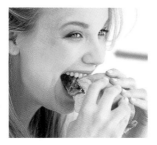

Eating 65 beats per minute

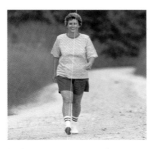

Walking 100 beats per minute

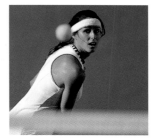

Tennis 110 beats per minute

The heart and its illnesses

One of the problems with heart and blood vessel disease is that it may develop slowly over many years without causing symptoms. What is more, symptoms that are relatively minor may be attributed to some other cause. Women may be slower in seeking help and in recognizing their symptoms than men are.

Too often they can be thought to be the inevitable consequences of getting older rather than important indicators of an existing problem. A prime example is recurrent indigestion, which may be an atypical symptom of angina in some women. An increased awareness of your own level of health will help you take steps if necessary to reduce your risks. It also helps to be aware of the forms heart disease can take.

ANGINA

The condition's full medical name, angina pectoris, simply means pain in the chest and it occurs because some muscle fibres in the heart are not receiving the oxygen they need. This happens as a result of narrowing of the arteries, but people don't usually get any symptoms until the problem is advanced—when the arteries have narrowed by more than 70 percent and blood flow to the region of the heart they supply is drastically reduced. Chest pain caused by angina often comes on when the heart's

demand for oxygen increases even slightly and exceeds the blood supply to the heart, so relatively minor exercise like walking uphill, going out into cold air or a strong wind or sexual activity can trigger the pain. When you stop whatever you are doing and rest or go into a warm environment, the pain should gradually ease within 10 minutes. Once the condition has been diagnosed, you will be prescribed medication to stop it even faster. If it doesn't go away or comes on when you are resting or even asleep, you should go back to your doctor as this may mean the condition has become unstable and could culminate in a heart attack.

Normally, angina does not damage the myocardium (heart muscle) itself, which recovers once its oxygen supply is restored.

HEART ATTACK

A heart attack happens when one of the coronary arteries becomes blocked by a thrombus (clot), which is why it is referred to as coronary thrombosis. Clots can develop in an artery which has narrowed from atherosclerosis and no blood or oxygen can reach the area of the heart supplied by that artery. If the blood supply is not restored, that part of the muscle will die within five to 10 minutes—this is called a myocardial infarction (MI). The extent of the damage to the heart depends on the size of the blocked artery and whether it is the only blood vessel supplying that part of the myocardium.

It may not be easy to distinguish the pain of a heart attack from that caused by severe indigestion, particularly in the early stages. The pain may be felt in the centre of the chest or on the left side and sometimes spreads into the shoulders and upper arms or into the neck and jaw. A person having a heart attack will look pale and sweaty and may also feel faint and sick. Don't hesitate to call an ambulance as prompt treatment is vital. Sometimes a severe heart attack can disturb the normal rhythm and result in the heart stopping altogether (cardiac arrest).

ABNORMAL RHYTHM

Many people have felt at one time or another that their heart is not beating regularly or seems to miss the occasional beat. In fact, this is quite common, although not everyone notices when

WHAT HAPPENS IN A HEART ATTACK

When a coronary artery is narrowed or blocked by fatty deposits on the artery wall, or by a blood clot, blood supply to the heart is restricted or stops and the heart muscle tissue "suffocates" through lack of oxygen. Cardiac muscle fibres begin to die, which causes chest pain. Clot-busting therapy, using drugs as fast as possible, reinstates blood flow in 60 to 90 percent of heart attack sufferers.

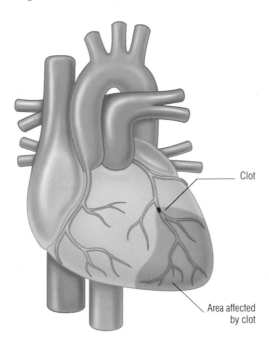

Clot

Area affected by clot

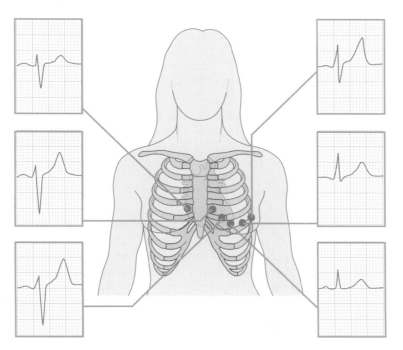

MONITORING THE HEART

An electrocardiogram (ECG) picks out rhythm abnormalities, detects old or recent heart attacks and provides information on whether the heart is working under strain because of disease or enlargement. It is done in a doctor's surgery or a hospital, is painless and takes about 10 minutes. Electrodes are placed on the chest, arms and legs to chart the pattern of electrical energy on a graph. Using many electrodes means most parts of the heart can be evaluated.

it happens, and it is not a problem provided you have no other symptoms such as chest pain, nausea, lightheadedness, sweating or loss of consciousness. It is most likely to happen when you are under severe stress or is sometimes brought on by drinking too much alcohol or caffeinated drinks such as coffee, tea or cola.

Arrhythmias (abnormal heart rhythms) are a possible complication following a heart attack (they can also be a symptom of an overactive thyroid gland). If the myocardium has been damaged it can affect the heart's electrical pacemaker, causing it to beat so that blood is not pumped in and out properly. Called ventricular fibrillation, it can affect the atrial (upper) or ventricular (lower) chambers of the heart. As it may be fatal, drugs may be prescribed to control it. Arrhythmia can sometimes cause the heart to stop completely. Immediate use of a device called a defibrillator, which delivers a short sharp electric shock, can restart it.

Another condition, Wolff-Parkinson-White syndrome, is characterized by arrhythmia known as tachycardia (rapid and irregular heartbeats) and may be treated by surgery.

HEART FAILURE

While this term means that the heart is no longer capable of pumping sufficient blood around the body to supply its normal require-ments it doesn't mean that the heart has given up altogether. A person may live for many years thanks to modern treatments, especially drugs, that can be used for heart disorders.

The problem may arise as a consequence of diabetes or blood pressure being too high for a long period, which makes the heart thickened and stiff. More often, it is a result of coronary heart disease. In an attempt to compensate for damage to large parts of the myocardium, the heart can enlarge but is unable to pump as efficiently as before. This can cause the lungs to fill up with fluid and water, which leaves the person breathless and causes legs and ankles to swell because of fluid retention.

VALVE DISORDERS

The four heart valves play a vital role in ensuring that blood flows in one direction only and in the right amounts. If they become damaged, they may prevent sufficient blood being pumped with each heartbeat, or they may allow blood to flow back in the wrong direction.

Some people are born with defective valves, but this does not always cause problems with the heart. A bout of rheumatic fever in childhood may affect the valves later in life, as can bacterial infection. Symptoms include breathlessness and angina, but their severity depends on the valves affected.

Living with heart disease

Women with cardiovascular problems need to be as vigilant about their health as they would be if their husbands or sons were diagnosed with heart disease. Treatment and prevention of further risks are important and it is worth you finding out as much as you can about both so you know what is involved.

DEALING WITH THE PROBLEM

Recovering successfully from a heart illness may involve confronting and dealing with emotions that your physical situation has brought. Apprehension and anxiety are commonplace, as are anger and depression. You may be especially aware of similar feelings in members of your family who may never have thought of women being susceptible to problems that for so long have been male-related. They too will need guidance about what can be done to improve your chances of returning to health.

With greater understanding of the way women are affected, more help is now provided by national bodies, usually charities, which have a countrywide support network. Cardiac rehabilitation groups and clubs provide a back-up service with information and advice. Some may offer counselling and stress management classes to show you and your family coping strategies. Sharing experiences with others can bring reassurance and making advised changes can prevent additional problems developing.

You may have many questions—about relationships, resuming sexual activity, returning to work, responses you may have to surgery or drugs, what you are physically capable of doing or not doing. Those involved in rehabilitation understand your needs and will take time to answer your queries. There may be a programme available that encompasses a range of aspects of recovery, from medication and diet through to exercise and stress management. Each of these is important. Physical activity, built into everyday life in combination with a low-fat, low-salt diet, can restore the quality of life which heart disorders threaten to take away.

STARTING AFRESH

The purpose of rehabilitation is to get you to identify which changes may be most beneficial to you, an approach which may be summed up as "heart-smart concepts". You need to pinpoint the areas of greatest stress in your life and discover ways to deal with them. Reducing their effects on you may be the most immediate way to improve your health. In turn this may help you conquer other heart-related problems, such as overeating, an unbalanced diet or smoking.

Physical activity, even if you are overweight, is health giving. In heart rehabilitation, a physiotherapist or exercise specialist can work out an exercise programme that is geared to you and your individual circumstances, helping you to reach a suitable level that will let you relax, breathe well and stretch muscles. All of these benefit blood flow and blood pressure and lift your spirits, encouraging well-being.

WIDENING YOUR ARTERIES
Modern surgery can expand arteries after they have become narrowed by fatty plaques. A catheter (fine tube), is inserted through your skin into the femoral artery in the leg.

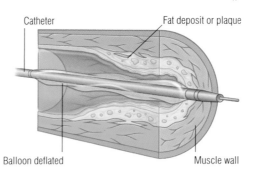

Catheter | Fat deposit or plaque
Balloon deflated | Muscle wall

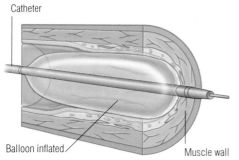

Catheter
Balloon inflated | Muscle wall

The catheter is threaded through the body to the coronary artery. Inside the catheter is a tiny balloon which the cardiologist can inflate at the point of constriction to clear the bore or lumen to improve blood flow through the artery.

To prevent the artery collapsing or being blocked again by fat deposits, the balloon is deflated and a coronary stent is left in its place. This is a fine mesh of stainless steel that can be expanded to brace the muscular wall.

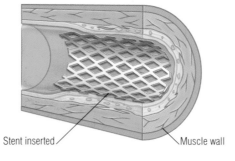

Stent inserted | Muscle wall

TREATMENT FOR HEART CONDITIONS

The aim of your medical team will be to alleviate the disorder to return you to health and improve your life expectancy. Treatment for any heart condition will be planned on an individual basis, but this chart lists some of the most common medical and surgical options for women as well as men.

Condition	Medical treatment	Surgical treatment
Angina	Drugs to reduce the amount of oxygen needed by the heart and/or dilate the blood vessels to improve the flow; aspirin or nitroglycerine (GTN) placed under the tongue to relieve symptoms. Also, daily aspirin and cholesterol-lowering drugs.	*Angioplasty (see opposite): inserting an expandable balloon into the narrowed artery to stretch it; sometimes a stent (wire mesh) is left inside to hold the walls apart. If severe, coronary artery bypass graft (CABG) may be done.*
Heart attack	Aspirin to make blood platelets less sticky; thrombolytics ("clotbuster" drugs) to dissolve clot within 12 hours; beta blockers to slow heart; ACE inhibitors to dilate blood vessels; statins and other drugs to lower cholesterol; nitroglycerine (GTN) to relieve angina attacks.	*Angioplasty or coronary artery bypass graft (CABG) operation to bypass the blocked section with either a piece of vein or artery from the chest wall or one from an arm or leg. May be single or multiple bypass.*
Abnormal rhythm	Drugs such as digoxin, beta blockers, amiodarone or other antiarrhythmia drugs.	*Implantable defibrillator or pacemaker for recurrent ventricular fibrillation.*
Heart failure	Drugs to relieve congestion and fluid retention, such as diuretics (water tablets); ACE inhibitors; nitroglycerine (GTN) to relieve angina, and other drugs.	
Heart block (upper and lower chambers of the heart out of synchronization)		*Operation to place electronic pacemaker under the skin of the chest to help heart muscle contract.*
Valve disease	Drugs to treat symptoms of heart failure. Prophylactic antibiotics. Drugs to reduce stress.	*Operation to stretch narrowed valves or replace damaged valves with synthetic or tissue ones.*
Mitral valve prolapse	Common in women but most cases are mild. Tests include ECG and echocardiography to reveal extent of the prolapse so management may be determined. Drugs to help with arrhythmia or murmur and possibly anxiety. Prophylactic treatment to protect the heart may include oral antibiotics before and after surgery, dental work and procedures such as biopsies and endoscopies.	

See also:

1/BEING A WELL WOMAN
Essentials of good health
pp. 16–21

3/GENERAL HEALTH ISSUES
Blood and the circulation
p. 120

4/HORMONAL HEALTH
Pregnancy pp. 172–173

5/ILLNESSES & EMERGENCIES
Urinary system problems p. 189

6/TREATMENTS & THERAPIES
Treatment plans pp. 262–269
Conventional treatments
pp. 272–277

High blood pressure

The medical name for blood pressure (BP) that is consistently above a recognized norm is hypertension. It is directly associated with increased risk of stroke and heart disease. Hypertension usually affects the middle-aged and elderly, with a markedly higher incidence in those with a family history of the condition.

When the heart muscle contracts to pump blood through the body, pressure in the arteries is at its peak. This is called the systolic pressure. The muscle then relaxes before the next contraction and the pressure drops to its minimum, the diastolic pressure. When your blood pressure is measured, it is expressed as two figures, for example, 150/85—the higher systolic and lower diastolic pressures, respectively.

THE SILENT THREAT

There is usually no way you can know whether your blood pressure is high without having it measured—you can't feel it, because hypertension does not have any symptoms until it gets very high. However, if it stays high, it causes serious and progressive damage to the blood vessels, making the linings rough and causing narrowing and thickening of the artery walls.

Eventually, these changes can lead to coronary heart disease (CHD), stroke and eye damage from bleeding in the retina (particularly in diabetics). Women who take oral contraceptives, who smoke and those over the age of 40 should have their blood pressure checked yearly. Ideally, it should be less than 140/90. Elderly women often have systolic readings above 140, a condition called isolated systolic hypertension, which should be treated.

WHAT YOUR DOCTOR CAN DO

You will need medication if your BP readings are high on two or three separate occasions, in spite of attempts to lower it by lifestyle changes. Modern drugs are effective and can reduce the risk of stroke by 35 to 40 percent and CHD by 20 to 25 percent. Diuretics or beta blockers can be used to slow the heart, and various drugs can open up blood vessels. You must take them as prescribed, even though you may feel well. If you have side effects, don't stop taking the medication. Consult your doctor who may prescribe a different drug. Medication will control but not cure hypertension and you will need to continue to take it for the rest of your life.

CONTROLLING YOUR BLOOD PRESSURE

Most doctors will encourage a self-help programme for mild hypertension. The basics are:
♀ Don't smoke.
♀ Limit your intake of salty processed foods and snacks and don't add salt to your food when you are cooking. Consuming a lot of salt significantly raises the risk of hypertension.
♀ Keep your weight within a healthy range for your height.
♀ Exercise every day.
♀ Don't have more alcohol than the recommended maximum weekly amount for a woman and avoid binge drinking. Moderate drinking (a glass of wine a day) may help to keep blood pressure down.

♀ Eat fruit, vegetables and low-fat dairy products, since these contain potassium and calcium which help control blood pressure.
♀ Analyse your lifestyle and make changes to reduce chronic stress.

♀ You may need a 24-hour blood-pressure monitoring to determine whether treatment is needed. This may also be used to monitor response to treatment.

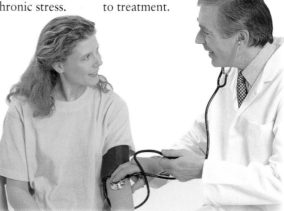

MONITORING
Having blood pressure measured is quick and painless. Even so, BP often goes up when you visit your doctor—so-called "white coat hypertension".

Hyperlipidaemia

See also:

1/BEING A WELL WOMAN
Essentials of good health
pp. 16–21
Helathy body systems p. 34

4/HORMONAL HEALTH
Endocrine problems pp. 136–137

Many women do not realize that cardio-vascular disease (CHD) is their greatest potential health problem. They, as much as men, can benefit from identifying their risk factors and reducing them. It is even suggested that women from the age of 20 should assess their risks and be screened for hyperlipidaemia (excess fat in the blood).

Checking the level of lipids (fats) in the blood, one of which is cholesterol, is one of the foremost indicators of the health of the heart. If hyperlipidaemia is left untreated, it increases a woman's risk of developing CHD, especially after the menopause. Establishing a healthy eating pattern—using the pyramids as a guide (p. 19) and the accompanying advice on serving sizes and total fat content—is considered the first step for women concerned about living well and living longer.

THE CAUSES

In most cases, hyperlipidaemia is caused by excessive consumption of dietary fat and cholesterol, combined with a lack of physical activity. Changes in lifestyle to reduce weight and cholesterol-lowering therapy are the major steps in helping reduce levels of blood fats in women who smoke, are overweight or obese (pp. 190–191), and have high blood pressure and/or diabetes. Other medical problems, such as liver or thyroid disease, excessive alcohol intake and undiagnosed diabetes can also cause increased lipid levels in the blood.

Two further important risk factors are premature menopause (before the age of 45) that is not treated with oestrogen or hormone replacement therapy (HRT) and a family history of premature CHD in a close relative (especially in a mother under the age of 65 or a father under the age of 55).

Women with these risk factors who have hyperlipidaemia or hypercholesterolaemia (sometimes familial, meaning inherited) will generally be placed on a restricted diet for a trial period of three to six months. The saturated fats found in butter, lard, cheese, meat and meat products and trans fats found in hard margarines and products made from them, such as biscuits and pastries, should be reduced and/or replaced by polyunsaturated fats in, for

Cholesterol

One of the essential components of cell walls is cholesterol, a natural waxy substance which is made in the liver and carried around the body in the blood. High levels of cholesterol in the blood are a risk factor for heart disease. Surplus cholesterol settles on the walls of the arteries, forming plaques that narrow the space through which blood flows. The excess in the blood comes from the way the body processes animal (saturated) fats in the diet.

Vegetable fats (unsaturated, polyunsaturated and monounsaturated) are chemically different from saturated fat and metabolized in a different way. They do not cause the same problems. The amount of fat eaten daily—of any type—should be kept to a minimum.

Cholesterol has three measurements: total, HDL (high density lipoprotein) and LDL (low density lipoprotein). The British guidelines are that healthy women should have less than 5 mmol/l (millimoles per litre) of total cholesterol of which at least 1 mmol/l should be HDL (good cholesterol). A measurement below 5 total cholesterol is desirable; a figure significantly above is too high. If HDL levels are too low, have your LDL (bad cholesterol) checked. It should be less than 3 mmol/l.

Your doctor may use the term cholesterol ratio, which is the total cholesterol divided by the HDL. The optimal ratio for women is 3.5 to 1; above 5 to 1 is a health risk.

example, sunflower, soya and fish oils and monounsaturated fats in, for instance, olive oil, rapeseed oil and nuts.

The restricted diet will be followed, if necessary, by treatment with lipid-lowering drugs. Women will be advised on a course of exercise activities to help them achieve and maintain their desirable body weight. Oestrogen replacement therapy can reduce LDL (bad cholesterol) and increase HDL (good cholesterol), and may occasionally be recommended for post-menopausal women who do not have existing cardiovascular disease.

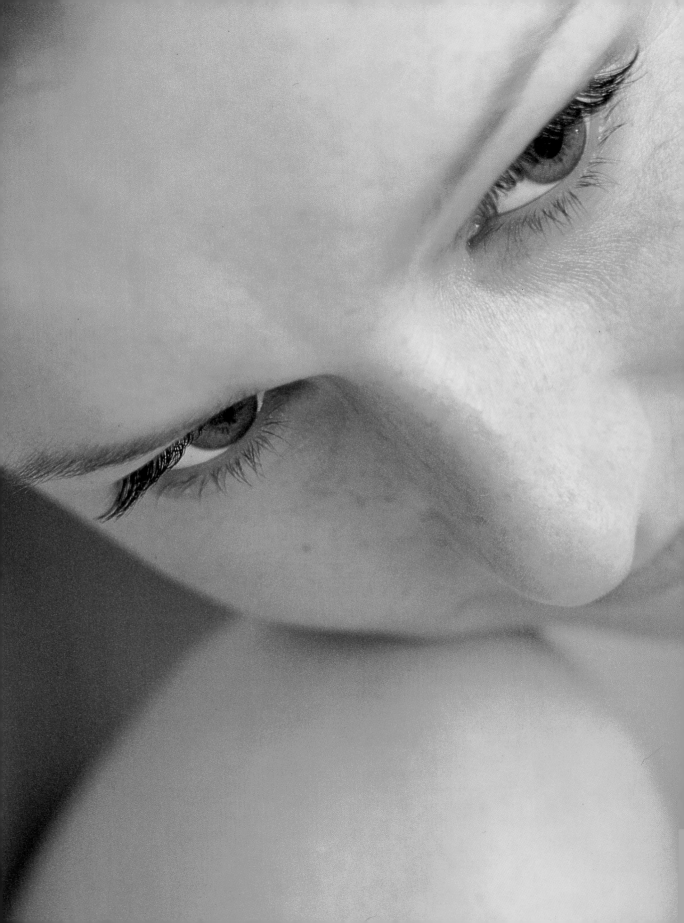

HORMONAL HEALTH

A woman's hormones are the fuel of her life. Their influence starts at birth and extends well into old age. The hormones govern the way she develops, her responses to stimuli and her reactions to a variety of situations. Keeping the various hormones working well, with the right balance throughout all the organs of the body, promotes a woman's wellness. Understanding their role and power is a constant challenge for the medical profession. Only in recent years has research shown that the hormones play a vital protective role in a woman's body. If this function is interrupted, then all aspects of her life and health may be under threat.

ENDOCRINE SYSTEM PROBLEMS

The endocrine system consists of various glands that secrete hormones into the bloodstream to regulate bodily processes. For a woman, the endocrine system is the hormonal system that most affects her whole life, governing her monthly cycle and the stages of pregnancy.

Diabetes

The hormone insulin is produced by the pancreas to enable the cells in your body to make use of the fuel they need, by processing the glucose in the blood. When someone has diabetes—type 1 or type 2—there is either not enough insulin or it is not being used properly, or both. Any interruption of the insulin supply results in glucose levels in the blood becoming too high. All brain and red blood cells need a constant supply of glucose, but too much is life threatening.

Diabetes mellitus is the fastest-growing illness in Western countries, yet it is not understood why some people get it and others don't. Genetics play a role in susceptibility, as do excessive weight and inactivity in type 2. Currently, there is no cure for the condition, but it can be controlled effectively by a treatment programme.

If the condition arises quickly, it suggests that the insulin-producing cells in the pancreas have stopped working, an auto-immune problem caused by the body attacking itself. This is type 1 or insulin-dependent diabetes, also called juvenile diabetes, though it can affect adults. If diabetes occurs gradually, "insulin resistance" is developing. This means that the cells are prepared for blood glucose to enter, but it is unable to, making the insulin ineffective. Called type 2 diabetes, it only occasionally begins before

Symptoms of diabetes in women

♀ Constant thirst and a dry mouth.
♀ Increased appetite.
♀ Need to empty your bladder frequently.
♀ Extreme tiredness.
♀ Blurred vision.
♀ Unexplained weight loss.
♀ Frequent vaginal infections.
♀ Genital itching.

WHO IS AT RISK?
Diabetes can strike at any age, from birth to old age. If you have parents with diabetes or are overweight (for type 2), you are more likely to develop the illness. You are also susceptible if you have elevated blood pressure, you are pregnant or have polycystic ovary syndrome (mostly under the age of 40).

TEENAGERS

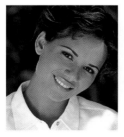

The genes inherited from your parents may play a part in whether you get diabetes. In young people the disease may be triggered by a virus.

20S AND 30S

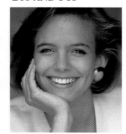

In this age group both types of diabetes may occur. The sudden onset of symptoms is likely to indicate a halt in insulin production.

PREGNANT WOMEN

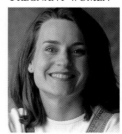

About 3 percent of women develop gestational diabetes. It will be picked up in antenatal tests after the 24th week of pregnancy.

OVER 40

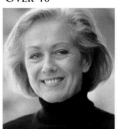

Type 2 diabetes is the most common in this age group, perhaps because of weight gain—a major contributory factor.

the age of 40—hence its former name, adult-onset diabetes—and is more common than type 1. Type 2 diabetes is associated with obesity and may be familial. It is prevalent in South Asian and Afro-Caribbean women. Symptoms may go unnoticed for as many as nine years. In the UK diabetes occurs in 2 to 3 percent of the population, though of these a third may be undiagnosed. Screening on an empty stomach every three years is advised for women over 45 without risk factors, or over 40 if they are over-weight or have a family history of diabetes.

HOW DIABETES IS TREATED

Lifelong regular injections of insulin are current-ly the main treatment for type 1, although diet is also essential to all diabetes management. Among the diagnosed type 2 diabetic population over a third manage their diabetes by diet alone. Sometimes this needs to be combined with pills that can help make better use of the insulin the body does produce or slow down the speed at which sugar is absorbed. Some type 2 diabetics may need insulin. Following a low-fat, high-fibre diet with plenty of vegetables, fruit, wholegrain foods and pulses and minimum consumption of refined carbohydrates and sugar—which quick-ly raise the blood glucose level—benefits every-one who suffers from diabetes.

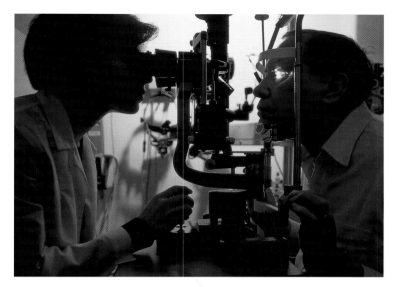

Diabetes in pregnancy

When you are pregnant, your urine is tested for any trace of sugar. This can appear, usually after the 24th week, because hormones from the placenta may affect the body's response to insulin, making it less effective. Glucose in the bloodstream rises and overflows into the urine. This condition is known as gestational diabetes. If nothing is done, the baby may grow too large—resulting in a difficult delivery—and may develop hypoglycaemia (low blood sugar). Often a change of diet may be enough to solve the problem, but some women may need to be treated with insulin until giving birth. Once the placenta is delivered, the diabetes usually disappears, but 30 to 50 percent of women may develop type 2 diabetes later. A woman with gestational diabetes is more at risk of urinary tract infections and preeclampsia. A baby whose mother had gestational diabetes may have a greater risk of diabetes.

AVOIDING COMPLICATIONS

The main long-term risk for people with diabetes is its association with high blood pressure and hyperlipidaemia, which leads to blood vessel damage and in turn to coronary heart disease or a stroke, can affect eyesight and damage the peripheral nerves, especially in the feet. Kidney disease is another common result of diabetes.

You should try to maintain blood glucose lev-els. Monitoring your blood sugar level regularly using a glucometer is essential so treatment can be adjusted if necessary. You can reduce chances of complications by healthy eating and control-ling your blood pressure and cholesterol levels.

HOW INSULIN IS SUPPLIED

Insulin is destroyed by the digestive system if taken by mouth. Insulin is most often injected into the fatty layer under the skin—a quick-acting form of insulin by day to counter the rise in blood sugar from food; a longer-acting one at night. As many as four injections in a 24-hour period may be needed. You can use a syringe, a pen with disposable cartridges or a jet injector that uses pressurized air. Those whose blood sugar fluctuates irregularly can use a pump taped to the skin, which injects insulin continuously. A new method— through an inhaler—is now available for some people with type 2 who are unable to inject themselves.

EYE TESTS

Many people who have undiagnosed type 2 diabetes find out during a routine eye exam: the ophthalmologist may notice changes in the retina. Damage to blood vessels at the back of the eye can cause loss of sight and even blindness. Laser treatments can stem, but not stop, the damage.

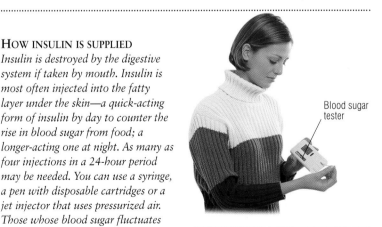

Blood sugar tester

! Caution

If you have diabetes, you should always be wary of over-the-counter medicines and supplements, since some can increase blood sugar levels. Check with the pharmacist or your doctor.

Thyroid diseases

Women are particularly susceptible to the problems of metabolism caused by autoimmune disease. For example, hyperthyroidism (overactive thyroid) is 10 to 15 times as common in women as in men. If the thyroid gland doesn't work properly bones, nerves and other body tissues suffer.

The thyroid gland, about the size of a small plum and located in the front of the neck, is under the control of the pituitary gland, which is connected by a stalk to the brain, and responds to signals from a part of the brain called the hypothalamus.

For reasons possibly related to oestrogen as menstrual irregularities are often symptomatic, the thyroid gland may become overactive or underactive—conditions known as hyperthyroidism and hypothyroidism. Both are usually autoimmune disorders.

Symptoms of hypothyroidism

Underactive thyroid:
- ♀ Weight gain.
- ♀ Dry, brittle and thinning hair.
- ♀ Dry skin.
- ♀ Forgetfulness and mental sluggishness.
- ♀ Lack of energy and constant tiredness.
- ♀ Depression.
- ♀ Scanty or irregular periods.
- ♀ Increased sensitivity to cold.
- ♀ Constipation.

DIAGNOSING HYPOTHYROIDISM

Because iodine in the diet is essential to the manufacture of thyroid hormones, shortage of it is the most common reason worldwide for people to develop hypothyroidism. In Western countries today, the cause is more usually an autoimmune disorder called Hashimoto's disease: in this, white blood cells take over thyroid tissue, which is then attacked by antibodies.

Hashimoto's disease progresses reasonably slowly and is not always promptly recognized. Sometimes the condition is mistaken for depression, which is in reality a symptom. Also, an expected side effect of treatment for hyperthyroidism can be hypothyroidism, as not enough tissue remains. The symptoms of hypothyroidism in its severe form, known as myxedema, might be due to psychological problems or ageing.

Routine screening is sometimes given after the menopause to measure the levels of thyroid stimulating hormone (TSH): too little means an overactive thyroid, too much and it is underactive. Another test identifies antithyroid antibodies, indicating an autoimmune link.

TREATING HYPOTHYROIDISM

In principle, this condition can be corrected by hormone replacement, using a synthetic form of the thyroid hormone thyroxine to bring levels back to normal. There may, however, be a certain amount of trial and error to find the right dose. Your doctor will normally start you on a low dose which can be increased if necessary (that is, if symptoms recur or if blood tests indicate abnormal levels), and you will have to continue taking the pills for the rest of your life.

Regular testing of TSH levels is needed to ensure that the treatment is not causing hyperthyroidism which can then affect bone density and result in osteoporosis. Women who are hypothyroid have an increased risk of atherosclerosis and heart disease because they tend to have high levels of blood fats (including cholesterol) which cause deposits in the arteries. Other causes of hyperthyroidism are: iodine deficiency; congenital (babies are tested at birth); previous thyroid treatment; drugs: lithium carbonate (used to treat manic depressives) and amiodarone (used for irregular heartbeat).

THYROID AND PARATHYROIDS
These important glands consist of two thyroid lobes on either side of the trachea (windpipe) and four parathyroids. The parathyroid lobes are found behind the thyroid gland.

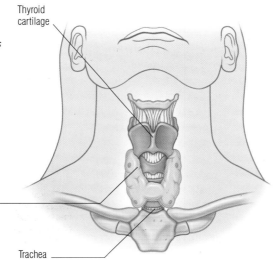

Thyroid cartilage

Left and right thyroid lobes

Trachea

Who is at risk?
Women are more likely than men to have a thyroid disorder. During the reproductive years prolonged menstrual cycles may indicate hypothyroidism, scanty or lack of bleeding can be a symptom of hyperthyroidism. The disorder may appear after giving birth and may be mistakenly diagnosed as post-natal depression.

Children

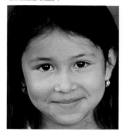

Girls as young as five can get Graves' disease. This is a very common disorder which can be diagnosed through a blood test.

20s to 40s

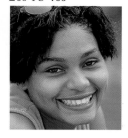

Women may not realize that their symptoms perhaps relate to thyroid excess or deficiency. Both can affect the menstrual cycle and fertility.

over 60

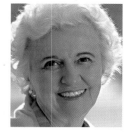

Hashimoto's disease may affect 1 in 10 women over the age of 60. They are 10 times more likely than men to develop a goitre in the neck.

Symptoms of hyperthyroidism

Overactive thyroid:
- ♀ Sweating and feeling too hot all the time.
- ♀ Anxiety and nervousness.
- ♀ Restlessness and insomnia.
- ♀ Weight loss despite increased appetite.
- ♀ Palpitations, racing heartbeat.
- ♀ Diarrhoea.
- ♀ Trembling hands.
- ♀ Bulging eyes.

DIAGNOSING HYPERTHYROIDISM

Through questions and close scrutiny your doctor will pinpoint the symptoms and confirm the diagnosis with a blood test for TSH. Graves' disease causes the disorder in around 80 percent of people. This is an autoimmune disease in which the body's own antibodies attack the thyroid gland and stimulate it into releasing excess hormone and thus speeding up the metabolic rate. It is not known why this happens, although there may be a genetic link. In the other 20 percent, the cause is thyroid malfunction.

TREATING HYPERTHYROIDISM

The doctor may prescribe antithyroid drugs to suppress hormone production, but these don't work for everyone. Another treatment—though not for pregnant women—is radioiodine, taken as a drink, which destroys thyroid tissue. Assessing the correct dose can be difficult; some people need more than one treatment while in others so much tissue is killed that they then have to take thyroxine pills to compensate. Alternatively, or if neither of these treatments work, most of the thyroid gland can be removed surgically; some people may need to take thyroid hormone replacement after such surgery.

OTHER THYROID DISORDERS

Thyroid cancer is rare and is treated by thyroidectomy (surgical removal of the gland). Most types have a high cure rate.

Subclinical hyperthyroidism, usually affecting women over 60, develops from toxic nodules which form on the gland. These may have no symptoms but can cause bone density loss, irregular heartbeat and make heart problems such as angina worse. Radioiodine or surgery are the usual treatments.

HOW BONES ARE AFFECTED

Hypo- and hyperthyroidism can affect bone mineralization. Parathyroids (four tiny glands found near the thyroid gland) regulate the levels of bone-building minerals—calcium and phosphorus—in the blood. Any treatment that affects the healthy functioning of the thyroid or parathyroid glands and their hormone production can influence the strength of your bones and teeth. Parathyroid overactivity is picked up by blood calcium screening, or if osteoporosis is diagnosed.

COMPLICATIONS OF THE EYES

Graves' disease can cause protrusion of the eyes. Eye disease can happen at any point, even after the thyroid is back to normal. The changes are irreversible and require steroid treatment, or in some cases surgery.

Premenstrual syndrome

See also:

1/BEING A WELL WOMAN
Healthy body systems p. 38

4/HORMONAL HEALTH
Reproductive problems
pp. 146–169

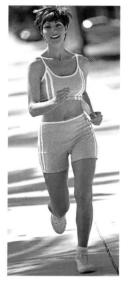

AEROBIC EXERCISE
Exercise releases feel-good hormones in the brain, which can ease depression. It also improves digestion, which can reduce feelings of bloating.

Approximately 80 percent of women are affected, to a greater or lesser extent, by premenstrual syndrome (PMS) at some time in their lives. The impact may be mild and infrequent or frequent and disabling.

For PMS to be diagnosed, only one of the following symptoms is required: mild psychological discomfort, bloating and weight gain, breast tenderness, swelling of hands and feet, various aches and pains, poor concentration, sleep disturbance and change in appetite. The symptom or symptoms occur in the second half of the menstrual cycle—that is, the 14 days before the beginning of the next period. They peak shortly before menstruation and usually stop when the menstrual flow begins. They may be at their worst in the week immediately before menstruation and may continue for the first couple of days of bleeding.

Although the range of physical, behavioural and emotional symptoms ascribed to PMS is enormous—as many as 150—the most common can be roughly classified into four groups:

Mood swings Feelings of anxiety, tension and irritability.

Fluid retention Giving rise to weight gain, swollen ankles and fingers, a bloated feeling in the abdomen and breast discomfort.

Depression Tearfulness, forgetfulness, confusion and insomnia.

Cravings For carbohydrates and especially sweet foods, increase in appetite, palpitations, faintness, dizziness and headaches.

Although the cause is clearly related to cyclical fluctuations in hormones, no one is sure precisely how symptoms are triggered or what determines who gets which ones. It may be that some women are naturally more sensitive to hormonal influences or become so as they get older and changing hormone levels build up over time. The menstrual cycle may also affect food metabolism, meaning that some women can control PMS symptoms by regulating their intake of carbohydrates and fats.

IDENTIFYING THE SYMPTOMS

Symptoms that come and go without any pattern or that trouble you in the first half of your menstrual cycle are unlikely to be related to PMS and will need medical evaluation to find the cause. Anxiety and depression, for instance, may have nothing to do with PMS, and your doctor will want to rule out causes such as an underlying physical disorder or a personal problem such as an abusive home situation or adverse sexual experience. Recurring pelvic pain is not a PMS symptom and needs full investigation.

Some women may experience PMS symptoms for the first time as they approach menopause, when the levels of reproductive hormones decline. But any problems that are the direct result of menopausal changes are likely to respond better to specific treatments such as hormone replacement therapy (HRT). Discuss this with your doctor or gynaecologist.

To see if there is a link between your symptoms and the onset of your period, your doctor will probably suggest that you keep a daily diary for two months. You will be asked to record when symptoms occur, what they are, the level of severity, how long they persist and whether they prevent you from performing normal activities. You may be given a self-rating form called COPE (calendar of premenstrual experiences), which is easy to complete.

EASING YOUR SYMPTOMS

Try reducing your consumption of salt, which encourages fluid retention, and avoid tea, coffee and most fizzy drinks, which contain caffeine and can exacerbate tension and anxiety.

Plan to have several small meals a day based on complex carbohydrates such as wholegrain bread, brown rice and pasta, cereals and pulses, and keep fatty and sugary foods to a minimum. This should prevent large swings in blood glucose levels, which may contribute to both physical and psychological symptoms.

Eat plenty of fresh fruit and vegetables every day to help balance blood glucose and prevent

Supplements packaged to help

Evening primrose and sunflower oils both contain gamma linoleic acid—an essential fatty acid—and are sold as a health supplement to assist the body in countering the effects of hormones. You can buy either oil on its own or combined with vitamin B6 (pyridoxine), which may also help relieve PMS symptoms such as fluid retention, or with chromium and magnesium, nutrients commonly deficient in young women.

If you decide to try these expensive supplements, keep a daily record to see whether they are having a beneficial effect. You should speak with your doctor before taking any herbal supplements.

constipation. Foods with the amino acid tryptophan (see chart below) increase serotonin, which controls the "feel-good" factor.

Exercise that makes you slightly out of breath and sweat will boost production of endorphins, the body's natural opiates, which ease aches and pains and lift your mood.

Gentler forms of exercise such as yoga and t'ai chi will help you relax and relieve anxiety. Taking time to care for yourself is essential in helping you manage PMS symptoms.

PMS OR PMDD?

While PMS is usually diagnosed by your doctor or obstetricians/gynaecologists, premenstrual dysphoric disorder (PMDD) is diagnosed by psychiatric and mental health professionals. As well as PMS symptoms, a woman may have mood changes that are severe enough just before her period starts to interfere with her ability to function at home or at work. The effect is similar to that of major depression and needs treatment with drugs.

PMS TREATMENTS

Therapy	Method	Action
PMS self-help		
Vitamin B6 and Oil of Evening Primrose	Taken in capsule form, these are available at healthfood shops or on prescription.	*Reduces sensitivity to hormones and can help with relaxation.*
Aerobic exercise	Increase heart rate for 20 minutes daily.	*Produces endorphins that relieve symptoms.*
Diet changes	Cut down on caffeine, salt, alcohol and chocolate. Eat more complex carbohydrates and foods containing tryptophan (sunflower, pumpkin and evening primrose seeds) and potatoes.	*Improves mood and assuages cravings.*
Relaxation exercises	Meditation, yoga.	*May alleviate tension or depression.*
Massage	Whole body or hands/feet (reflexology).	*Relaxes and stimulates self-healing.*
Aromatherapy	A few drops of lavender, chamomile, juniper or geranium oils added to a warm bath.	*Relieves anxiety and irritability.*
Herbs	Teas of chasteberry, Chinese angelica (dong quai) or black cohosh.	*May act by balancing hormones.*
Drugs prescribed for PMS		
Combination oral contraceptive pill	Controls the body's hormones.	*Regulates the 28-day cycle.*
Antidepressants	Pills to treat depression or tearfulness. This method appears to have the most effective results.	*SSRIs (selective serotonin reuptake inhibitors) raise the level of the feel-good brain chemical, serotonin.*

The menopause

KEEPING ACTIVE
Get into the habit of regular weightbearing exercise before the menopause and continue to enjoy it afterwards. Getting out into the fresh air— playing golf, or tennis, or walking—slows bone loss and maintains muscle tone, helps to prevent weight gain and keeps your cardiovascular system healthy.

Women react to what is often called "the change of life" in different ways, both physically and emotionally. Some welcome the absence of periods and not having to think about contraception any more; others regret the loss of their fertility and may feel less of a woman. The most positive see it as the start of a new phase in their life.

For the vast majority of women, the monthly cycles stop around the age of 50, after years in which bleeding has varied from heavy to scanty, or been irregular. With the decline in the amount of the female hormone oestrogen being secreted by your ovaries you ovulate less frequently, so conception and pregnancy become increasingly unlikely in that time known as peri-menopause. After 12 months without bleeding you can accept you are postmenopausal.

The time span is usually about four years though it may be longer or in some cases abrupt. Some women have a premature menopause, either naturally or as a result of medical or sur-

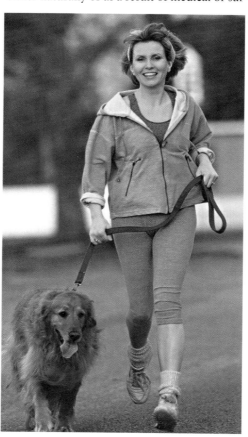

gical treatment involving either the removal or destruction of the ovaries.

Women under 40 will be advised on the benefits and risks of hormone replacement therapy (HRT), which will reduce their risk of developing osteoporosis. Without oestrogen they are also at increased risk of heart disease. Menopausal symptoms can appear two or so years earlier in women who smoke. A few women will go through the menopause with few or no problems, but the majority experience some symptoms which can range from being a minor nuisance to quite troublesome.

A RANGE OF SYMPTOMS

Hot flushes, which can occur at any time, are the most common problem and one which many women find difficult to cope with simply because of their unpredictability. Insomnia— often made worse by night sweats—leaves you feeling tired and lethargic. You may lose confidence and get more headaches than you used to. Another common symptom is mood swings, especially irritability and depression, although both may have more to do with other changes happening in your life at this time rather than with the menopause as such.

You may find you "leak" urine when you cough, laugh, sneeze or run. Lack of oestrogen can affect the cells lining the vagina, so that it becomes drier and lacks lubrication, making intercourse uncomfortable or even painful. You may lose interest in sex, perhaps even find it difficult to respond to your partner and you may not want your children near you.

It is important to reassure yourself that what you are going through is a natural life event, that there is nothing unusual in what is happening to you, that you are healthy and the symptoms can be alleviated. Find someone to talk to. Your doctor may be the one to help you get through this time or you may find a menopause counsellor more useful. Sharing your thoughts with your partner or a friend may help you clarify problems and give you perspective on the solutions.

BABY-SAFE AT THE MENOPAUSE

"Change of life" babies are usually born to women who thought that they could not be

Changing your life

For some women, the changes which occur at the menopause may coincide with changes in their personal lives. A relationship may go wrong, working women may be made redundant or reach the peak of their career ambitions, and those who have devoted most of their energy to their families may feel at a loss when their children leave home or need less of their mother's support.

It is not unusual for women to put on weight around this time and you may feel less attractive as wrinkles and other skin changes become more noticeable because of oestrogen loss. Putting yourself first will help you be positive about making the necessary changes that will carry you into and through the postmenopausal years.

If you feel you can't handle what is happening to you, seek support. Talk to your doctor about counselling, psychotherapy or possibly antidepressants.

pregnant again. If you haven't been sterilized, continue contraception for two years after your last period if you are under 50, or for one year if over 50. HRT treats symptoms of the menopause but does not restore fertility.

Most women will be past their menopause by 54 which is when "bleed-free" HRT (treatment that stops all bleeding) can be prescribed. It can be difficult to know when you have reached the menopause if you are taking the combined contraceptive pill or progestogen-only pill, have been using HRT for several years or been fitted with the intrauterine contraceptive system, all of which may prevent you noticing symptoms. At 50, you should ask your doctor if changes need to be made to your prescription.

SELF HELP AT THE MENOPAUSE

Keep moving. Run up stairs, walk instead of driving or taking the bus. Regular exercise that causes you to breathe more deeply, to take in more oxygen and increase your heart rate is known to help reduce mood swings and hot flushes and improve concentration and energy levels. Start slowly—30 minutes at least three times a week—and build up to five or more days.

Running, brisk walking, dancing (line dancing especially), tennis, golf and badminton are weight-bearing activities that benefit bone strength.

If you are very overweight, talk to your doctor and a dietician about a weight-loss diet combined with physical activity that will gradually help you reach an acceptable weight.

Take control of your diet. Include plenty of calcium-rich foods, especially low-fat dairy foods, green leafy vegetables and pulses (see box below) and oily fish.

Spend at least 20 minutes a day outdoors so that your skin is able to make the vitamin D needed to absorb calcium efficiently. Remember to use skin protection—it won't hinder the process of vitamin making, but it will protect your skin from the risk of skin cancer and the drying, wrinkling effects of photoageing.

OESTROGENS IN PLANT FOODS

There is a theory, although not yet proven, that Asian women are less likely to report menopausal symptoms. This is thought to be related to their high intake of phytoestrogens, substances found in many plant-based foods. If eaten regularly it seems they may compensate for declining oestrogen levels and decrease cholesterol levels. The two main groups are lignans and isoflavones; they block the uptake of normal oestrogen (for example, in breast tissue).

Opt for soy products (beans, milk, tofu, miso), pulses (black beans, mung beans, alfalfa sprouts), whole grains (rice, wheat, barley), fennel, celery and rhubarb.

Supplements including ginseng, red clover and linseed are said to ease hot flushes. Tea made from wild yam and liquorice, and herbal extracts such as black cohosh, blue cohosh, false unicorn root and yarrow are all prescribed by herbalists to stop menopausal symptoms. Do not take any herbal preparations without discussing them with a herbalist as some may have side effects in people with certain conditions. Take note that the possible long-term effects of phytoestrogens are not yet fully known.

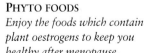

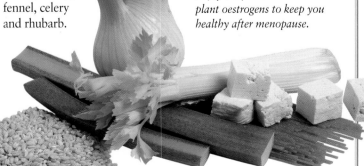

PHYTO FOODS
Enjoy the foods which contain plant oestrogens to keep you healthy after menopause.

Hormone replacement therapy

At and after the menopause, which occurs on average around the age of 51, a woman's own natural hormones are no longer needed for reproduction. However, one in particular, oestrogen, is also vital to the health of other parts of the body. Hormone replacement therapy (HRT) aims to offer protection from the effects of reduced oestrogen—to treat symptoms premenopausally or replace hormone levels after the menopause.

During the reproductive years it is thought that your own natural oestrogen gives you protection against coronary heart disease and loss of bone strength and density (osteoporosis). Once your ovaries stop producing eggs and your hormones (oestrogen, progesterone and testosterone) are reduced, your risk of heart disease increases almost to that of a man and fast calcium loss from bones makes fractures more likely. Laboratory-produced hormones (that is, oestradiol/oestrione/oestriol, all names for oestrogens, and progestogen/progestin, both progesterone) in the form of HRT, and a new type called selective oestrogen-receptor modulators (SERMs) may be able to reduce both risks.

Remaining as well as you can be will be one of your prime concerns after the menopause, for this ensures your independence in the 30 or more years that may lie ahead. If you are contemplating HRT, it should be an informed choice, based on what is known about its short- and long-term use. Working with your doctor, you should be involved in the decision-making, know how the therapy could affect you, and evaluate the benefits against the risks.

You should know, for example, that the amount of oestrogen in HRT is about one-fifth of that in the contraceptive pill. Even so, there may be a hormonal surge that may cause side effects such as nausea and breast tenderness at first. Usually your prescription will be for a trial period of two to three months so that you can monitor the effects. If you do not feel any different on the type tried, discuss further options with your doctor. You are more likely to benefit from the therapy if you have confidence in it, have realistic expectations and have the backing of people interested in your well-being.

TAILORING HRT

If you have your uterus you will initially take both oestrogen, for menopausal symptoms and your bones, and progestogen to protect the uterine lining. You will have regular period-like bleeds, although not necessarily every month, depending on the HRT formulation. When you are postmenopausal and have been free of natural periods for two years (or when you reach 54), you can change to bleed-free therapy (continuous combined). If you have had a hysterectomy you can receive oestrogen only.

A woman in her 60s or 70s is not precluded from HRT. It may be an option to take HRT for symptoms during menopause and postpone long-term use until later when risks of heart disease and osteoporosis increase, or if vaginal problems occur. You may need to try different types and dosages to find the one that suits you.

Designer oestrogen

Raloxifene is an oestrogen alternative, used in postmenopausal hormone therapy. Its purpose is to confer oestrogen's alleged heart and bone-preserving benefits, without the risks of breast or uterine cancer.

Raloxifene is a SERM—selective oestrogen-receptor modulator—which mimics oestrogen in some tissues while blocking the hormone in others. Taken as a pill, a SERM may meet the needs of older postmenopausal women who cannot, will not or should not use HRT but may be concerned about osteoporosis. Raloxifene improves bone density of the spine, and stops bone loss without affecting the breast and uterus. It does not, however, treat menopausal symptoms; in fact, in the first few months you may have side effects such as mild leg cramps and hot flushes.

Although it is an oestrogen from a plant source, it is not hormone replacement and so will not alleviate a menopausal problem such as vaginal dryness. While oestrogen in HRT is known to boost the levels of HDL or "good" cholesterol and to lower LDL, the "bad" form, raloxifene has no effect on HDL and only lowers LDL. Raloxifene is not advised for women with a personal or family history of thrombosis (blood clots) as there may be an increased risk.

WHO CANNOT TAKE HRT?

HRT may not be suitable for anyone who has had breast or uterine cancer, heart disease or deep-vein blood clots, or who has a family history of any of these conditions. An obstetrician or gynaecologist will want to ensure that a woman who is overweight, has hypertension, diabetes, gallstones or fibroids is managing her condition well before thinking about taking HRT. Specialist consultation and treatment may be needed if a woman has or has had endometriosis, breast problems or osteoporosis caused by long-term use of steroids. However, if a woman is not able to take HRT, plant oestrogens found in soy products may provide alternative help.

THE TYPES OF HRT

Whether you attend a menopause clinic or consult your doctor, it is important to get as much information as you can about the various types of HRT so that you can find out those which are most suited to you and your symptoms. Take time to discuss your health and lifestyle before deciding which to try.

Treatment	Method	Points to consider
Oral: *oestrogen and progestogen*	Pills are taken by mouth, absorbed through the stomach, broken down by the liver and distributed in the blood. Can be sequential or, postmenopausally, continuous combined.	*Simple to take. Side effects may include nausea, breast tenderness. Need to take as prescribed, as lapses negate the effect. Must not be taken by women with liver disease. Breakthrough bleeding may occur.*
Oral: *tibolone*	A synthetic steroid that treats menopausal symptoms, prevents bone loss and improves libido and mood. Does not affect breast and uterus.	*Only for postmenopausal women.*
Transdermal patches	See-through shapes containing either or both hormones, applied to buttocks or thighs. Hormones are absorbed through the skin into the blood so are not initially metabolized by the liver.	*Can be either sequential (oestrogen for so many days, progestin for so many days) or continuous combined (for period-free, postmenopausal women, but breakthrough bleeding may occur). Patches are visible, don't always adhere to dry skin, can cause allergies, can leave telltale adhesive marks when changed (either once or twice weekly).*
Vaginal therapy	Direct treatment for vaginal and urinary symptoms.	*Wide range of methods: creams, pills, suppositories or silicone ring replaced every three months. Vaginal therapy is not licensed for prevention of osteoporosis. Intravaginal progestogen also needed for women with uterus.*
Intrauterine device	Releases progestogen and provides contraception for perimenopausal women.	*Must be fitted by a doctor. May be used with oral oestrogen. Lasts up to five years.*
Implant	Pellet inserted under skin in groin or buttock (done with local anaesthetic). Releases oestrogen as body demands. Testosterone may be added for libido.	*Must be inserted by a doctor. Used with oral progestogen to prevent thickening of endometrium (women with uterus). Lasts about six months.*

REPRODUCTIVE PROBLEMS

From adolescence on, a woman's reproductive system has a major impact on her life. The complex demands made on her body by hormonal changes, from her periods to childbearing to menopause, can lead to health problems. A woman needs to be able to recognize the warning signs so that she can seek medical help as early as possible.

Menstrual disorders

Menstrual problems and pains are common. Many women will experience a menstrual cycle disorder of some kind at least once in their lives.

THE NORMAL MENSTRUAL CYCLE

Unless a woman is pregnant, her menstrual cycle takes place about every month, from menarche (the first period, occurring between the ages of about 10 and 17) to menopause (the last period, occurring in the late 40s or early 50s). In most women the cycle is from 28 to 30 days long, but anything from 24 to 35 days may be considered normal. The purpose of the menstrual cycle is to prepare the uterus for a

UNDERSTANDING THE MENSTRUAL CYCLE

Menstruation, when bleeding occurs, is the actual period and signals the fact that a fertilized egg has not implanted in the uterus. Blood flow that is absent, scanty, infrequent or too frequent, heavy or accompanied by pain, are all typical of disorders.

possible pregnancy. The cycle is controlled by the complex interaction between hormones, starting with gonadotropin releasing hormone (GnRH) secreted by the hypothalamus in the brain which stimulates the endocrine system's master gland, the pituitary.

The first phase of the menstrual cycle is known as the proliferative or follicular phase. At this stage several eggs, called ova, begin to ripen in follicles in the ovaries. This process is governed by two hormones secreted by the pituitary gland, follicle stimulating hormone (FSH) and luteinizing hormone (LH). The action of both is affected by the female sex hormone, oestrogen, produced by the ovaries.

As the oestrogen level rises it inhibits further production of FSH and stimulates the release of LH. This in turn causes the release of just one mature egg around the middle of the menstrual cycle, bringing this phase to an end. The body temperature rises slightly and, under the influence of oestrogen, starts to thicken the

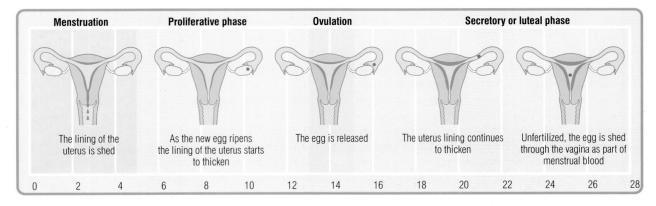

Menstruation	Proliferative phase	Ovulation	Secretory or luteal phase	
The lining of the uterus is shed	As the new egg ripens the lining of the uterus starts to thicken	The egg is released	The uterus lining continues to thicken	Unfertilized, the egg is shed through the vagina as part of menstrual blood

0   2   4   6   8   10   12   14   16   18   20   22   24   26   28

IRREGULAR PERIODS

At various times in your life your periods may change their usual pattern. This may not be something to worry about but, if menstrual irregularities bother you or you have pain, you should discuss the problem with your doctor.

POST PUBERTY

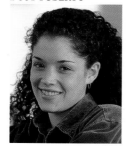

Periods can be irregular for the first couple of years. It may take some women until after they are 20 for their hormonal cycles to be fully established.

ATHLETE

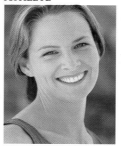

Excessive exercise with a marked decrease in body fat can stop your periods or make them irregular. This is reversible but may cause osteoporosis due to low oestrogen levels.

AFTER PREGNANCY

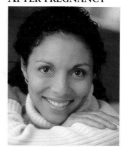

Normal periods usually resume about two months after giving birth if the mother is not breastfeeding. However, if she is it may take longer.

PERIMENOPAUSE

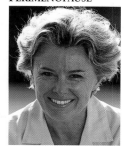

Irregular bleeding is one of the symptoms which indicates that hormones are becoming less influential. This stage can last for several years.

---

endometrium (uterus lining). After ovulation, the ovaries secrete the other female sex hormone, progesterone, to complete the preparation of the endometrium which is thickened for a possible pregnancy. The medical term for this is the secretory or luteal phase. If the released egg is not fertilized by sperm the levels of oestrogen and progesterone begin to drop and about 14 days after ovulation the unfertilized egg is shed through the vagina, together with the endometrium, as a menstrual period.

The loss of blood is described as menses. It may last from three to seven days with a varying amount of blood—the average loss is about 60 ml (2½ fl oz). It may be less if taking oral contraceptives. When menstruation begins, for many young women it takes a couple of years for periods to settle into a regular cycle. Minor fluctuations are normal at every age and the cycles may shorten in women over the age of 35.

ABSENT PERIODS

If menstruation doesn't start by the age of 16, or stops in a woman who is not pregnant or is approaching menopause, the medical term for this is amenorrhoea. If your periods become irregular (called oligomenorrhoea)—that is, they arrive less often than once every 35 days or stop altogether—it is important to see your doctor. Persistent lack of menstruation may affect your ability to become pregnant and weaken your bones, leading to osteoporosis later in life.

Late puberty is the commonest cause of primary amenorrhoea, or it may be due to a fault in the endocrine and reproductive systems. This may be because of poor nutrition (girls must reach a certain body weight before menstruation can start), hormonal disorders or a genetic disorder such as Turner syndrome in which one of the female sex chromosomes is absent.

Secondary amenorrhoea can have several causes—such as stress, weight loss and diet. Often periods can be stopped temporarily by excessive exercising and dieting (lowering the body fat to below 15 percent)—common in athletes, dancers, models and anorexic women. Illnesses, such as the bowel disorder, Crohn's disease, or thyroid problems, may all affect menstruation.

Another common cause of secondary amenorrhoea is polycystic ovary syndrome (PCOS. In this disease irregular ovulation is linked to an excess of male hormones produced by the ovaries or the adrenal glands or by premature menopause.

If your periods have not started at all or if they have started and subsequently stopped, the doctor will want to do a careful medical history. A test will be carried out to ensure you are not pregnant, the most common reason for amenorrhoea in the reproductive years.

The doctor will want to know whether you are taking any prescribed drugs that may be affecting your menstrual cycle. Blood tests will evaluate your hormone levels to determine whether your pituitary and thyroid glands are functioning as they should. If none is found to be a cause, the doctor may refer you to a ▶

See your doctor

The menstrual cycle is especially sensitive to external upsets such as lifestyle changes, which may be stressful or unusual (for example, prolonged travel), or an illness. However, you should see the doctor if:
♀ Your periods become unusually heavy.
♀ Your periods become irregular, are infrequent or stop altogether.
♀ You have bleeding between periods or after intercourse.
♀ You experience severe pain or heavy bleeding that interferes with your normal life.
♀ You start bleeding any time after menopause (usually defined as when you have been without periods for a whole year).

gynaecologist to check that your ovaries are functioning as they should, and whether there are any other underlying factors. In cases where the cause is not obvious, no specific treatment may be given. Your doctor may suggest waiting a few months to see if your periods establish a regular cycle. If blood tests find that there is an underlying hormonal imbalance the doctor may prescribe drugs to correct the problem or to induce ovulation. This, however, is only done when you want to conceive.

PAINFUL PERIODS

Abdominal pain or cramping—medically called dysmenorrhoea—is common during a period. The pain, which can vary from mild to severe, is generally in the lower abdomen and may spread to the lower back and thighs. Severe pain may be accompanied by bowel disturbances such as constipation or diarrhoea, as well as nausea, dizziness, faintness and vomiting.

Most women experience a painful menstruation at some point. Pain in the mid-abdomen, called *mittelschmerz*, occurs in ovulatory cycles (when an egg is released) and not in anovulatory ones (when no egg is released).

The mild cramp-like abdominal pains typical of primary dysmenorrhoea rarely begin after the age of 20. Once believed to be a psychosomatic symptom, the pains are actually caused by muscular contractions of the uterus which are similar to—but not as intense as—labour pains. Natural, hormone-like substances called prostaglandins are involved in uterine contractions. They are produced by the cervix and also help to seal blood vessels in order to prevent excess blood loss as the endometrium is shed.

More severe pain that may be caused by various conditions is known as secondary dysmenorrhoea; it may occur at any age. The pain is usually recurring and may be a symptom of: endometriosis, in which fragments of the endometrium are found in other parts of the pelvic cavity and bleed cyclically; an infection of the Fallopian tubes or of the ovaries; the presence of fibroids, which are benign tumours that tend to grow within the uterine wall, especially in women over the age of 30; and ovarian cysts. In some women the presence of an IUD (intrauterine contraceptive device or "coil") can cause such pain.

SELF-HELP WITH PAINFUL PERIODS

♀ Moderate physical exercise can be beneficial, but do not attempt it if the pain is severe. Gentle yoga-type stretches done through the day may help. Deep-breathing exercises will also help to alleviate the pain.

♀ Hugging your knees or lying on your back with your knees elevated may provide more comfort from menstrual pains.

♀ Heat can have a soothing effect —have a warm bath or shower or place a hot water bottle over your abdomen.

♀ Well-balanced meals containing plenty of fruit and vegetables can improve matters.

♀ Essential fatty acids (EFAs), especially from fish oils, have an anti-inflammatory effect which may ease pain.

♀ Aromatherapy can help with painful periods. Antispasmodic oils such as clary sage, cypress and lavender can be used with gentle abdominal massage.

♀ Acupuncture and acupressure may provide relief from backache and cramps.

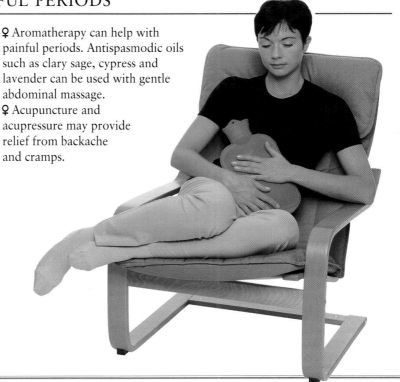

The type of dysmenorrhoea decides the treatment. The doctor compiles a history of the symptoms, when they began and occur and how long they last. A pelvic examination may also be carried out.

Primary dysmenorrhoea can usually be treated by a simple painkiller such as paracetamol, and by rest and relaxation techniques, as well as taking gentle exercise. There are also various medications that have been developed specifically for treating period pains. If this fails or the pain is more severe, your doctor may prescribe a three to six months' trial of nonsteroidal anti-inflammatory drugs (NSAIDs) that inhibit prostaglandin production. The more powerful NSAIDs include mefenamic acid, ibuprofen and ketoprofen. Hormonal treatment such as the oral contraceptive pill may also be suggested.

HEAVY PERIODS

About 1 in 10 women of reproductive age have heavy periods—called menorrhagia—in which the total blood loss exceeds 90 ml (3 fl oz) during one cycle. It is impossible in practice to measure how much blood you lose but, if you are menorrhagic, you may experience flooding, which soaks your underwear or bedclothes, may pass large blood clots, have to change sanitary towels or tampons frequently (more than every two hours) or have to wear extra absorbent tampons or double protection. Your periods may be so heavy that they limit your ability to live a normal home or work life.

Some women always have heavy periods and provided they are not anaemic and the effects of the periods are not intolerable there may be no need for any treatment. Periods can be heavier if you have recently given birth, have just stopped taking the oral contraceptive pill or have had an IUD inserted. Periods may also become heavier due to the development of a thicker endometrium as the menopause approaches. Irregularity caused by changes in the body's hormonal balance is also common at this time.

Other causes of heavy periods include fibroid tumours, polyps, endometriosis, pelvic inflammatory disease (PID), as well as a thyroid or blood clotting disorder. Sometimes an isolated heavy period may be an early miscarriage that occurred before the woman knew she was pregnant. In other cases, the problem is caused by changes in the blood clotting

mechanism in the uterus, changes in the concentration of prostaglandins or by changes in the body's hormonal control of periods. However, quite often no cause can be detected at all.

The doctor will perform a pelvic examination to check for fibroid tumours, polyps or any other abnormalities of the uterus and may refer you to a gynaecologist for further treatment. A cervical smear may be carried out, and if other symptoms include fatigue and breathlessness a blood sample may be tested for anaemia. If you have an IUD the doctor may suggest that you try changing your method of contraception to see whether this helps, although sometimes periods become more normal after a few months with an IUD in place.

The usual drugs prescribed include mefenamic acid and tranexamic acid, which can help reduce flow and provide pain relief. Other options for medical management are hormonal drugs such as the oral contraceptive pill, or progestogen preparations such as medroxyprogesterone, norethisterone and dydrogesterone which can reduce blood loss and regulate irregular periods. Mirena may also be used to control heavy periods. While they all may be effective you should know what side effects to expect before starting treatment.

Your gynaecologist may recommend an ultrasound scan to check for abnormalities in the uterus, or perform a hysteroscopy and uterine biopsy in which a special telescopic instrument is used to examine the uterus and to obtain endometrial tissue for lab analysis.

BREAKTHROUGH BLEEDING

Bleeding from the uterus between periods, called metrorrhagia, can be experienced for a variety of reasons. It is normal in some women throughout their reproductive life. It may be due to the presence of an IUD or occur while taking the oral contraceptive pill. It can also be a symptom of many vaginal or uterine disorders, such as fibroid tumours or polyps and may be a side effect of some types of hormone replacement therapy (HRT). If you have breakthrough bleeding, you should discuss it with your doctor.

> ### Endometrial ablation and resection
>
> These are surgical procedures in which the endometrium is destroyed either using a thermal balloon (diathermy) or a hot revolving metal ball (roller ball) or a laser, to burn away tissue. This reduces blood loss for around half to three-quarters of women with heavy periods. These treatments are not suitable for women with a very large uterus or those wanting to become pregnant.

BREAST CARE

The breasts are one part of the body which a woman finds almost impossible to ignore. They can play a crucial role in your sexual identity as well as in your nurturing role as a mother. They tend to change size and shape as you progress from puberty to old age. It is important to know which of these changes may need investigation.

See also:

1/BEING A WELL WOMAN
Healthy body systems
p. 33; p. 38

2/SEX & SEXUALITY
Discovering your sexuality p. 54

4/HORMONAL HEALTH
Endocrine system problems
pp. 140–145
Pregnancy and motherhood
pp. 170–179

See your doctor

Even if you do have fibrous tissue or cysts on a regular basis you should never ignore new lumps or any other changes to your breasts because there is always the possibility that a cancerous growth is present. It's important to remember that the earlier breast cancer is diagnosed the greater the possibility that it can be prevented from spreading.

Benign breast changes

There is an almost infinite variety in the shape and size of women's breasts. For example one can be bigger than the other. They can be rounded and full or rounded and small, stand away from the chest wall or hang down. Some nipples are prominent, others are inverted, and some women have extra nipples on the chest wall. All of these describe "normal" breasts which develop from puberty under the influence of the female hormone oestrogen, their shape depending on fatty and fibrous tissue surrounding the network of milk-secreting glands. Usually fully formed by the age of 20, breasts have no muscles but are supported by the pectoral muscles of the chest.

Few women go through life free from breast discomfort, whether it is pain before a period begins or tenderness which heralds the onset of a pregnancy. Some women regularly find lumps in their breasts but the majority of these are benign. In women under 25 these are almost always growths of harmless fibrous tissue, called fibroadenomas. Between 30 and 40 a woman is more likely to develop breast cysts which are full of fluid and can be painful. After consulting a doctor, the usual treatment is for the cyst to be drained using a needle and syringe, and the fluid sent for analysis to ensure that the cells are not cancerous. Cysts rarely need treatment.

BREAST PAIN

Medically known as mastalgia, breast pain is common and rarely a sign of serious disease: in fact, breast cancer is rarely accompanied by pain in the breast. In most women breast pain varies in severity through the menstrual cycle. It is usually worse just before a period when the breasts also tend to be lumpy. Most find that the pain disappears after the menopause. Starting hormone replacement therapy (HRT) may cause cyclical pain in the first months.

Some noncyclical pain has no known cause; it may be due to the weight of the breasts, muscle strain, a cyst or infection, even ill-fitting bras. If you have breast pain see your doctor. A breast examination and mammography may be done and your doctor may suggest you keep a pain diary. Noting when the pain occurs, its severity and details such as what you have eaten or just done (run for a bus, lifted a heavy weight, played sport) and stressful events will help you see after a few months whether your pain is cyclical and if anything makes it better or worse.

Breast pain can often be dealt with by simple changes. Make sure, for example, that your bras fit you properly. You should be measured by a trained bra fitter. If you play sport or do any form of vigorous exercise, wear a sports bra. You may need to alter your eating pattern to reduce your intake of caffeine and salt and foods containing fat, particularly those high in saturated fats. If you smoke try to stop. Try patches or gum or join a support group. Take up regular aerobic exercise.

For persistent pain your doctor may prescribe danazol, a hormonal drug which reduces oestrogen levels. However, it can have troublesome side effects such as weight gain and acne. Gamolenic acid can be useful and with its lack of anti oestrogenic side effects may be preferred by younger women who wish to continue on an oral contraceptive.

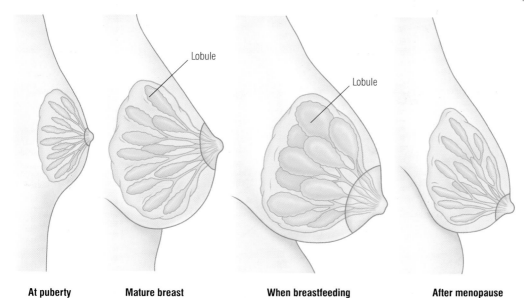

Lobule

Lobule

At puberty   **Mature breast**   **When breastfeeding**   **After menopause**

BREASTS AS YOU AGE
Mature breasts are composed of glandular tissue made up of 15 to 20 lobules. Milk-producing tissue becomes active in the days before a period starts when some women have tenderness and lumpiness. In pregnancy the breasts enlarge, the milk-duct system expands with more lobules formed. After the menopause, the glandular part shrinks as the proportion of fat increases, making the breasts less dense.

BREAST INFECTIONS

A breast abscess is a collection of pus which forms a firm, painful lump. It develops if mastitis, or inflammation of the breast caused by bacterial infection, is not treated promptly with antibiotics. Infective mastitis most commonly occurs during breastfeeding in the first six months when bacteria in the baby's mouth can enter the breast through a crack in the nipple.

Infections are characterized by redness and tenderness; you will have a raised temperature and feel unwell with flulike symptoms. Your doctor may prescribe antibiotics and you should continue to feed from the infected breast—which may be uncomfortable or painful—as the regular emptying of the breast reduces the likelihood of an abscess developing.

If an abscess does develop it will need to be drained, either with a fine needle or through a small incision made in the skin.

LUMPS IN THE BREAST

Many women have lumpy breasts, with the lumps becoming more obvious just before a menstrual period. (This tends to improve from around the age of 40, when fat starts to replace breast tissue.) This is known as fibrocystic condition and is a normal response to the hormonal changes of the menstrual cycle. Tenderness is often a feature of this condition.

Women with fibrocystic breasts are not at increased risk of breast cancer though the condition may make it more difficult for new lumps to be noticed. Regular self examinations (see next page) will make you familiar with the usual texture of your breasts so you are more likely to pick up changes if they occur. Cysts are ▶

Nipple problems

Some women are born with inverted nipples which may be corrected over several weeks by drawing out the nipple between finger and thumb. If a nipple suddenly becomes inverted, consult your doctor.

It is common for breasts to discharge a little, often before a period—particularly if you take the oral contraceptive pill—and this is not usually a cause for concern. Milky discharge is often present in the later stages of pregnancy and may persist for weeks or months after stopping breastfeeding.

Even women who have never been pregnant may produce a small amount of discharge if they squeeze their nipples. This may be due to an excess of prolactin, the hormone that stimulates milk secretion, or may be caused by aprolactinoma, a non-cancerous tumour in the pituitary gland at the base of the brain.

Yellow or bloodstained discharge may be due to a non-cancerous tumour in a milk duct. This needs investigating by your doctor. Discharge containing pus usually indicates an infection for which antibiotics will be needed. Clear discharge does not generally need treatment.

filled with fluid but may be felt as smooth lumps. They are sometimes painful. One in two women who have a cyst will have further ones; they do not necessarily need treatment, but you should always get them checked by your doctor.

Another type of lump, a fibroadenoma, is firm, painless and tends to move around easily when the breast is felt. They are most common in women aged between 15 and 30 and can get bigger during pregnancy and breastfeeding. They do not usually require any treatment and many disappear within a year or two. However, if you are worried or the lump is large, you should discuss it with your doctor who may recommend that it is removed.

HOW LUMPS ARE INVESTIGATED

If you notice a new lump in your breast see your doctor immediately. Imaging tests such as mammography or ultrasound scanning may be arranged. Fine needle aspiration may also be performed, a procedure in which a small syringe needle is inserted into the lump to withdraw cells. This may be uncomfortable but it doesn't take long to do. If the lump is solid, the cell samples will be sent for lab analysis.

KNOW YOUR OWN BREASTS

Breasts are influenced by hormonal variation, which can make them sensitive, over-heavy, over-full, tender or lumpy. Every woman should know her own breasts well, how they look and feel at different times of the month so that she is confident about what is normal for her. A self-examination is recommended for every woman from the age of 20: once a month five to seven days after the start of her period. Menopausal women should examine their breasts at the same time each month.

You can lie down or examine yourself while in the shower. Place one arm behind your head and with the flat of your fingers of the opposite hand, feel all over the breast and armpit, first gently and then more firmly. Don't prod or push or squeeze. Also look at your breasts in a mirror. Notice any changes such as dimpling or puckering of the skin, whether the nipples look as usual without any sign of discharge, bleeding or a rash.

It is also worthwhile reminding yourself that most women will not develop breast cancer and that if you do find a lump, nine out of 10 that are discovered are benign.

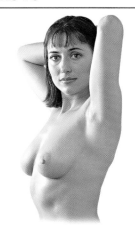

1 *Stand in front of a mirror, raise your arms above your head and lean forward so you can see the shape of your breasts and how they move from side to side.*

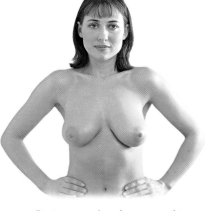

2 *Put your hands on your hips so that your chest muscles tense. Look again, then turn sideways so that you can see the contours of your breasts from every angle.*

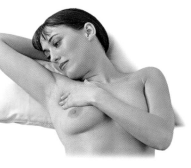

3 *Now lie down with one arm behind your head. Use the flat of the fingers of your other hand to feel for any lump or thickening.*

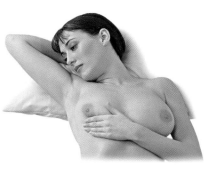

4 *Work your way around your breast in a spiral, covering the whole area. It is also important to feel the armpits, but don't prod.*

The presence of fluid determines that the problem is a cyst and usually all fluid will be withdrawn. A sample may be sent for analysis, as very rarely cancer can develop in the wall of a cyst.

You are bound to be anxious if you do find something during self-examination, but keep reminding yourself that nine out of every 10 lumps are benign—in other words, they have nothing to do with cancer.

Your doctor may be able to reassure you that there is nothing to worry about but if there is the slightest doubt you may ask for an appointment at a breast clinic where the problem can be investigated with tests such as a mammogram or by a biopsy—taking a sample of cells for microscopic examination in the laboratory. The odds are that you will have something minor like a cyst, but even if abnormal cells have been found and cancer is suspected, the earlier it is diagnosed and treatment begun, the better the chances that the treatment will be effective.

MAMMOGRAPHY

The national screening programme offers women from the age of 50 to 65 a mammogram —a breast X-ray—every three years. After 65, an invitation to be screened may not be sent but you can request it through your doctor. If a woman had early menopause or has a family history of breast cancer she may have a mammogram as recommended by her doctor, in some cases every two years. Generally, screening is thought not to be suitable for women under 50 as their breasts are denser, making mammograms harder to "read", also because breast cancer is not common in this age group.

The aim of mammography is to detect cancer at a very early stage before it has a chance to spread. As the incidence of breast cancer increases with age (1 in 14 by age 70, 1 in 10 at 80) women who are in these age groups may consider annual mammograms a worthwhile investment. Mammography can also be used to investigate breast abnormalities.

Mammography picks up most, but not 100 percent of, cancerous tumours. Although you can feel reassured by a normal result, you should continue to check your breasts regularly.

HOW MAMMOGRAPHY IS DONE

You must remember not to use deodorant or powder in the underarm or breast area. The radiographer will ask you to undress to the waist and will then position each breast in turn between a Perspex cover and the X-ray plate so that the breast tissue is compressed. Two pictures of each breast will be taken.

The test may cause mild discomfort, especially if you are small-breasted, but lasts only a few minutes. It is easier for the radiographer to position your breasts in precisely the right way if you can relax.

You will be asked to wait, usually for about 10 to 15 minutes, while the film is processed to ensure the image is clear. The X-rays are analysed by a radiologist who gives the result to your doctor or may contact you direct if the picture was not clear (you may have moved during the X-ray) and it has to be repeated.

Who is at risk?

Between five and 10 percent of women have an increased risk of developing breast cancer at an early age due to a genetic link. A woman with one first degree relative— mother or sister—with breast cancer has a slightly higher risk than other women. If two of her first degree relatives have had the disease the risk is greater. Women who fall into this category may wish to have a gene test and counselling to determine what this might mean. Having the gene does not mean that you will develop the cancer.

The risk of developing breast cancer in women taking long-term HRT is less than that reported from drinking two glasses of alcohol a day, smoking cigarettes or being obese after menopause. Studies show that after five years on HRT, there are two extra cases per 1000 women; after 10 years, six extra cases per 1000; after 15 years, 12 extra cases. There is no evidence there are more breast cancer deaths. The increase in risk also reduces after stopping HRT—after four years it is not significantly elevated.

Breast cancer is both age- and oestrogen-related. In particular, the less time a woman is exposed to her own hormones (from puberty to menopause), the lower her risk. In the population as a whole, risk estimates show that for women aged from 50 to 54, the risk is 1 in 450; from 55 to 59, 1 in 386; from 60 to 64, 1 in 292; and from 65 to 69, 1 in 244.

A national study of hormone therapy and mammography is not due to be completed until 2005.

! Caution

Your breasts will have to be squeezed briefly to flatten them in order to produce a good image on the mammogram, which is an X-ray photograph. The flattening may be uncomfortable but is not dangerous. If your breasts have been augmented with an implant, do inform the radiographer as this may make a difference to the way the X-ray is taken and analysed by the radiologist.

Breast cancer

Women can still be reluctant to go to their doctor when they first notice a lump. But time is important because many forms of cancer can be cured or at least controlled if they are diagnosed and treated early.

Treatment is likely to be more effective when it is provided by doctors who are experienced in dealing with a particular form of cancer. Those cancers that only affect women are best treated by gynaecological oncologists, specialists in both gynaecology and cancer. Talk to your doctor about the various options available.

WHAT ARE THE RISK FACTORS?

Some women may be more susceptible to developing breast cancer than others as a result of their genetic inheritance or lifestyle although many individuals who have several or even all of the risk factors listed below will never do so.

Being over the age of 50 Although younger women do get the condition, three-quarters of those affected are in the older age group.

A family history of breast cancer This is especially relevant if it developed at a relatively early age. Having one first degree relative (mother or sister) with breast cancer doubles the risk; having two multiplies it five-fold.

Having no children, or a first pregnancy after the age of 35 These women have about double the risk of a woman who has her first child before the age of 20. Women who choose not to breastfeed may also be at greater risk.

Beginning your periods before the age of 12 and having late menopause (after the age of 50) The longer the time between menarche and menopause the greater the risk. In China where there is a low incidence of breast cancer, the average age for a girl to begin her periods is 17 years, compared with 12.5 years in the UK.

Inheriting one or both of the genes (known as BRCA1 and BRCA2) These are associated with an increased susceptibility to breast and ovarian cancer; 50 to 60 percent of women with this genetic inheritance will develop breast cancer. However, only 5 to 10 percent of all breast cancer is thought to be genetic in origin.

Regular high alcohol consumption, a diet high in saturated fats and an inactive lifestyle In all countries where a sedentary lifestyle and fatty food predominate the incidence of breast cancer has increased drastically.

WHEN CANCER IS DETECTED

Breast cancer is identified either by biopsy—taking a sample of tissue for analysis, or by CT scan, computer-assisted tomography, in which a three-dimensional X-ray picture of the breast is built up. Large-needle core biopsy is now an alternative to excision for some breast abnormalities which are non-palpable (not able to be felt by examination). A sample of tissue is extracted very accurately with a needle, under local anaesthetic. The operation can be done on an out-patient basis and you get the results quickly. The most important factor in analysing the tissue is whether the cancer is invasive or not. Invasive disease means cancer that is spreading out of the duct or lobule in which the lump was found. Most breast cancers are of this type.

Non-invasive disease describes cancer that grows in just one place inside the duct or lobule—called carcinoma in situ. Abnormal cell growth is called atypical hyperplasia; some types may be premalignant and may be regarded as a warning sign that cancer may develop.

Other rarer types of cancer include Paget's disease, where a slow-growing cancer produces

---

> **! Caution**
>
> It is difficult to say with certainty what the outcome will be for a particular treatment and individual. You need to get your information from someone who can explain what any statistics mean in your particular case. The specialist should talk you through your treatment options, answering any questons you may have.

SENTINEL NODE MAPPING
The technique of sentinel node mapping is used to detect whether cancer has spread to the lymph nodes. The "sentinel node" is the first lymph node draining a tumour. It is identified by injecting the tumour with a radioactive dye. The first node found to contain dye is removed and sampled (a biopsy). If there are no cancerous cells found, there is a 98 percent certainty that the cancer has not spread to the lymph node in the armpit.

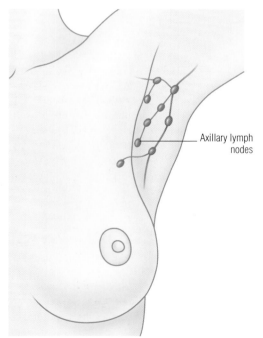

Axillary lymph nodes

changes in the nipple; cystic carcinoma, a cancer growing within a cyst; and inflammatory cancer which causes swelling, redness and pain, spreads quickly and has no evident lump.

Two crucial questions have to be answered before treatment is decided. Is the chance of spread to other parts of the body high or low? What can be done to reduce that chance? There are many factors doctors look at before making a choice: they want to know whether the tumour has spread to the lymph nodes, and if so how many are involved; they look at the size of the original tumour when removed by surgery, compared to what it was before the operation. Blood tests are carried out to measure substances called CEA, CA153, CA199 and others. Rising levels may indicate cancer is recurring or spreading).

THE AIMS OF TREATMENT

Treating breast cancer has three aims: to remove the primary tumour, to reduce the chance of the cancer returning in the breast or armpit, and to reduce the chance of the cancer establishing secondaries in the body (called distant spread).

The medical team's recommendations will consider all the factors that might affect you, including the emotional, social, spiritual and financial aspects of treatment as well as the physical. It is important that you are actively involved in the discussion and understand as much as possible about the proposed treatment.

SURGERY AS TREATMENT

The aim of surgery is to effect a cure where the disease is confined to the breast, to achieve local control of the disease, to prevent complications such as skin ulceration, to determine the existence and extent of lymph node involvement, and to obtain sufficient tumour to assess further treatment and prognosis. The options are:

Total or simple mastectomy The removal of the entire breast, but no chest muscle.

Modified radical mastectomy The removal of the entire breast and pectoralis minor muscle to allow removal of axillary lymph nodes.

Subcutaneous mastectomy Sometimes used with high-risk precancerous conditions, most tissue is removed, leaving skin and nipple intact. The breast is reconstructed with an implant.

Lumpectomy The local excision of the lump. The lump is located with magnetic resonance imaging (MRI) and removed along with surrounding tissue with an electrical "pencil" in a technique called mono-polar cautery, which seals off the blood vessels as it goes.

Quadrantectomy Similar to lumpectomy but more tissue, the entire quadrant (a quarter of the breast), is removed.

Lymph gland (axillary nodes) removal This may follow sentinel node mapping which checks for spread of cancer cells.

Breast reconstruction Sometimes this is done at the same time as mastectomy, sometimes much later (pp. 156–157).

ADJUVANT THERAPIES

Two types of therapies may be used, either before or after surgery, depending on where the cancer is.

Radiotherapy Normally following surgery, radiation aims to destroy any cancer cells which were not removed during the operation. It may be done externally, with the radiation targeted through the skin, or internally by inserting radioactive material into the affected tissues under a general anaesthetic. The average course is five days a week for five or six weeks, starting one month after surgery when you are able to move your arm and shoulder again.

Chemotherapy Sometimes given in pill form, more often chemotherapy involves giving cytotoxic (cell-killing) drugs through an intravenous drip, over several weeks. This type of treatment may be suggested for women under 50, especially where tests show cancer cells in the axillary nodes. It is usually done following surgery, but may be given to shrink a large tumour before an operation to remove it. An alternative is to give half the chemotherapy, pause for radiotherapy, then complete the treatment with more chemotherapy.

INTRA OPERATIVE RADIOTHERAPY

A new treatment is being developed, called "Breast Cancer Wand". During surgery to remove a tumour, a probe is placed into the resulting cavity. A device delivers X-rays to the tissue immediately around where the tumour was found. ▸

Getting a second opinion

It is important not to rush into making a decision about treatment until you are assured you have as much information as possible. While breast cancer treatment can be very successful, there is no such thing as the ideal treatment for all women.

Much research is being done to develop new treatments and to refine and improve existing ones. Build up a clear picture of the pros and cons. Questions which you might ask your doctor include:

♀ How long has this treatment been in use?

♀ What is the success rate for your patients?

♀ Are there any side effects and how common are they?

♀ How long does the treatment take?

♀ How much time should I take off work?

HORMONE THERAPY

Many breast cancers grow in the presence of the hormone oestrogen. In breast cancer, hormonal treatments are designed either to alter oestrogen levels or to prevent the tumour from taking it up. Tamoxifen, the best known of these treatments, is mostly given to women who are past the menopause as it can cause menopausal symptoms. It is never offered to pregnant women who also have breast cancer. A newer drug called toremifene, which works in a similar way, is an alternative for women who experience side effects such as hot flushes. Other hormonal treatments such as progestogen, aromatase inhibitors and LHRH analogues which also inhibit oestrogen production may be used if a woman develops a resistance to tamoxifen.

REMOVAL OF THE OVARIES

Surgery to remove the ovaries (a bilateral oophorectomy) or radiation used to destroy them (an ovarian ablation), may be done to alter the levels of hormones in the body. This procedure is necessary due to the fact that the hormones have an effect on the way breast cancer behaves.

BREAST RECONSTRUCTION

Women who have a breast removed may be offered a breast reconstruction, either at the time of the mastectomy or later. This can be done using an implant or with tissue taken from a muscle in the back or from the abdomen. If you are considering this option, discuss it with your breast surgeon and a plastic surgeon. While a reconstructed breast may never look exactly the same as before surgery, many women are happy with the results, but this type of surgery is not right for everyone. Prostheses (artificial breasts) worn inside a bra can look natural under everyday clothes; there are also ranges of beach, swim and sportswear designed for women who have had mastectomies.

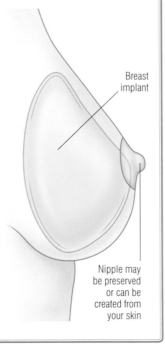

Breast implant

Nipple may be preserved or can be created from your skin

There may be an option to have an oophorectomy instead of, or as well as, chemotherapy. The disadvantage is that it causes an immediate menopause. Women at high risk of recurrence may choose to give up their ability to have children or more children to improve the chances of a cure. An injection of ovary-supressing drug, goserelin, induces a reversible menopause in younger women.

COPING STRATEGIES

Having a serious illness is stressful and you may find that even the most caring doctors and nurses may not be able to help you think straight about the choice you make and what lies ahead. It is common to feel uncertain and alone. At the same time, it is important to remember that decisions rarely have to be made immediately. Seek the assistance of a psychologist or specialist counsellor who can help you develop the skills to cope and get through this critical time. Your partner, children and parents may be scared too and may need reassurance and support.

Mind and body medicine is not a cure, but provides you with tools for managing anxiety and discomfort. These include relaxation techniques, guided imagery, cognitive restructuring and assertiveness training. Find out at the hospital whether there is a group you can join where you can meet others with breast cancer.

As with any disease, you should avoid any complementary therapy or alternative practitioner claiming to offer you a cure. There is no evidence that such a possibility exists. Wise use of complementary approaches, such as visualization, massage, aromatherapy and yoga, however, can make you feel better during treatment for the cancer. You should always think carefully before deciding to discontinue any orthodox treatment while it still has something to offer you.

AFTER THE OPERATION

You will be encouraged to get out of bed as soon as possible after surgery. There is no need to be in pain—you can take painkillers if necessary. Your arm movement will be restricted at first but exercise will help restore it. Stitches are usually taken out within two weeks and the scar will heal in two to four weeks. There may be problems with the flow of lymph after surgery to the lymph nodes or radiation therapy which can cause the arm to swell (lymphodema). Tubular compression garments can be made to help with this. The usual treatment is massage to encourage lymph drainage, use of a mechanical pump to reduce swelling and exercises, such as those below, which involve raising the arm. Discuss it with your doctor if it continues or worries you.

CARING FOR YOURSELF

Once your treatment is finished, it could be a good time to adopt a healthy eating programme. Building a regular exercise routine into your life will benefit your overall health and can improve your psychological well-being.

POST-OPERATIVE EXERCISE

You should start exercising to regain arm movement as soon as you feel able to do so, usually the day after the operation. Do exercises 1 and 2 only for the first five days, then add in exercises 3 to 6 and continue them until you can move both arms equally well. Try to use your affected arm as normally as possible; use it when brushing your hair or doing light housework. Build up gradually to heavier activities, but stop if it causes pain. There may be discomfort at first; it may help if you take painkillers 30 minutes before exercising.

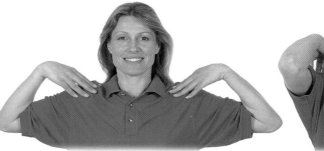

1 *While sitting, hold your hands relaxed in your lap. Shrug your shoulders up to your ears, then push them down. Next pull your shoulders forward, then brace them back. Repeat five times, twice a day.*

2 *Stand with your arms by your sides then raise them to shoulder level. With your fingertips on your shoulders circle both shoulders back, then forward. Repeat five times twice a day.*

3 *Standing or sitting, rest your fingers lightly on your shoulders. Slowly lift your bent arms up in front, then lower them. Repeat 10 times, three times a day.*

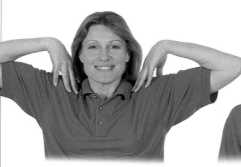

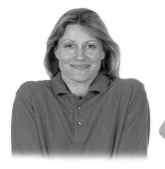

4 *Keeping your hands on your shoulders, move your elbows out to the side. Slowly lower your arms to your waist then raise them up again to shoulder level. Repeat 10 times, three times a day.*

5 *Raise your affected arm to shoulder level, then slowly lift your hand to behind your neck. Stretch the arm out again, then reach behind your back, with your hand at bra level. Repeat 10 times, three times a day.*

6 *Stand with your affected arm stretched out to shoulder level. Gradually lift it above your head, then lower it slowly. Repeat the exercise with your arm straight out in front. Repeat 10 times, three times a day.*

CERVICAL PROBLEMS

From the time a woman becomes sexually active, staying well and ensuring good reproductive health requires regular checks on the genital area. Any changes that do occur in the cervix or surrounding tissue can be detected by a simple test, and treated.

See your doctor

Any vaginal bleeding after menopause should be discussed with your doctor in case further investigation is needed. It may simply be caused by vaginal dryness, which can be treated with various lubricants.

Screening for health

When you turn 18 or when you become sexually active, you should ensure that you have a cervical smear on a regular basis; this is usually done in conjunction with a pelvic examination. If you have more than one sexual partner most doctors recommend both tests be done yearly, along with practising safe sex. If you are not sexually active, or are in a monogamous ongoing relationship, the doctor may consider three- or five-yearly screening satisfactory.

There is increasing incidence of cervical cancer in younger women who are smokers, have nutritional deficiencies or a sexually transmitted disease (STD). The cervical smear is the most efficient method of detecting the human papillomavirus (HPV), the common STD known to be involved in cervical cancer. The test

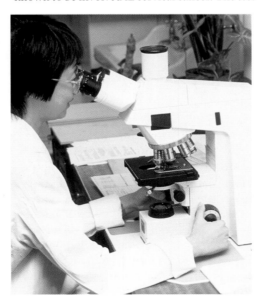

is done at the doctor's surgery, midway through the menstrual cycle (if you have not yet had the menopause), about two weeks after the start of your last period.

Changes in the cervix—the neck of the uterus—or the surrounding tissue can range from very minor ones affecting the epithelial (surface) cells in the membrane covering the cervix, to actual cancer, with many grades in between. Treatment can be given if necessary to get rid of abnormal, precancerous cells and even if cancer is found it can be effectively treated if it is picked up at an early enough stage. You may need to have repeat tests if the results of the previous cervical smears were ambiguous or not completely normal.

CERVICAL SMEAR AND PELVIC EXAMINATION

To improve the test accuracy, in the week before your appointment you should avoid vaginal creams, foams or suppositories; in the 24 hours before do not douche, have sex or use tampons.

Nobody enjoys this examination but it is completed quickly and if you can relax it should not be painful. The doctor will ask you to remove clothes and underwear below the waist and to lie on your back on an examination table. An instrument called a speculum will be inserted to part the walls of the vagina so that the cervix can be seen and checked for any sign of

HOW CERVICAL SMEARS ARE ANALYSED
In the laboratory the glass slide is examined through a microscope by a cytologist, a specialist in cells of the body, or analysed by computer. There is a routine for checking the cells for changes in shape or colour.

irritation or disease. The doctor will scrape some cells from the covering of the cervix and the cervical canal which will be smeared onto a slide and sent to a laboratory for microscopic analysis.

The speculum will be removed and the doctor will inspect the vulva and vagina, then use a gloved hand to check that your ovaries, uterus and Fallopian tubes are healthy.

Women over 50 may be advised to have a yearly pelvic examination as a precautionary measure against ovarian cancer. Your doctor may also check the wall separating the rectum and the vagina, using a gloved and lubricated finger. This is common practice in women over 40.

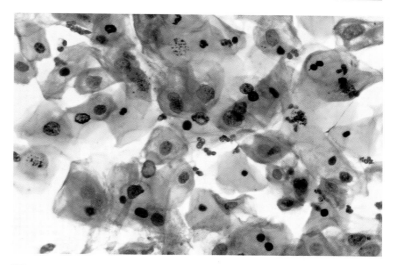

CHECKING THE RESULTS

You will be sent the results of your cervical smear, in which your doctor will let you know if it is normal or has shown abnormal cells. If the test needs to be repeated it should not be a cause for concern—sometimes the cell sample is unsatisfactory for a technical reason and a second check is required. If your results show anything other than normal cells you will need to discuss this with your doctor.

Whether further investigations and treatment will be required depends in part on the changes that have been found.

Abnormal cells are classified as CIN1, 2 or 3, depending on how deeply the changes have affected the covering cell layer in the cervix. CIN stands for cervical intraepithelial neoplasia, which may also be referred to as cervical dysplasia or precancerous changes.

CIN1 Mild, with only one-third of the cell layer thickness affected.

CIN2 Moderate, affecting two-thirds of the cell layer thickness.

CIN3 Affecting the full thickness.

CIS This fourth category stands for carcinoma in situ, but despite the name it does not necessarily mean that cancer is present.

Doctors do not always agree on whether treatment is needed for CIN1 and CIN2, as the cells can sometimes return to normal on their own in time. The most usual procedure is to have a repeat cervical smear, and then another in three or six months, to check whether this has happened. Antibiotics may also be prescribed. If the test following this is abnormal a tissue sample will be taken, followed by a colposcopy (p. 160).

WARNING SIGNS

Early, precancerous changes rarely cause any symptoms and one stage can move to the other over years. It is known that dysplasia is most common between the ages of 25 and 35, carcinoma in situ between 30 and 40 and invasive cancer between 40 and 60. The symptoms of cervical cancer are often ignored because women may regard them as a normal part of life and don't bother to mention them to their doctor.

Especially if you are a smoker, it is worth seeing your doctor if you experience vaginal discharge that doesn't go away, especially if it smells unpleasant or shows traces of blood. If you feel pain or discomfort during sex or bleed after sex this may also be a warning. Usually a cervical smear will be done to determine the health of the cervix so that appropriate treatment can be decided.

OTHER CERVICAL CONDITIONS

There may be possible causes other than CIN for discharge or pain:

Cervicitis Inflammation of the cervix, may be both acute and chronic. It can be caused by infection of a cervical tear in childbirth but more usually is associated with STDs (chlamydia, gonorrhoea, genital herpes and trichomoniasis).

Cervical incompetence Premature opening of the cervix during pregnancy, creating a high risk of late miscarriage or premature birth.

Cervical cysts These form when a mucus gland on the cervix is blocked. They require no treatment and clear up by themselves.

Cervical polyps Benign growths which may cause irregular bleeding and discharge. They can affect fertility and may be removed surgically.

CELLS OF THE CERVIX
For close examination, cells are seen at a greatly enlarged size through a microscope. The cytologist will look for the presence of STDs and in particular HPV which can cause cervical cancer. HPV incidence is highest in women aged from 18 to 28.

> **! Caution**
> After cervical treatment, it's advisable to wash or shower every day and use sanitary towels or liners rather than tampons. You should not have long, hot, soapy baths, use soap inside the vagina or use "feminine hygiene" products such as sprays. Avoid wearing synthetic, tight-fitting clothes (such as tights and stretch trousers). Choose cotton underwear and clothing in preference to other types of fabric.

Cervical cancer

When precancerous changes in cervical cells are found tests will be carried out to find out how far they have spread. The first test is likely to be a colposcopy which involves shining a light on to the cervix and looking at its surface through a magnifying lens. Tissue and cell samples can be taken from any area which looks abnormal using a technique called a punch biopsy. A colposcopy usually takes about 15 minutes and should be only a little more uncomfortable than having a cervical smear.

If this test reveals a more serious abnormality the next step may be a cone biopsy in which a section of the central lining of the cervix is removed under general anaesthetic. This may get rid of all the abnormal cells and no further treatment will be needed. The tissue which was removed will be examined in a pathology lab and you are likely to have to wait for a week or so for the results.

POSSIBLE TREATMENTS

The three main types of surgical treatment to remove precancerous cells can all, except diathermy, be carried out in an outpatient clinic under local anaesthetic.

Laser evaporation A concentrated beam of light of a specific wavelength is used to "burn away" the cells.

Cryotherapy A metal probe, cooled to the temperature of about -160°C, is used to freeze and therefore kill the abnormal cells.

SUPPORT AT A DIFFICULT TIME
Accept as much support from friends and your medical team as you can. It may be difficult to remember all that has been discussed in a meeting with your doctor, so taking a friend or member of your family with you may help.

Questions for your doctor to answer on cervical cancer

♀ Will I experience any side effects from the treatment?
♀ Are there any complications I should expect, such as anaemia?
♀ When is it safe to resume sexual relations with my partner?
♀ Are my periods likely to be affected?
♀ Should I be using sanitary towels rather than tampons?
♀ Is it possible to consider pregnancy in the future?
♀ What is the likelihood of recurrence of the disease in my particular case?
♀ When should I come back for my first check-up after treatment and for how many years should I return for regular check-ups?
♀ How often should I have a cervical smear now that I have had cervical cancer?
♀ Will I be able to use hormone replacement therapy?

Large loop excision A thin wire is applied to the surface of the cervix to cut the cells away.

Diathermy An electrical current is applied to the cells to burn and destroy them.

The other treatments are radiation therapy and chemotherapy. They may be given in various combinations.

It is unusual for cervical cancer to spread beyond the nearby tissues; it is also unlikely to provoke secondary tumours in relatively distant parts of the body.

Your doctor will discuss with you what treatment he or she thinks is most appropriate in your case and why, and you should also be told about any potential side effects which you may experience. Unless the cancer has reached a very advanced stage by the time it is first detected, treatment is often completely successful.

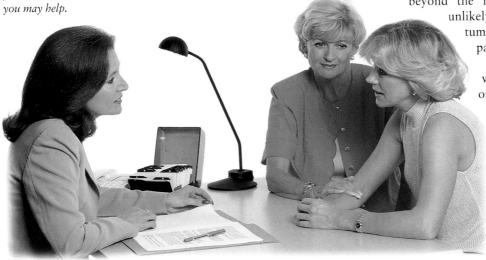

SURGERY

If tests indicate that the cancer is confined to the cervix itself or has only just begun to spread beyond it, it may well be possible to get rid of it completely with surgery. This may mean removal of the uterus, cervix and possibly the nearby lymph nodes, or a more major operation known as a radical (or Wertheim) hysterectomy which involves removing the uterus, cervix, the upper part of the vagina and some adjacent tissues.

An operation of this type can be a most upsetting prospect for a woman to face and she may need help to come to terms with it. Many hospitals and cancer support groups offer counselling services that can also explain aspects of the surgery and the effects on your body. Although physical recovery takes only weeks, it may take much longer to get over the psychological consequences, particularly if part of the vagina has been removed.

RADIOTHERAPY

This form of treatment is likely to be recommended if the cancer has spread any further than beyond the cervix itself, because it offers a greater chance of cure than an operation. It works by targeting the rapidly dividing cancer cells and destroying them.

Radiotherapy (also called radiation therapy) can be given externally—much the same as having an X-ray—or internally, feeding radioactive material through a tube leading directly into the affected area. Many women are treated with both in turn. Either way, the dose of radiation needs to be relatively high to be fully effective, and this means that there is a risk of side effects as a result of damage to healthy tissue during treatment. A premenopausal woman should be informed that the treatment will bring her instant artificial menopause as the ovaries stop working. There may be other side effects later, such as bowel and bladder problems and it is essential to find out as much as possible about the potential risks from your medical team.

CHEMOTHERAPY

When a cancer has grown to the point where surgery or radiotherapy would be difficult, a course of chemotherapy may be recommended to shrink the tumour first. It may also be needed following radiotherapy to reduce the chances of the cancer recurring.

TYPE AND STAGE OF CANCER

Tests include blood tests, X-rays, pelvic ultrasound and body scans—CT (computer tomography) or MRI (magnetic resonance imaging). A pelvic examination under anaesthetic may be performed. Alternatively an intravenous urogram (IVU) is carried out, in which a dye is fed into your arm through an IV drip to enable the doctor to check for any abnormalities in the kidneys or urinary system. There are several stages of cancer of the cervix:

Stage	What is happening
Stage 0	Carcinoma in situ, a very early cancer.
Stage I	Cancer cells have penetrated the cervix but have remained confined to the uterus.
Stage II	The cancerous cells have spread to other parts of the pelvis, such as the tissues around the cervix and the upper part of the vagina.
Stage III	There is evidence of cancerous cells throughout the pelvic area, down to the lower part of the vagina and perhaps blocking the ureters which connect the kidneys to the bladder.
Stage IV	The cancer has spread into the bladder or outside the pelvis.

The most common type of cervical cancer is known as squamous cell carcinoma and affects the covering of the cervix. A rarer form, called adenocarcinoma, may affect the glandular cells in the cervix. Only when all the tests have been completed will your doctor be in a position to discuss the most appropriate form of treatment.

Anticancer (or cytotoxic) drugs are given in liquid form as an intravenous drip or injection, or as a pill. The different doses and combinations of the drugs depend on each individual circumstances. Your doctor will explain how the treatment will be done and make you aware of possible side effects such as fatigue, increased susceptibility to infection and the effect on bone marrow. With modern treatment, the doctors will endeavour to reduce the nausea, sickness and hair loss which are toxic effects of chemotherapy.

UTERINE PROBLEMS

The uterus is an adaptable, muscular organ at the core of the reproductive system. In order for it to provide the life support system for a foetus it must be kept healthy. However, it can be prone to a variety of problems.

Changes in the uterus

The uterus lies behind the bladder and in a woman who is not pregnant is the shape and size of an upside-down pear: approximately 7.5 cm (3 in) long and 5 cm (2 in) at its widest point. The upper, wide part of the uterus is known as the body and the lower, narrow neck which leads into the vagina is called the cervix. Before pregnancy, the cavity of the uterus is small and narrow. Its muscular walls have a thick middle layer known as the myometrium and an inner vascular lining called the endometrium.

The endometrium thickens every month under the influence of hormones in preparation for the implantation of a fertilized egg. If pregnancy does not occur, the endometrial cells degenerate and the uterus sheds them through the process of menstruation.

ENDOMETRIOSIS

In this disease cells similar to the type that normally line the uterus become established outside it. The cells may travel anywhere in the pelvic area—on to one or both ovaries, the Fallopian tubes, the bladder, the uterus, the bowel, the peritoneum—the membrane lining the abdominal cavity—or on the pelvic wall. These cells then respond to the hormonal changes of the menstrual cycle. During part of the month they grow and when the lining of the uterus is being shed the endometrium breaks down and bleeds in the same way. Because these cells are trapped inside the pelvic area, they become raw when they bleed and spread, joining organs to each other, or to the pelvic wall. These areas of tissue are called adhesions. They can form swellings which fill with dark blood. Because of this appearance, doctors call these chocolate cysts.

Endometriosis is a complicated and difficult disease, with symptoms such as abdominal pain, backache, cramps and sometimes nausea and dizziness. It often goes undetected, as women—and sometimes their doctor—attribute the symptoms simply to painful periods. However, not only is it a common condition, it is also a leading cause of infertility. One in 20 women

UTERUS POSITION
20 percent of women have a retroverted uterus. This is when the uterus tilts backward rather than forward. It is a harmless condition. A retroflexed uterus is tilted back even further. If this is as a result of disease, it may be uncomfortable.

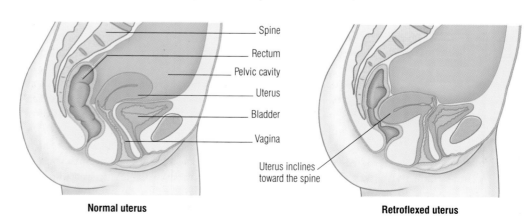

Spine
Rectum
Pelvic cavity
Uterus
Bladder
Vagina
Uterus inclines toward the spine

Normal uterus

Retroflexed uterus

Ways to cope with pelvic pain

♀ Keep a pain diary: record in it your pain levels every day, three times a day (morning, noon and bedtime).
♀ Describe what you were doing at the time: watching TV, working, socializing etc.
♀ Rate the pain on a scale of 1 to 10: from not too bad to very painful.
♀ Rate any distress (anger, frustration, sadness) you feel because of the pain: from 1, little distress, through to 10, the worst possible distress.

Keep the diary for a week and then analyse it. Are your pain ratings lower than your distress? If so, reducing distress may affect the pain. Any method which brings relaxation will help you to gain control.

of childbearing age referred to gynaecologists has endometriosis.

The cause of the disease is unknown. One theory is that it is related in some way to the malfunctioning of the immune system. "Reverse" menstruation is another theory: in this, endometriosis starts when a small amount of the menstrual flow goes up the Fallopian tubes (instead of down). The blood enters the pelvic cavity and then reaches the whole abdominal cavity where the cells implant and spread—in some rare cases it may go as far as the lungs, brain and legs.

There is no known way of preventing endometriosis, although studies show that the oral contraceptive pill and pregnancy both protect against the condition.

METHODS OF DIAGNOSIS

The most usual symptom of endometriosis is severe pain—at the time of periods, at ovulation, when emptying the bowels and during sexual intercourse. Inability to become pregnant is also common and tests for infertility may be the way its presence is discovered. It can sometimes be difficult to distinguish the symptoms of endometriosis from those of pelvic inflammatory disease (p. 164).

At present endometriosis may only be diagnosed by laparoscopic examination—a minimally invasive surgical procedure in which a tube with a tiny camera at one end is inserted just below the navel into the pelvic area. It is performed under general anaesthetic.

BENIGN TUMOURS

The most common uterine problems are polyps and fibroid tumours, benign tumours with no known cause. Polyps occur in the cervix or endometrium and are usually harmless. A cervical polyp may cause a watery, blood-streaked discharge between periods, after sex, or postmenopausally. The discharge may be smelly. Polyps may be removed surgically.

Fibroids, made up of bundles of muscle fibres that grow in the wall of the uterus, can be pea or grapefruit size. They occur in 20 percent of women over 30. Some have no symptoms, however an urgent need to urinate, severe cramps, constipation and infertility are common factors.

Sometimes, heavy menstruation results in anaemia.

A physical examination, ultrasound scan or a hysteroscopy can be carried out by a gynaecologist. Local anaesthetic is injected into the cervix and the doctor uses a lighted tube to view the uterus. Some fibroids can be removed through the hysteroscope. Out-patient surgery is an option with general or regional anaesthesia. Other treatments include TCRE (transcervical resection of the endometrium, in which the cells are shaved with a wire loop), drug therapy (to reduce oestrogen levels and shrink the fibroids), myomectomy (p. 164) and hysterectomy (p. 165).

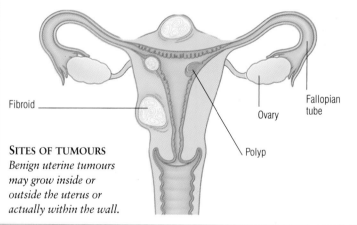

Fibroid

Ovary

Fallopian tube

Polyp

SITES OF TUMOURS
Benign uterine tumours may grow inside or outside the uterus or actually within the wall.

POSSIBLE TREATMENTS

Treatment should be discussed with your doctor. Oral contraceptives are sometimes successful, however the two main treatments are drug/hormone therapy and surgery. Drug therapy often has side effects, such as menopausal symptoms. A surgeon may remove adhesions using laser or cautery with laparoscopy. In very severe cases of endometriosis, a hysterectomy may be needed. A new treatment, the thermal coagulator, uses helium gas ionized by an electric current to dry out the sticky endometriotic cells. It is regarded as quick, safe and accurate.

! Caution

Women who have continuous pelvic pain should not accept any diagnosis that "it is all in the mind". Endometriosis should be suspected. It is a real, sometimes disabling condition and every effort should be made to find a gynaecologist who specializes in this condition. A mind / body counsellor may also help.

Treatment for uterine problems

Certain conditions can occur which affect the uterus including congenital disorders, sexually transmitted infections and a prolapse. These can be dealt with in different ways, either surgically or through medication.

PELVIC INFLAMMATORY DISEASE

Known as PID, pelvic inflammatory disease involves inflammation of the pelvic area, which includes the uterus, Fallopian tubes and ovaries, due to bacterial infection. Bacteria enter the body through the vagina and work their way up the cervix into the pelvic cavity. The bacteria responsible for gonorrhoea and chlamydia are thought to be the chief causes, although other bacteria, particularly some that normally exist harmlessly in the bowel or the vagina, may play a part too. It can occur as a consequence of childbirth, miscarriage, termination of pregnancy, the fitting of an IUD and of sexual intercourse with an infected partner.

PID can range from a mild condition with virtually no symptoms other than an inability to become pregnant, to a serious, occasionally life-threatening, disorder.

Constant abdominal pain, which may become severe, or discomfort, weakness, fatigue, fever and very heavy and painful periods are the most common symptoms. The pain usually manifests itself within a matter of hours and it feels like a dull ache across the lower abdomen. It may be so severe that the woman cannot move.

PID can cause infertility and women who suffer with PID may have seven times the risk of ectopic pregnancy. The scar tissue caused by PID can increase the risk of recurrent infection and it can cause pain during sex.

To diagnose PID, the doctor will do a physical examination, taking swabs to look for any signs of infection. A laparoscopy may be recommended, to confirm the findings. PID is frequently detected when a woman undergoes tests to discover the reasons why she has been unable to conceive. The symptoms of the disease can be mistaken for endometriosis (p. 162) and appendicitis.

PID is usually treated with antibiotics, given in hospital intravenously or in oral form as an outpatient. Sufferers are advised not to use tampons (which may introduce bacteria into the cervix) and to practise safe sex. Women with an IUD should be checked regularly for symptoms.

PROLAPSE OF THE UTERUS

The forward or downward displacement of an organ caused by weakness of the muscles is known as prolapse. The uterus and the vagina are the most common organs to be affected, particularly postmenopausally when the muscles and ligaments slacken as a result of hormonal changes. The direct cause of prolapse may be vaginal and for this reason it is important to do pelvic floor exercises regularly.

The most usual symptoms include discomfort, backache and incontinence. The cervix can be felt in the vagina or may become visible at the vulva. In minor cases, losing weight and regular exercise may succeed as treatment but in serious cases surgery may be required in order to tighten the ligaments. It is important to get the best possible advice as the risks of surgery may outweigh the benefits. After the menopause a hysterectomy is a treatment option.

HYSTERECTOMY

The surgical removal of the uterus, necessary for some because of uterine disorders or disease or menstrual problems, is known as a hysterectomy. As it involves major surgery, it is performed under general or regional anaesthetic.

> **! Caution**
> If a hysterectomy is recommended make sure you receive counselling and good advice. Losing your uterus and/or ovaries may have psychological effects which you may need to come to terms with in order to regain full health.

> **Myomectomy**
> The myometrium is the thick muscular wall of the uterus. A myomectomy is the removal of anything—such as fibroids, for example—from this wall while leaving the uterus intact. Under general anaesthetic a cut is made into the wall of the uterus, the fibroids are removed and the uterus sewn up. There remains an above 50 percent chance of successful pregnancy after a myomectomy. There are, however, a number of possible complications with this procedure. These include: weakening of the uterus wall, heavy bleeding, scarring or adhesions, backache, pain during sexual intercourse. It may be the case that there is no alternative to a hysterectomy (p. 165).

Hospitalization is required for up to a week after an abdominal hysterectomy has been performed, followed by a recuperation period of six to eight weeks. A vaginal hysterectomy is done during a two-night hospital stay, followed by four weeks for recuperation.

The most common reasons a hysterectomy may be recommended include severe, uncontrollable uterine bleeding (also known as flooding); severe and uncontrollable pelvic infection; cancerous growth in the vagina, cervix or uterus that cannot be managed with other treatments; or as part of surgery necessary to deal with a life-threatening disorder (such as cancer) elsewhere in the abdominal cavity, for example, in the ovaries or bladder. Other reasons a hysterectomy may be performed include painful, recurrent attacks of pelvic inflammatory disease (PID), extensive endometriosis that does not respond to treatments, and uterine fibroids.

The two definite consequences of a hysterectomy are that periods cease and the woman can no longer bear a child. The impact either of these have may vary according to the age of the woman and understanding the ramifications should be an essential part of gynaecological care. A woman should also be advised about the ovaries, their function and how her body might be affected if they remain or are removed.

HOW A HYSTERECTOMY IS DONE
A hysterectomy can be performed through an incision in the abdomen—either a bikini line cut leaving a small, neat scar, or a vertical midline cut (used perhaps in the case of large fibroids). In cases where existing adhesions from previous infection or surgery, or large fibroids are present, an abdominal hysterectomy may be the only option.

A vaginal hysterectomy leaves no visible scar. It is generally less painful, causes less bleeding and has less chance of adhesions. It may be assisted by a laparoscopy—keyhole or minimally invasive surgery through the navel and two small incisions.

TYPES OF HYSTERECTOMY

There are a number of different types of hysterectomy. The most common is called the total (or simple) hysterectomy, in which the uterus and the cervix are removed. Sometimes the Fallopian tubes and the ovaries are removed in addition to the uterus. This is known as a total (or simple) hysterectomy with bilateral salpingo-oophorectomy. A radical hysterectomy, where the uterus, the cervix, part of the vagina and the pelvic lymph nodes are all removed, is used to treat stage II of cervical cancer. It is preferred especially for treatment in young women, due to the fact that the ovaries may be left in place.

A hysterectomy may be performed through the abdomen or the vagina. In the cases of a total hysterectomy with bilateral salpingo-oophorectomy and a radical hysterectomy, the operation cannot be vaginal as the ovaries are not able to be removed in this way. With a total hysterectomy this is possible.

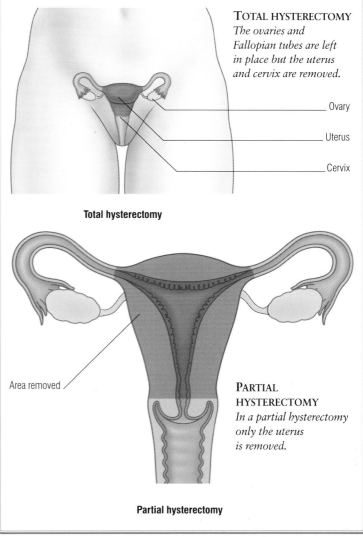

TOTAL HYSTERECTOMY
The ovaries and Fallopian tubes are left in place but the uterus and cervix are removed.

Ovary

Uterus

Cervix

Total hysterectomy

Area removed

PARTIAL HYSTERECTOMY
In a partial hysterectomy only the uterus is removed.

Partial hysterectomy

Uterine/endometrial cancer

Cancer of the uterus predominantly affects women in Western countries and being seriously overweight is the main risk factor. It is probable that carrying a lot of excess fat increases oestrogen levels, which can cause the uterine lining to overgrow and sometimes to become malignant.

A woman who is still having periods in her early to mid-50s is also at increased risk, as are postmenopausal women with diabetes, high blood pressure or a history of infertility. Around 80 percent of women who develop the condition do so after menopause. A cervical smear, which screens the cervix for cancer, can in some cases detect uterine cancers before symptoms develop, hence the recommendation that it should be performed yearly from the age of 40.

SYMPTOMS AND DIAGNOSIS

Irregular bleeding of various kinds is the primary indication. The most important symptom of uterine cancer is vaginal bleeding after menopause. Similarly, bleeding between periods should be reported to your doctor if you are premenopausal. Total absence of periods for months in premenopausal women also increases the risk of uterine cancer and should be reported to the doctor.

The doctor will take a sample of tissue from your uterine lining either in a uterine biopsy or in a minor operation known as a D & C (dilatation and curettage). This sample is examined under a microscope to confirm the diagnosis. Other possible tests include transvaginal ultrasound or a biopsy taken by inserting a flexible instrument called a hysteroscope (p. 163) through the vagina and into the uterus.

TREATMENT AND AFTERCARE

In the majority of cases a hysterectomy in which the ovaries are also removed will offer a cure. If the cancer has spread or there is a suspicion that it might recur, you may also need radiation therapy. This can be done either externally or by inserting a radioactive tampon into the uterus for 24 to 48 hours, or both. Sometimes treatment with synthetic progestogen either in pill or injection form may be necessary if there is a risk of the cancer coming back or if it does so following surgery.

After the operation and treatment you may want to discuss with your doctor how often you will need to be checked and ways of maintaining good health. Whether you are pre- or postmenopausal, the doctor is unlikely to prescribe any drugs containing oestrogen because the hormone may be implicated in triggering the development of the cancer. However, other treatments which offer similar protection against heart disease and osteoporosis may be an alternative and oestrogen in the form of a vaginal cream or ring may be recommended if vaginal dryness is a problem.

SUPPORT GROUPS

Being diagnosed with cancer can bring a range of emotions which you may need help to deal with. Counselling will especially benefit women who are premenopausal and now have to face the fact that they can no longer bear children. Find out from your hospital or medical team the support that is available to you. You and your partner may want to discuss alternatives such as the possibility of finding a surrogate mother to carry a baby for you.

Hormone therapy

For hormone-dependent cancers, anti-hormone therapy may be part of the treatment. The cancer shrinks because it is no longer receiving the amount of hormone it needs. Endometrial cancer as well as precancerous changes in the uterine lining may respond to anti-hormone therapy and it is therefore particularly useful in cases in which surgery is risky or unwarranted.

One of these therapies, tamoxifen, best known for the effective treatment of breast cancer, slightly increases the risk of endometrial cancer. However, the risk of recurrent breast cancer is much greater than that of endometrial cancer, which is usually curable by surgery or radiation therapy.

Anti-hormone therapy should not be confused with hormone replacement therapy (HRT). It is believed that combined oestrogen/progestogen HRT poses minimal risks for developing uterine or endometrial cancer—the benefits far outweigh the risks.

OVARIAN PROBLEMS

The ovaries are under the influence of hormones and their role in the menstrual and reproductive cycles is beyond your control. The ovaries are well protected inside the body but they can be susceptible to disorders which affect your health.

Cysts and syndromes

See also:

1/BEING A WELL WOMAN
Healthy body systems p. 33;
pp. 37–39

3/GENERAL HEALTH ISSUES
Problems of the mind pp. 98–99

4/HORMONAL HEALTH
Reproductive problems
pp. 146–149

The two ovaries, normally about walnut size, are responsible for producing eggs and oestrogen throughout a woman's reproductive life. The efficiency of both actions can be affected by cysts, tissue sacs which form on or inside the ovary. It is not known what causes ovarian cysts but they are more common in smokers than non-smokers. There are many different types, varying in size and in content. Usually a cyst is filled with fluid. If the growth is solid, it is known as a tumour and may be benign (harmless) or malignant (cancerous).

Often there are no symptoms, especially when the cyst is small. Some types grow to a large size—as big as an orange—and may cause swelling of the abdomen. A cyst or cysts may put pressure on the bladder or bowel, making bathroom visits more frequent. Other symptoms include periods becoming irregular, or heavier, lighter or stopping, bleeding between periods, pelvic pain, growth of facial and body hair and gradually deepening of the voice.

Questions to ask your specialist

♀ Is it possible to have a laparoscopic fenestration rather than a laparotomy? If not, why not?
♀ Are you removing only the cyst/tumour, or the whole ovary?
♀ What are the risks of leaving my other organs?
♀ Might it be necessary to remove my uterus?
♀ What am I agreeing to on the consent form for surgery?
♀ Will this treatment affect my sex life and, if so, in what way?
♀ How does this affect my fertility?

Oophorectomy

The removal of one ovary is called an oophorectomy; the removal of both is termed bilateral oophorectomy. If the uterus is also removed, the operation is known as a hysterectomy. The removal of both ovaries will cause an abrupt premature menopause (p. 168) if the woman has not yet reached it. In this case, hormone replacement therapy (HRT) may prove beneficial—it is a subject for you to discuss with your gynaecologist.

TREATMENT

After the diagnosis the doctor may adopt a watch and wait attitude as some cysts disappear of their own accord within a few months. If this isn't the case, surgical removal may be recommended to prevent the cyst or cysts increasing in size and damaging surrounding healthy tissue or to assess the possibility of ovarian cancer.

SURGICAL OPTIONS

Various operations can be carried out to remove ovarian tissue. Laparoscopic fenestration is a keyhole operation to drain the cyst, after which the contents are sent for laboratory analysis. With a laparotomy the entire cyst is removed by abdominal surgery using a bikini line cut and the cyst is sent for analysis. For an oophorectomy and hysterectomy see left. In a salpingectomy both ovaries and Fallopian tubes are removed.

Polycystic ovaries

The word polycystic literally means many cysts. Medically speaking, a polycystic ovary is one that contains at least 10 cysts that lie just below the surface, causing the ovary to become enlarged. The covering of the ovary thickens which makes ovulation—the release of an egg—increasingly difficult or can prevent it from happening at all. More than 20 percent of women have this condition and generally it has no adverse effect. However, if certain symptoms are evident polycystic ovaries may then become a problem.

These symptoms—which indicate that the production of hormones by the ovaries has been disrupted—include irregular or absent periods, infertility, miscarriage, hair growth on face, chest, abdomen, arms and legs, acne, weight gain, pelvic discomfort and feelings of depression. Women with polycystic ovaries are also abnormally resistant to insulin and therefore have high levels of blood sugar.

The condition is brought about by a malfunction of the pituitary gland in the brain. In this case the pituitary gland produces too much luteinizing hormone (LH) and too little follicle-stimulating hormone (FSH). The ovaries are therefore subjected to excess stimulation and produce abnormal amounts of male hormones (androgens).

DIAGNOSIS AND TREATMENT

The first step to diagnosis is a physical examination, followed by blood tests to check hormone levels, ultrasound scan and sometimes a laparoscopy (p. 167). Polycystic ovaries are a common cause of infertility and may be discovered during investigation for that.

Treatment varies according to symptoms and which are most troublesome, your age and if you have already had children, or want them. Hormonal drugs or oral contraceptives may be given to correct hormone imbalance and stimulate ovulation, or laparoscopic ovarian drilling may be done. This involves using diathermy or a laser to make tiny holes on the ovary surface. This process or drugs may precede an IVF treatment cycle. Weight loss may also help to correct polycystic ovaries.

Premature menopause

In most women, menopause occurs naturally over a period of about two years between the ages of 45 and 55. For some unknown reason a few women experience it prematurely in their 20s or 30s. In young women it is usually sudden with symptoms such as hot flushes, night sweats, insomnia, mood changes, anxiety, irritability, poor memory, poor concentration, loss of self-esteem, vaginal dryness, no interest in sex, genitourinary infections, aches and pains, incontinence and depression.

Premature menopause can also be caused by certain drugs, notably chemotherapy, radiation therapy and surgical procedures such as a hysterectomy.

In order to deal with the symptoms you are experiencing in premature menopause, you should seek help and advice from your doctor. The loss of ability to have your own biological children and to assess your risks for long-term problems such as the increased likelihood of heart disease and osteoporosis, will need to be discussed with your doctor who can explain preventive measures. He or she may, for example, recommend dietary changes to reduce cholesterol level. You should also talk about hormone replacement therapy (HRT) and the risks and benefits of its long-term use.

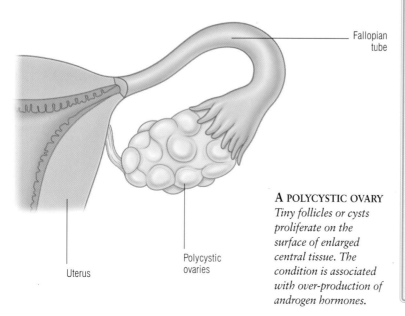

Fallopian tube

A POLYCYSTIC OVARY
Tiny follicles or cysts proliferate on the surface of enlarged central tissue. The condition is associated with over-production of androgen hormones.

Polycystic ovaries

Uterus

Ovarian cancer

Most women who develop this form of cancer are over the age of 45, with the majority of women between 65 and 74 when it is diagnosed. It is more common in Western countries than in places such as Japan, though the daughters and granddaughters of Japanese women who move to the West seem to become susceptible, suggesting that environmental factors must play some as yet unrecognized role in triggering it.

In some cases genetic inheritance may be involved: a woman who has a close relative with ovarian cancer and others with either breast cancer or colon cancer diagnosed at a relatively early age may be at increased risk. Having children appears to offer some protection, as does the oral contraceptive pill. Women who have never had a baby and those who have never taken the pill seem to be more susceptible to ovarian cancer.

Women over the age of 35 with the above risk factors are advised to have regular screening by their doctor or health centre.

SYMPTOMS

One of the main difficulties with ovarian cancer is that it may cause few symptoms especially in the early stages, and even when they do appear they are often ill-defined.

Bearing in mind that they may well be caused by other conditions that have nothing to do with ovarian cancer, it is worth making an appointment with your doctor if you experience particular symptoms. You may, for example, notice a change in your usual bowel habits so that you become constipated or suffer diarrhoea for more than a few days. Perhaps you experience indigestion and feelings of nausea and bloatedness or a loss of appetite. Other symptoms can be a swollen abdomen or pain in the lower abdomen. You may have unexpected vaginal bleeding, although this is relatively uncommon.

Because the ovaries have plenty of space in which to become enlarged several times their own size by the tumour, it may be a long time before symptoms are observed. Generally, symptoms appear when the increasing size of the tumour exerts pressure on other organs of the body. If you are in middle or later life, it

may be worth questioning a new diagnosis of irritable bowel syndrome as the symptoms can be similar to those of ovarian cancer.

TESTS AND INVESTIGATIONS

You will be referred to a hospital clinic and may need a number of different tests including blood tests, X-rays, ultrasound and/or CT or MRI scans, among others. A sample of abdominal fluid may be taken under local anaesthetic and the doctor may also decide to look inside your abdomen under a general anaesthetic. The most common ovarian cancer, epithelial cancer of the ovary, starts in the covering (epithelium). Other types can start in other components of the ovary: cancers of ovarian tissue are known as sarcomas, and cancers that start in the ova-producing part of the ovary are known as germ-cell tumours.

TREATMENT

Treatment will depend on your age, general health, type and size of tumour and the extent of spread. Surgery may be performed with chemotherapy and radiotherapy as further options. Chemotherapy is very effective for ovarian cancer. Treatment sometimes combines two of the three options, starting with an operation to remove the ovaries and uterus, plus tissue samples from nearby lymph glands and, if necessary, the surgeon will remove as much as possible of any cancer elsewhere in the abdomen.

See also:

1/BEING A WELL WOMAN
Healthy body systems p. 33;
pp. 38–39

2/SEX & SEXUALITY
Contraception pp. 62–67

3/GENERAL HEALTH ISSUES
Anxiety-related disorders
p. 108

4/HORMONAL HEALTH
Endocrine system problems
pp. 144–145
Reproductive problems
pp. 146–147
Pregnancy pp. 170–179
Conception problems
pp. 180–185

? Did you know?
It is important, as in all cancers, to do everything you can to boost your immune system. Lifestyle changes that you can make include healthy eating, regular exercise in the fresh air, sufficient sleep and drinking at least eight glasses of water a day.

SCREENING

Levels of a chemical marker in the blood, known as CA 125, may be raised in a woman with ovarian cancer but this has not yet made earlier diagnosis possible. Trials are in progress to try and develop a reliable screening method, possibly using a combination of blood tests and ultrasound scans, so that the disease can be identified at an early stage.

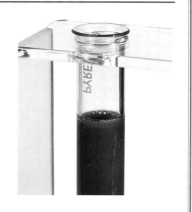

PREGNANCY AND MOTHERHOOD

From the moment you become pregnant your body, relationships, feelings and life will be forever changed. Learning all you can about pregnancy, childbirth and raising a family will help prepare you for the different aspects of giving birth and being a parent. You should work together with your doctor to make sure that all goes smoothly.

See your doctor

Find out if your doctor runs a programme of antenatal care, or get yourself referred to one who specializes in pregnancy and childbirth.

Pregnancy planning

The ideal situation is to be in the very best of health before attempting to conceive so that you can maximize your chances of the safe and successful delivery of a healthy baby. In essence, this means:

Stopping smoking By far the single most important thing you can do for a healthy baby.

Toxins Cutting out alcohol and illegal drugs and limiting tea and coffee to 1–2 cups a day.

Healthy eating Plenty of nutrient-rich foods such as fruit and vegetables.

Folic acid Eating foods rich in folic acid and taking a dietary supplement to lessen any risk of bearing a child with a central nervous system disorder—400 mcg daily is advised.

Weight watch Eating to gain weight if you are underweight and cutting down on high-fat foods as well as improving the overall quality of food that you eat if you are overweight.

Exercise Getting plenty of exercise several times a week in the fresh air.

Sleep Getting enough sleep.

Water Drinking at least eight glasses of water every day in order to encourage the elimination of toxins from the body.

Contraception Changing to a barrier method of contraception if you are taking the oral contraceptive pill, so that your periods are reestablished before attempting to conceive.

Rubella Checking your immunity for rubella by means of a simple blood test at your doctor's surgery or local hospital.

STDs If you feel that you may be at risk, getting tested for chlamydia or any other sexually transmitted diseases.

Teeth Having any necessary dental work done so that you won't need X-rays or anaesthetic while you are pregnant. Good dental health is important as both teeth and gums can be adversely affected during pregnancy.

CHECK OUT YOUR PAST

Your family medical history and individual medical history are significant in prepregnancy planning, as may be the family and individual medical history of your partner. In your case, menstrual problems, infections, STDs, preexisting health problems (for example epilepsy, hypertension, diabetes) will need to be taken into account by you and your doctor as part of your care.

If you or any of your family have any condition, for example cystic fibrosis, that may be a risk factor for pregnancy, you should see a genetic counsellor (through your doctor) to discuss and assess the level of risk for you and how to manage it.

ADJUSTING PSYCHOLOGICALLY

Having a first baby involves an enormous life change and in the months before conception you should take the opportunity to talk through possible problems or attitudes with your partner. It is perfectly normal to experience a range of emotions, some of which may be conflicting. Both the woman and the man, about to be parents, may rework old relationships (with their mother and father, for instance, friends who don't have children, with colleagues at their workplaces) and their feelings may veer from

Risk factors for pregnancy

The following factors should be discussed with your doctor. Remember that more than 97 percent of pregnancies result in the safe delivery of a healthy baby. It helps the hospital team to identify any risk factors in your pregnancy so that they are fully prepared for any complications.

- ♀ Younger than 18.
- ♀ Older than 36 if already have children.
- ♀ Over 34 and no previous children.
- ♀ Have four or more children.
- ♀ Have an IUD in place.
- ♀ Vaginal bleeding after last period.
- ♀ Previous stillbirth or neonatal death.
- ♀ Previous Caesarean delivery or myomectomy.
- ♀ Previous very small (less than 1.3 kg/3 lb) or very large (over 3.6 kg/8 lb) baby.
- ♀ Two or more previous miscarriages.
- ♀ History of premature labour, cervical stitch, late miscarriage or abortion, two or more abortions.
- ♀ Congenital abnormality in previous baby.
- ♀ Antibodies in previous pregnancy which could harm foetus, such as rhesus antibodies.
- ♀ Preeclampsia, hypertension or proteinuria in a previous pregnancy.
- ♀ Severe bleeding after giving birth or removal of placenta in previous pregnancy.
- ♀ History of very short labour (under two hours) or long labour (over 12 hours).
- ♀ Postnatal depression after birth of previous baby.
- ♀ Uterine problem such as fibroids or cysts.
- ♀ Blood disorder.
- ♀ Family history of diabetes or congenital foetal abnormality.
- ♀ Smoking.
- ♀ Drinking two or more units of alcohol a day before pregnancy.
- ♀ Inability to stop drinking while pregnant.
- ♀ Illegal drugtaking by either parent.
- ♀ Several different sexual partners, anal intercourse or bisexual partner.
- ♀ Hepatitis B, HIV or AIDS.
- ♀ High blood pressure (over 140/90, after you have been lying down for five minutes).
- ♀ Over or underweight or under 1.5 m (5 ft) tall.
- ♀ Protein in urine.
- ♀ Heart murmur.
- ♀ Pelvic or abdominal abnormalities.
- ♀ Vaginal bleeding at any stage in pregnancy.

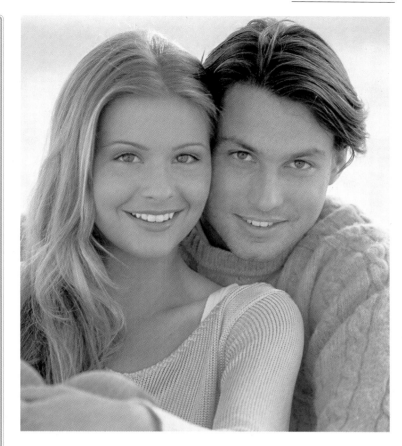

elation and excitement to anxiety. Both of you may enjoy knowing that you are carrying on the family line but may also have concerns about finances, job security and personal freedom.

As a couple, over the months that lie ahead you may make new discoveries about each other. You will be sharing the joys and discoveries of being parents but more negative feelings will also arise and you should be prepared for them. Worries and hidden anxieties about meeting the demands of parenthood may surface. There may be unhappy memories from the past to deal with. Your feelings for each other may be tested by crises, such as problems with the development of the foetus. If tests show the likelihood of impairment you may even need to make the most difficult decision of all, to terminate the pregnancy. You may disagree about what should be done and need good support from family, friends and counsellors in this situation.

Antenatal groups provide a good forum for airing feelings and raising subjects that concern new parents. Information and friendship found in support groups can be of longstanding help to the new mother and her partner.

TIME OF ADJUSTMENT
Preparing yourself for pregnancy is both physical and emotional —two people looking together to the future with a child who will make you a family.

! Caution

If in the past you have suffered from mood disorders (depression or generalized anxiety in particular) or eating problems (such as anorexia nervosa or bulimia) you should talk to your gynaecologist or GP. You may need special treatment during pregnancy as you and the developing foetus may be at significant risk.

Stages of pregnancy

See also:

1/BEING A WELL WOMAN
Essentials of good health
pp. 16–25
Healthy body systems
p. 33; pp. 38–39

> **! Caution**
> Special precautions need to be taken to prevent a woman with HIV passing the virus to her child. Careful obstetric management is essential to prevent premature birth and rupture of the membranes more than four hours before delivery by Caesarean section. The obstetrician will also advise on using an adequate alternative to breastfeeding.

VIEWING THE WOMB
Ultrasound scanning is a painless procedure. It is done when you have a full bladder which pushes your uterus up so the technician gets a clearer image. You and your partner will be able to see the monitor—and will be given a printout of what you saw.

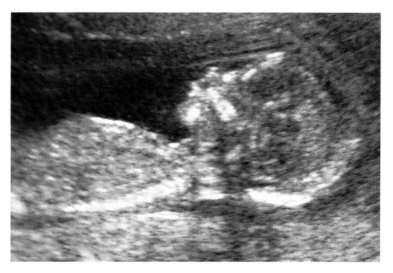

Some women know very quickly whether or not they are pregnant but most may need something more than a missed period to be sure. You can obtain a pregnancy test at your doctor's surgery or family planning clinic or you can buy one over the counter from a pharmacist. Pregnancy testing can be reliably carried out four weeks after the last monthly period. Pregnancy can be confirmed by a positive pregnancy blood or urine test result, a physical exam and/or an ultrasound scan.

By this stage you may be experiencing common early signs of pregnancy which include feeling sick, tired, needing to urinate more frequently than usual, swollen and tender breasts, constipation, disliking foods that you normally relish and craving foods that you don't usually care for and a significant absence of the irritability associated with PMS.

THE FIRST TRIMESTER
In the first 13 weeks of pregnancy (counted from the first day of your last menstrual period), the changes occur at an astonishing rate:

Weeks 3-4 The embryo is no more than the size of a grain of rice, as it attaches to the uterus.

Weeks 4-5 The body structures are starting to develop.

Weeks 5-6 The head is beginning to form and the heart is beating. This can be seen on an ultrasound scan.

Weeks 6-8 All internal organs are formed and the embryo is now about 2.5 cm (1 in) long.

Blood and other tests
Your antenatal care will probably include these tests:

♀ Blood test to find your blood group (in case you are later in need of a blood transfusion) and to determine whether you are rhesus positive or rhesus negative, (p. 175).

♀ Blood test to see whether or not you are anaemic.

♀ Blood test to check for your immunity to rubella.

♀ Blood test to ensure that you are free of hepatitis B and to check for HIV if you agree to the test.

♀ Blood test for syphilis.

♀ Blood test to see if you are at risk of any of a large number of disorders, which include sickle cell disease, B-thalassaemia, cystic fibrosis, Down's syndrome.

♀ Urine test in order to check for kidney disease, diabetes and urinary tract disease such as cystitis.

♀ Cervical smear, unless one has already been carried out recently.

♀ Gonorrhoea and chlamydia tests of your cervix, if you are at high risk.

The limbs, no more than tiny buds at first, are now visible.

Weeks 10-11 The foetus moves around (although you will not be able to feel it yet); eyes are formed; fingers and toes are forming.

Weeks 12-13 External genitals are forming; facial features are distinguishable; muscles are increasing in strength; movements are becoming more vigorous. Length is 7.5 cm (3 in).

WHAT YOU CAN EXPECT
The first antenatal visit is usually scheduled for around 12 weeks. An ultrasound scan may be done to confirm the age of the foetus, checking for a heartbeat and for more than one foetus. Antenatal care in the first three months involves a range of tests (see box, above) and is intended to identify any unknown risk factors (p. 171). Your doctor will discuss the results with you and your partner.

You will experience fatigue and more fatigue. Do everything you can to rest your body and give it the fuel it needs for the developing baby. Eat regularly and well at least three times a day, and avoid junk food and alcohol. If you can, eat five or six smaller meals a day rather than three big ones. Avoid foods that may harbour dangerous organisms: unpasteurized milk, soft mould-ripened cheese (Brie, Camembert, blue-streaked), soft ice cream from machines, fish and meat stored unwrapped at a deli, precooked or preroasted poultry and cook-chill foods.

For constipation and morning sickness, both common at this time in pregnancy, eat as much fruit and vegetables and wholegrain products as possible. Drink at least eight glasses of water a day. Get out of bed very slowly, use deep breathing and relaxation techniques to overcome morning sickness (which may, in fact, occur at any time of day). Indigestion and heartburn tend to be facts of life during pregnancy. Allowing plenty of time for digestion after a meal will help this.

There are many ways in which you can help and nurture yourself that may benefit you during this stage of pregnancy. It may help to go to a yoga class for pregnant women to learn relaxation techniques and muscle control; continue to exercise if you exercised before. If you didn't exercise, ask your doctor how to start safely in pregnancy. You must take care not to become overtired as it is more difficult to recover when you are pregnant. You can also use meditation techniques to restore energy. ▶

A TIME OF CHANGE
While no two women are alike, some experiences of pregnancy will be similar. There will be days when you don't feel or look your best, on others you will be blooming. Keeping in touch with what is happening to you and your body helps you work in partnership with your doctors.

ANTENATAL SCREENING AND TESTS

You may be offered one or more of these procedures if you are at risk. Discuss in advance the implications if your baby is found to have one of these conditions.

Procedure	When	To identify condition
Chorionic villus sampling	between weeks 9 and 11	*chromosome abnormality*
Alphafetoprotein blood test	between weeks 15 and 22	*foetal abnormality, including spinal cord defects*
Amniocentesis	between weeks 15 and 20	*chromosome abnormality*
Ultrasound scan	from 18 weeks	*defects of spinal cord, other foetal abnormalities. Check growth and well-being*
Cordocentesis (foetal blood sampling)	from week 20	*rhesus negative mother with antibodies that may destroy baby's blood cells*

! Caution
The organism that causes toxoplasmosis may be present in uncooked or undercooked fish or meat and in cat faeces. A mother may already have immunity which will protect the foetus, but if she catches toxoplasmosis while pregnant the effects on the baby can range from jaundice to blindness and mental disabilities.

THE SECOND TRIMESTER

Weeks 14-16 The foetus is fully formed, has all vital organs and is gaining weight fast. It can stretch, turn its head, open its mouth, yawn and frown.

Week 18 First movements may be felt by the mother as the foetus kicks, bumps, twists, turns and pushes against the springy uterus wall.

Week 20 Teeth are starting to form in the jawbone and head hair is growing. The foetus is now 25 cm (10 in) long. Ultrasound to screen for any abnormalities.

Week 24 Fingernails have formed, thumb-sucking and hiccups begin (to coordinate sucking and swallowing needed for feeding after birth). The eyes open occasionally. The length is now 33 cm (13 in).

Week 27 Body fat is forming, the body is coated with waxy vernix, which prevents its skin from becoming soggy in the amniotic fluid. The length is now 37 cm (14½ in).

Seek medical help immediately if:

♀ You don't feel movements for more than 12 hours after 24 weeks.
♀ You lose weight.
♀ You have vaginal bleeding.
♀ You have severe abdominal pain.
♀ You have a continuous and severe headache.
♀ Your temperature is 38.5°C (101°F) or more.
♀ You have blurred vision.
♀ Your feet and/or hands swell.
♀ You are vomiting.
♀ Your waters break (p. 176).

WHAT YOU CAN EXPECT

Indigestion and constipation may occur as in the earlier months, although choosing foods carefully will help, as will allowing plenty of time for meals as digestion will take longer now.

Make sure you take some time every day to do something that gives you pleasure, but remember also that you will feel tired very easily so you should have regular rests. Start pelvic floor exercises and continue to walk in the fresh air and swim. Stretch marks may also start to appear at this stage, however these may be minimized by massaging in vitamin E cream.

THE LAST TRIMESTER

Week 28 The foetus almost completely fills the uterus and may turn head down. You feel much kicking and fluttering of feet and hands.

Week 32 All parts are now developed and the lungs are maturing.

Week 36 The head will probably engage now if this is your first baby. Weight is gained for an efficient heat regulating system after birth. Irises are blue; hair may be 2.5 cm (1 in) and the cord, about 51 cm (20 in) and slippery, making it unlikely to knot during constant twisting and turning. Length is 46 cm (18 in).

Week 40 There's less space to move but movement continues. Eyes are sometimes open and light can be discerned through the uterine wall, as can sound vibrations and links with the mother's mood. The length is 51 cm (20 in).

Most babies are pointing head down by now: the head is the heaviest part of the body and its weight can stimulate labour. How the baby is lying determines how it will be born.

GETTING READY FOR BIRTH

When the baby's head engages—moves into the pelvis in preparation for birth—there is less pressure on your ribs and more on the urinary tract. In some it does not fully engage until labour starts. You may have mild "practice" contractions (Braxton-Hicks)—short and intermittent. In your breasts the lobules enlarge as protein and fat accumulate in the widened milk reservoirs.

Bladder

Problems relating to pregnancy

Anaemia This is common and will show up in routine blood tests. Fatigue is the prime symptom. You may be prescribed iron supplements so that you and the baby receive sufficient freshly oxygenated blood for healthy growth.

Anxiety and emotional ups and downs These are normal. Discuss any worries or feelings of depression that you have with your doctor, your hospital consultant or your midwife.

Backache Caused partly by the effect of the pregnancy hormones and partly by the weight you are carrying. Treat with warm baths, massage or a hot-water bottle to warm the bed at night. Strengthen your muscles with back exercises, regular walking and swimming. Try the Alexander Technique and yoga. Avoid high heels and maintain a good posture.

Bleeding gums Caused by pregnancy hormones. Use an electric toothbrush and dental floss morning and night to dislodge food particles and to massage the gums.

Breasts They become tender, enlarge and may leak. Wear a correct-fitting pregnancy bra from the first trimester.

Breathlessness This may come from the growing baby pressing on your internal organs or may be a symptom of anaemia. Consult your doctor. Try the Alexander Technique. Regular exercise will improve stamina.

Fatigue This is normal, but may be a sign of anaemia. Take short rests whenever you can. Make sure you get enough sleep.

Haemorrhoids These are caused by constipation. It will help if you eat more fibrous foods and drink more water.

Heartburn and indigestion Common during the second half of pregnancy when hormones soften the valve in the digestive tract so that acid rises up from the stomach. Cut down on acidic, spicy, very hot and very cold foods. Speed up your digestion by increased exercise and drinking plenty of liquids, especially water. Use antacids containing calcium.

Preeclampsia A medical emergency. Symptoms include high blood pressure, swelling of the face, ankles, wrists and sometimes the whole body and protein in the urine. Contact your doctor if you notice any swelling. It can prove fatal to the baby and/or the mother if the condition progresses to its severe forms.

Stretch marks Wavy, pinkish-silvery lines that may occur on the breasts, abdomen, thighs and buttocks as the skin stretches to accommodate the size of the growing baby. It is possible, though not proven, that massage creams and oils as well as regular exercise, may help reduce them.

Vaginal bleeding or discharge Contact your doctor immediately.

Varicose veins Common in pregnancy as a consequence of the effect of pregnancy hormones and of your increased weight. Walking helps to relieve the dull ache. Avoid constricting garments, such as knee-high socks, ankle socks with too-tight elastic, hold-up stockings, too-tight trousers and too-tight boots. When you are sitting, raise your legs on a stool or a chair whenever possible.

See also:

3/GENERAL HEALTH ISSUES
Skeletal system problems
pp. 84–85
Blood and the circulation
pp. 116–117; p. 122
Women and heart disease p. 132

4/HORMONAL HEALTH
Endocrine system problems
pp. 136–137

5/ILLNESSES & EMERGENCIES
Digestive system problems
p. 191; p. 196

The rhesus factor

Most people have blood that is rhesus positive (Rh+), but about 15 percent (1 in 6) are rhesus negative (Rh–). Rh+ blood cells possess an antigen that can stimulate the production of antibodies to fight alien blood cells. Rh– blood lacks this antigen.

Problems arise in pregnancy only if you are Rh– and the baby has the same blood group as you, but is Rh+: some blood cells that escape from its body into yours during pregnancy, especially during birth, provoke your body to make antibodies to destroy the alien cells. This does not usually harm you or the baby. However, if a subsequent foetus is again Rh+ and you now have antibodies to fight and destroy these cells, these can pass into the baby's circulation breaking down its cells, and possibly causing stillbirth, severe anaemia, heart failure, mental problems, spasticity or extreme jaundice.

Women with Rh– factor blood who have developed antibodies from a previous pregnancy may need special care to protect the baby. After an invasive procedure, such as chorionic villus sampling, cordocentesis and amniocentesis, she must be given anti-D gamma globulin injections. This should also be done after the birth of her first child and subsequent children to destroy the antibodies, and after a miscarriage occurring later than 12 weeks into a pregnancy.

! Caution
A woman with Rh– blood who is carrying a baby with Rh+ blood is at risk of developing antibodies against her baby's blood. Although the greatest risk occurs at delivery, it can also happen in pregnancy. Your doctor will advise you to get anti-D gamma globulin at 28 weeks and again at delivery to minimize the chances that you will develop antibodies.

Labour and birth

The waiting is over. It is time to put into practice the techniques you have learned to manage labour and birth. You will have much support from the medical team to ensure that the outcome will be health and well-being for you and your baby.

HOW YOU KNOW WHEN IT'S TIME

Regular, pronounced contractions Cramps and tightening in the abdominal area, once labour has started, are regular (every 10 minutes or so and getting closer) and last for 40 seconds or more. At worst, they can follow one another relentlessly, which is painful and exhausting, not letting the mother catch her breath and breathe into the next contraction. Use breathing techniques and pain relief (see opposite).

Show A discharge of pinkish blood, indicating that the gelatinous plug of mucus that has been blocking the cervical canal during pregnancy has been dislodged and that the cervix is beginning to stretch.

Your waters break A painless leakage of amniotic fluid, which can vary from a slight dribble to a heavy gush. It indicates that the membranes surrounding the baby in the uterus have ruptured.

VAGINAL DELIVERY

The process of birth consists of three stages, only the contractions continue throughout:

Stage 1 The uterus starts to contract at regular intervals until the cervix dilates to about 10 cm (4 in) in diameter. This is the longest stage of labour.

Stage 2 The cervix is fully dilated. Contractions and the mother's pushing move the baby down through the pelvic canal. This is usually a much shorter stage.

Stage 3 After the birth of the baby, the placenta separates from the lining of the uterus and further contractions expel it.

ASSISTED DELIVERY METHODS

If your doctor sees complications developing he or she will aid the birth process in the best way for you and your baby. If the baby's head is visible but the body cannot get through the

A multiple birth

If you have two or more babies, you may go in to labour earlier (usually around the 36th week) or your doctor may advise induction or Caesarean before the 40-week term to prevent the uterus being overstretched. You may also be at greater risk for high blood pressure. You will agree a birth plan with the medical team—doctor, midwife, anaesthetist and two paediatricians (one for each baby)—and ultrasound will reveal the way each twin is positioned. In a vaginal delivery they will be born sequentially. Each baby will usually weigh less than that of a baby from a single pregnancy.

HOW THE BABY LIES
Most babies are positioned head down by the time they are about to be born. Some, however, remain head up in what is known as a breech presentation. A baby positioned this way can be delivered vaginally but your doctor is likely to recommend that it is delivered by Caesarean section.

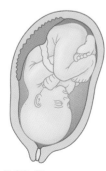

ROP: RIGHT OCCIPUT POSTERIOR
The baby is positioned head down, facing toward the front, crown slightly to the right.

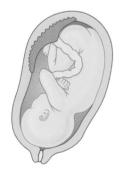

LOA: LEFT OCCIPUT ANTERIOR
Still head down, the baby is facing toward the back, crown slightly to the left.

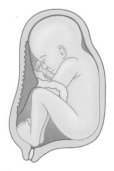

FOOTLING BREECH
Positioned head up, the baby is sitting in the pelvic cavity with a foot or feet extending toward the cervix.

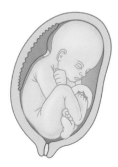

BREECH
The baby is sitting in the pelvic cavity, positioned head up, with bottom down and feet tucked away.

birth canal forceps may be used to help him or her out. Forceps are sometimes used to speed delivery if the mother or baby are in distress. A shortlasting anaesthetic is given and the doctor gently eases the baby out, maybe eliminating the need for an emergency Caesarean.

A Caesarean section is performed by making an incision along the bikini line and lifting the baby out. It is major surgery performed with an epidural (a screen is placed to obscure the mother's view) or, in an emergency when an epidural is not in place, under general anaesthetic.

An elective Caesarean is decided in advance, usually because the baby is breech, the mother is HIV positive or a Caesarean was necessary in a previous delivery. An emergency Caesarean is the same operation carried out when the woman is already in labour and there is an urgent need to deliver the baby quickly—either because the baby has turned and is in breech presentation, or becomes short of oxygen. In the mother reasons include severe preeclampsia or eclampsia, placenta previa, in which the placenta is lying across the cervix and would be ruptured if labour continued and cause potentially dangerous haemorrhaging, or pelvic tumours, such as fibroids or ovarian cysts, which could obstruct the baby's delivery. The great majority of deliveries, including emergency ones, are very successful.

Once the baby has been born the connective blood vessels close off, preventing excessive bleeding as the placenta comes out. This is examined by the medical team to ensure it is all there—that none has been left inside. The umbilical cord will be clamped and cut once it has stopped pulsating and the baby is breathing well.

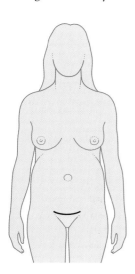

CAESAREAN SECTION
Some women are not able to give birth vaginally or may need help during delivery. In this safe surgical procedure a lateral incision is made through the abdomen into the uterus. It is possible to deliver another baby vaginally after having had a Caesarean; your doctor will be able to advise you.

COPING WITH CONTRACTIONS

Treatment	Action
Natural	
Controlled breathing	♀ Between contractions, relax and breathe in. On exhaling, push a little and imagine all the air in your lungs being emptied. ♀ As you feel a contraction coming breathe a little more quickly but don't empty your lungs. Continue breathing quickly. As the contraction ends revert to slower breathing. Take a long breath out. ♀ As contractions become intense they need concentration. Breathe in quickly, blow out and breathe in again. If you feel faint cup your hands over your nose and mouth and breathe deeply.
Relaxation	Close your eyes and imagine yourself in a peaceful place, contract and relax every part of your body. Start from your toes and work up to your head.
Visualization	Focus on something that makes you feel good and brings a sense of achievement. It doesn't matter what it is as long as it holds your concentration and helps you relax.
TENS	A machine which gives out a low-level electrical current to nerves which blocks the pain signals from the uterus.
Pharmacological	
Gas and air (entonox)	For stages 1 and 2, you breathe in a mixture of oxygen and nitrous oxide through a facemask or mouthpiece. Gives limited relief, may make you feel lightheaded.
Pethidine	A powerful synthetic analgesic injected into thigh or buttocks at stage 1. If done too early the effects may wear off. Also given for episiotomy, a cut made in the perineum (between anus and vagina) to widen the exit area for the baby.
Epidural	Spinal anaesthesia for stage 1 or Caesarean, to take away all feeling below the waist (numbness lasts several hours). A catheter is placed in the epidural space beside the spinal cord. If necessary, forceps delivery may be used.

Motherhood

You are at last handed your newborn baby and the joys and irritations of pregnancy and the pain of labour are behind you. In these first few minutes in the delivery room as you hold the baby close to you, a new stage of adjustment begins, the start of the bonding process. In the last stage of labour or after delivery, you may be given an injection of oxytocin. This stimulates the uterus to contract strongly to push out the placenta and later it also stimulates milk production.

WHAT'S NEXT FOR YOU

Immediately after birth you will be stitched if you had an episiotomy or tore during the birth. You will be given an anti-D gamma globulin injection if the rhesus factor applies to you (p. 175). Provided you are both in good health, the baby will be brought to you to be placed on your breast before he or she is washed (to remove any grayish vernix and blood). A baby's sucking reflexes can be strong in the first hour after birth and the sucking action stimulates the release of oxytocin from the pituitary gland, which helps your uterus to contract and return to normal size.

During the first few days after the birth your breasts will produce colostrum, a yellowish liquid rich in proteins, sugar and antibodies (lymphocytes and immunoglobulins). It may not seem much in quantity, but it is nourishing and helps protect the baby from infection.

BIRTH AND YOUR EMOTIONS

It is quite normal to experience an array of emotions during birth and after, responses brought about by excitement and your hormones and it may take some time for you to come down to earth. For the first-time mother especially, there may be a new intensity of feeling, balanced perhaps by the physical effects of childbirth which can leave you tired, sore and even shocked. Give yourself time. The adjustment process—of bonding with your baby and becoming a family—is gradual and evolves as you gain confidence.

Fluctuating hormone levels may cause you to feel dejected between three and seven days after the delivery, known to health professionals as the "baby blues" (p. 112). It may occur as your body is still recovering and you are tired from the unaccustomed new routine. No one

THE APGAR SCORE FOR YOUR BABY'S HEALTH

Your baby is assessed for the five factors shown below and then weighed. A baby scoring 7 or more points is in good general health. A week or so later, a blood sample from the baby will be analysed for vitamin K deficiency, phenylketonuria.

Sign	0	1	2
Respiratory effort	none	weak cry, slow breathing	strong cry
Pulse (heart rate)	none	slow, under 100 beats per minute	fast, over 100 beats per minute
Colour (pallor)	blue-pale	pink body with blue fingers and toes	all pink
Muscular tone	limp	some flexing of fingers and toes	active, fingers and toes flexing well
Response to stimuli (reflexes)	no response	grimace	cry

will think less of you for feeling weepy for what doesn't seem to be any real reason. Don't hesitate to talk about it. If these feelings persist see your doctor. You may need some help to get you through this time.

If you have any physical problems—the incision from a Caesarean delivery or stitches—get advice from your doctor or midwife. Do your postnatal exercises, including those for the pelvic floor. Use sanitary towels rather than tampons. Make sure you have a balanced and normal diet. You will have a postnatal check-up at six weeks and but can raise any concerns before then.

BREASTFEEDING YOUR BABY

If you are undecided, why not start breast-feeding and see how it goes? Putting your baby to the breast as soon as possible after delivery introduces the baby to your nipple and the surrounding areola. When the baby takes most of this into the mouth, called "latching on", a vacuum is created with the tongue. In the first few days colostrum is sufficient but this soon gives way to mature breast milk—at the right temperature and full of nutrients—stimulated by the baby's suckling.

If you have difficulties positioning the baby or with latching on, ask the midwife or a lactation consultant to help you. While breast-feeding may be natural, mothers and babies have to learn to do it. It may take a week or two for feeding to get going and longer for a pattern to be established. The baby's weight and mood are the best indicators of whether or not he or she is receiving enough food.

If your baby cries a lot, it may be that he or she is not getting enough milk or that you are not producing enough to satisfy him or her. Try to be positive. Don't rush it. Allow time for feeding. If you offer a breast when your baby cries for no reason you can discern, and he or she stays there for as long as he wants, he is almost certainly getting enough milk.

Looking after a new infant day and night brings its own pressures and you should try to ensure you get as much rest as you can—get back in touch with the relaxation techniques you practised in pregnancy.

Make sure that you eat well and that you drink plenty of water. This is very important while breastfeeding to replace fluids. Be advised by your health professional about establishing a feeding routine, but have faith in your own instincts. Learn to enjoy being close to the baby rather than becoming concerned. Cuddling and gentle stroking will relax you both. Accept that when the baby is hungry he or she will almost certainly eat.

If your breasts become engorged, express some milk to be used later. This will enable your partner to feed the baby too. Some women, despite all their efforts, suffer leaking and cracked nipples and infections such as mastitis, although the milk itself can help to heal them. Report bleeding nipples, fevers or painful breasts to your doctor or midwife.

BOTTLE FEEDING

You may decide to bottle feed, because you either don't choose to, or can't, breastfeed. This can have the advantage of allowing your partner to become involved in feeding the baby from the start. You can consult your doctor about preventing your breasts producing milk. It may be necessary to take tablets for a while. Ask for guidance so that you know the right formula for the size of your baby, and follow the instructions exactly.

CARE FOR YOUR NIPPLES
When you are breast-feeding take good care of your nipples. Wipe off all milk and dry them after feeding your baby. Wear pads inside your nursing bra to catch leaks. Change the pads as frequently as you change the baby's nappy.

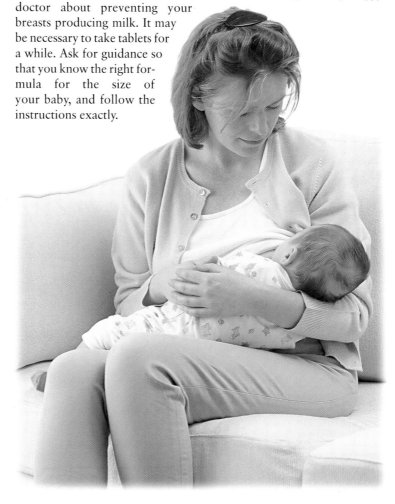

CONCEPTION PROBLEMS

A woman has a 25 percent chance of conceiving a baby every month and three out of four couples will be successful within six months of having regular unprotected sex. For some, however, sustaining a pregnancy and achieving a live birth might prove to be more difficult.

Miscarriage

The loss of a baby through miscarriage is more common than many people realize. Leading gynaecologists set the figure as high as 75 percent of all pregnancies, but as most occur within the first two months many women may not have been aware that they were pregnant. Miscarriage is much less likely after 12-16 weeks. The warning signs are vaginal bleeding, cramps and backache similar to those of a period, and absence of pregnancy signs such as tender breasts and morning sickness. Once a miscarriage starts, little can be done to halt it.

WHAT ARE THE CAUSES?

Miscarriage investigation is not done as a matter of course, although if it occurs late in the pregnancy it should be investigated by a gynaecologist. Most couples who lose a pregnancy do so for no clear reason and go on to have a healthy baby later.

While a miscarriage, particularly in the early months, does not mean an increased risk of another, some women do have repeated miscarriage and only after three are they generally referred for investigation. This may include referral to a genetic counsellor, notably if there has been foetal abnormality, to determine the level of risk and the best way forward. Antiphospholipid syndrome can be tested for. It is a cause for recurrent miscarriage and can be treated with aspirin.

Rubella, listeriosis or chlamydia are known common causes of miscarriage, as is a major abnormality in the foetus or abnormalities of the uterus, such as fibroids or polyps. An incompetent cervix—the cervix dilates instead of remaining tightly closed during pregnancy—can also cause it. A woman is at risk too if she has a pre-existing condition such as diabetes, epilepsy, asthma, kidney disease or high blood pressure and her pregnancy is likely to be more closely monitored.

Pregnancy complications

Complications that may prevent a full-term pregnancy or live birth:
♀ Preeclampsia (see right).
♀ Rhesus factor (p. 175).
♀ Antenatal haemorrhage (caused by serious problems with the placenta).
♀ Too much or too little amniotic fluid.
♀ Retroversion of the uterus (p. 162).
♀ Pre-existing disease.
♀ Foetal death.
♀ Stillbirth.

Testing for preeclampsia

Having your blood pressure checked regularly is essential during pregnancy. This detects the one in 20 women—usually first-time mothers—who has soaring blood pressure which puts her at risk for a complication of pregnancy called preeclampsia, also called toxaemia of pregnancy. When she retains fluid and starts to excrete vital proteins, she may need urgent drug treatment to reduce her BP or labour will be induced to prevent the progression to eclampsia, one of the leading causes of maternal death. If preeclampsia develops late in pregnancy, particularly after week 36, delivery is usually safely achieved. However if a woman falls ill before the third trimester, her premature baby might not survive.

A woman is susceptible if there is a family history of the condition or if she has existing hypertension, diabetes mellitus, autoimmune disorders or kidney disease. Research continues to find a blood test to be done in early pregnancy that might identify women at risk.

RISKS OF ANTENATAL TESTS

Certain antenatal tests carry a risk of miscarriage—these include chorionic villus sampling (1 in 100) and amniocentesis (1 in 200). CVS is done between 8 and 11 weeks using a fine needle inserted through the cervix or abdomen to remove uterine tissue that eventually becomes the placenta. This sample contains genetic information and may reveal whether the foetus has a chromosomal disorder (for example, Down's syndrome) or genetic one (such as sickle-cell). Amniocentesis, normally carried out between 16 to 18 weeks, involves a needle being inserted through the abdomen into the uterus and amniotic sac to obtain a cell sample which can reveal genetic, chromosomal and developmental disorders (such as spina bifida). It can also assess rhesus incompatibility and the foetus's lung maturity.

These invasive procedures are normally done after blood has been tested for: alpha-feto-protein (AFP), human chorionic gonadotropin (hCG) and unconjugated oestriols. Their levels may indicate an increased risk of chromosomal problems or neural-tube defects (as in spina bifida). The results will read as a "one in something" chance—for example, "one in 350" means that for every 350 pregnancies with the same result, 349 are likely to be normal.

You should discuss the implications of such tests with your doctor. They can cause anxiety and the 10-day wait for results can be emotionally upsetting. While most come back normal, you need to consider how you would feel if the test showed an abnormality and whether you would find a termination acceptable.

PLACENTAL DISORDERS

Severe vaginal bleeding in the third trimester is the symptom most indicative of placenta previa and placental abruption (placenta abruptio), disorders that need urgent attention. Both are far more likely in women over 35 and those who have had several children and similar problems in previous pregnancies. An emergency Caesarean is performed to prevent extensive blood loss in the mother and oxygen deprivation in the foetus.

> **! Ectopic danger signs**
> ♀ Sudden, sharp or persistent pain in one side of the lower abdomen.
> ♀ Pain that feels as though it is under one of the shoulder blades.
> ♀ Vaginal bleeding.
> Once an ectopic pregnancy is suspected or confirmed by ultrasound, a laparoscopy is carried out to remove the pregnancy and, sometimes, part of the Fallopian tube and part of the ovary as well. Women who have suffered one ectopic pregnancy are at greater risk of a subsequent one, but many women succeed in conceiving and achieving a normal pregnancy and delivery after an ectopic (although if a Fallopian tube has been removed there is less chance of conception).

ECTOPIC PREGNANCY

An ectopic or tubal pregnancy develops in the Fallopian tubes or occasionally elsewhere in the abdominal cavity rather than in the uterus. It is not known why this happens but it is more likely if either of the Fallopian tubes has been damaged. The most usual causes of damage are endometriosis, pelvic inflammatory disease (caused by chlamydia and other sexually transmitted diseases), pelvic adhesions, gonorrhoea, a ruptured ovarian cyst, tubal surgery or by a previous ectopic pregnancy. Risks are higher in women taking the progestogen-only contraceptive pill.

Ectopic pregnancy is a potentially fatal condition which requires emergency attention. The symptoms include severe abdominal pain, vaginal bleeding and collapse—see danger signs, right.

An ectopic pregnancy may be mistaken initially for appendicitis or the threatened spontaneous abortion of a normal pregnancy.

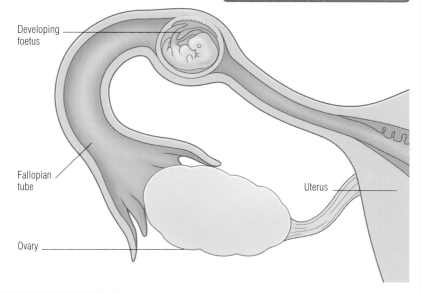

Developing foetus

Fallopian tube

Ovary

Uterus

Dealing with infertility

**INFERTILITY
COUNSELLING**
*An infertility specialist
will want to have a
complete history before
deciding on the right
course of action for a
woman who has
not become
pregnant after
a year of
regular sex.*

I nfertility is defined as the inability to become pregnant after more than one year of regular, unprotected sexual intercourse. It is estimated that just over 10 percent of women of reproductive age have problems in conceiving. In one-third of cases, the problem lies with the woman's reproductive system and in another third the problem lies with the man's reproductive system. In the remaining third the problem is with both partners or is not known. After specialist investigation of both partners and treatment, between 30 and 40 percent of couples achieve a pregnancy within two years.

CAUSES KNOWN AND UNKNOWN

Why some people should be unable to become pregnant is not yet fully understood but some causes have been identified. In women, it may be because the ovaries are not producing eggs (no ovulation or early menopause) or they are polycystic. Endometriosis and other hormonal disorders may be causes as can be damaged or blocked Fallopian tubes and pelvic inflammatory disease. In some women mucus around the cervix may be hostile to the partner's sperm.

In men, the most common cause is defective sperm (in quantity, motility or normality). In couples, the genetic make-up of one partner prevents the couple achieving a pregnancy naturally or occupational hazards (such as chemicals and working practices) are involved.

EVALUATING THE PROBLEM

The doctor may see the woman, the man and the couple on separate occasions. The woman will have a physical examination and a detailed personal history will be taken. Obesity, acne and menstrual irregularities will be noted and questions may be asked about eating disorders, stress, occupational hazards (working with toxins, for example), exercise methods, sexual pattern, previous contraception and lifestyle habits such as alcohol, smoking and prescribed or illegal drugs. Blood tests may be done to seek known reasons for infertility—an excess of prolactin (a hormone regulating menstruation), excess or deficiency of thyroid hormone or an excess of androgens (male hormones).

If a woman has endometriosis, uterine fibroids, polyps or ovarian cysts the doctor may refer her to a gynaecologist or reproductive endocrinologist for assessment before treatment is decided. In the partner's case, the doctor may suggest sperm analysis. Finding out early on that the man has too few sperm, no sperm at all or slow-moving or misshapen sperm may lessen the chance of a woman having to undergo invasive tests (although if she has other physical symptoms she may still need investigation as well).

If the doctor suspects that sexual problems could be a cause of infertility in the couple, a therapist may be recommended. If the actual issue of becoming pregnant is thought to be adversely affecting a woman's health, the doctor might recommend complementary therapies to aid relaxation.

INVESTIGATIONS

Various methods may be used to assess the condition of a woman's reproductive system. Laparoscopy is a minor operation involving a small incision in the abdomen through which a special endoscope can be inserted to view the uterus, Fallopian tubes and ovaries. Dye is passed through the neck of the uterus into the tubes to

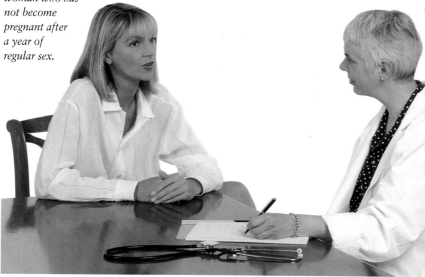

check for blockage or constriction. Depending on agreed consent before the operation abnormal growths or other problems may be dealt with by laser vaporization, electrocautery or excisional biopsy.

Hysteroscopy is similar to laparoscopy but no incision is required. A specialized endoscope, the hysteroscope, is passed through the neck of the uterus to check for adhesions (scar tissue) and other problems.

Hysterosalpingography, an X-ray technique, employs a contrast (radio-opaque) medium injected into the uterus to outline the reproductive organs. It identifies 75 percent of tubal blockages. It should be done in the first 10 days of a woman's menstrual cycle when she is least likely to be pregnant as radiation can harm a developing foetus. It may not be used in a woman with a history of pelvic infections, ectopic pregnancy or tubal surgery. It can cause abdominal cramps.

With hysterosalpingo-contrast sonography a contrast medium is injected through the neck of the uterus, and with the help of an ultrasound, a probe is guided through the vagina to enable detailed viewing of the woman's reproductive system. There is minimal discomfort.

RANGE OF TREATMENTS

If ovulation is the problem, drugs can induce it. Disorders such as polycystic ovaries, endometriosis and PID can be treated. Damaged Fallopian tubes can be repaired by surgery.

If the tubes are damaged beyond repair, a pregnancy may be achieved with in vitro fertilization; other assisted reproductive technologies may be considered for lack of ovulation or sperm problems. Artificial insemination with the partner's sperm is a treatment option in cases of infertility in which the sperm are too few or are insufficiently motile.

SELF-HELP FOR INFERTILITY

Preconceptual care is highly important. Excessive drinking, smoking, infections, obesity, anxiety and stress can each play a part in reducing fertility. You are advised to stop taking the contraceptive pill some time before attempting to conceive so that periods are reestablished, which may take some months. It is vital to understand your own monthly menstrual cycle so you know which days are optimum for sexual intercourse.

CHECKING UP ON OVULATION

To find out whether a woman is ovulating, she may be asked to keep a basal body temperature chart (BBT) on which she records her morning temperature on waking, along with the day of the menstrual cycle. She marks the days when bleeding occurs with a cross, and the days when intercourse occurs with a circle. During the menstrual cycle, the BBT is higher once ovulation happens—confirmed by an 0.4°C rise in temperature for three consecutive days.

Over-the-counter ovulation kits can be used to detect luteinizing hormone which surges just before ovulation. A blood test to measure progesterone levels can also confirm ovulation—the hormone is secreted around day 20, about a week after the egg is released, to stimulate the thickening of the uterus lining.

The doctor may do an endometrial biopsy toward the end of the menstrual cycle but before bleeding begins, to check that thickening of the uterus lining has occurred. The simple procedure is usually done at a clinic or fertility unit, without anaesthetic.

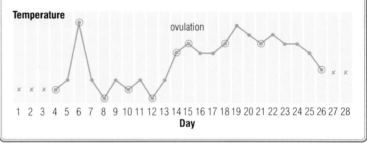

You can identify these by observing changes in vaginal mucus, by making a temperature chart and by calculating over several months the cycle's length.

There are three vital stages. Implantation takes place some seven days after fertilization and fertilization takes place within 48 hours of the woman ovulating. Ovulation takes place 14 days before the expected next period. This is not the same as saying that it takes place 14 days after the last period as menstrual cycles vary in length from 24 to 35 days—hence the need to identify the usual length of your own cycle.

Note changes in your vaginal mucus. Just before ovulation the mucus increases in quantity and becomes thinner and more elastic, jelly-like and transparent—a drop can be stretched into a long strand without breaking. After ovulation, it returns to a milky colour.

It is said that a man's sperm will be more vigorous and more in number if he ejaculates only every few days rather than every day.

Assisted reproduction technology

See also:

1/BEING A WELL WOMAN
Essentials of good health
pp.16–29
Healthy body systems p. 33;
pp. 38–39

6/TREATMENTS & THERAPIES
Treatment plans pp. 262–269
Conventional treatments
pp. 272–277; 284–289
Complementary therapies
pp. 292–293

Reproduction specialists today have a wide range of options which they can employ to help previously infertile people to have children. Known as ART (artificial reproduction technology), the techniques fall into two groups: artificial insemination and assisted conception. Each can either involve a couple's own eggs and sperm or those from a donor or donors.

The procedures are costly and labour intensive as they are carried out over several weeks and need a large number of trained medical and technical staff to do them. In some cases part of the costs, such as the drugs needed, will be covered by a health authority but generally ART is paid for privately. The chances of taking home a live baby are between 18 and 40 percent depending on the age of the mother and the age of the egg. Counselling about the procedures is usually made available by an infertility unit. Issues to be discussed should include side effects and risks of taking the drugs, the recommended number of treatment cycles and the legal implications of using donor eggs or sperm. Help may be needed to cope with your feelings should you fail to achieve conception or a live birth.

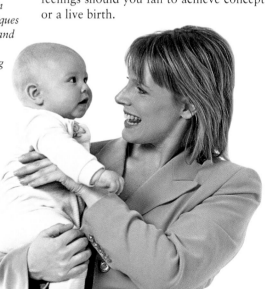

A BABY IS BORN
Modern advances in reproductive techniques mean that women and men who have difficulty conceiving a baby naturally can be helped to start a family. Ask to see a clinic's successful birth rates before agreeing to treatment.

A RANGE OF TECHNIQUES

AIH (artificial insemination) This involves a woman using a syringe to place her partner's sperm in her cervix during the time she is ovulating. This method is useful for couples who experience sexual difficulties such as male impotence and for unexplained infertility.

DI (donor insemination) A similar procedure to that above but in this case the syringe contains donor sperm. This method is used in cases of the male partner's impotence or if he has defective sperm.

IUI (intrauterine insemination) A specialist procedure in which sperm is introduced directly into the woman's uterus through the vagina and cervix. The sperm are treated first and the woman may be given drugs to help her produce more than one egg at the time of ovulation. These measures enhance the chances of conception by artificial insemination and are used when the woman's body makes antibodies to her partner's sperm, for male impotence or unexplained infertility.

IVF (in vitro fertilization) The so-called "test tube baby" procedure that fertilizes the woman's eggs with her partner's sperm outside the body in a hospital or clinic laboratory. First the woman takes drugs to stimulate her ovaries to produce fertilizable eggs. These are collected in the operating theatre—the woman is lightly sedated—and mixed with sperm. If fertilization occurs (it takes several days) the woman returns to the operating theatre where two embryos may be placed in her uterus and the remainder frozen in liquid nitrogen for later use. This technique is mostly employed in cases of poor quality sperm, when the woman's body makes antibodies to the sperm, unexplained infertility, blocked or scarred Fallopian tubes or irregular ovulation.

GIFT A suitable technique for women who have no problem with their Fallopian tubes. It is a variation of IVF—the eggs and sperm are collected as described above and placed in the Fallopian tube for fertilization to occur.

ZIFT A combination of IVF and GIFT, in which the woman's eggs are collected (as in IVF) and the eggs mixed with sperm in a test tube. Once fertilization has taken place the fused eggs and sperm—embryos—are placed in

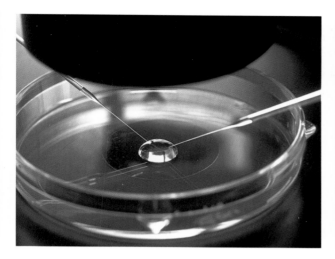

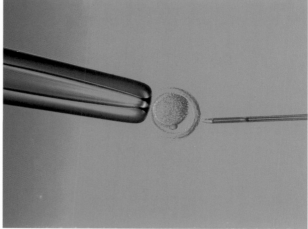

a healthy Fallopian tube, not in the uterus as in IVF. This technique is used when GIFT hasn't worked or is considered unlikely to work.

PROST Almost the same as IVF, but the technique is surgical. Using a laparascope, the specialist places the fertilized eggs in a healthy Fallopian tube rather than into the uterus through the vagina and cervix.

ICSI An acronym, the initials of "intracytoplasmic sperm injection" and a technique that may involve two actions. In men who are not producing sperm in their semen, sperm are retrieved surgically from the vas deferens. One sperm is then directly injected into an egg which has been retrieved from the woman as in IVF and placed in the woman's uterus. This technique may be especially suitable for those couples in whom sperm is of poor quality, has little movement (motility) or is unable to penetrate the egg. It is known that sons conceived with the aid of ICSI will have the same congenital abnormality as their fathers.

Egg donation This is key to conception when a woman cannot produce her own eggs or her own eggs are not fertilizable. Donor eggs from a woman aged under 35 have the highest success rate. The eggs are fertilized by the male partner's sperm as in IVF and one or two embryos are placed in the female partner's uterus. She is given hormonal drugs in order to maintain the pregnancy. The only alternatives to this technique are surrogacy or adoption.

Surrogacy This is rare. It allows one woman to give birth for another who is unable to carry a baby to term or who is unable to conceive. The surrogate either carries the other woman's fertilized egg or her own which has been fertilized by the father's sperm to full term and then hands over the baby at birth. This is a choice that is riddled with legal problems—including adoption of the newborn child—and loopholes, and needs all parties to conform with the law and to be fully aware and in written agreement about each aspect of the transaction.

Adoption This is an alternative for couples who have not found success with some of the options described here. The legal situation surrounding adoption is much clearer than that of surrogacy.

NEEDLE ACCURACY
Two common causes of infertility concern the inability of eggs and sperm to fuse and create an embryo. With modern help they are brought together to fertilize outside the body, above left, or, as with ICSI, above, sperm is injected into an egg.

Freezing eggs, sperm and embryos

The techniques of ART and the pursuit of a family are enabled by having a supply of eggs and sperm or embryos which can be used at any time. The medium is liquid nitrogen which "freezes" for storage at a fertility unit. Before use their quality is tested and only healthy ones are chosen.

Donor sperm is automatically frozen for six months while it is screened for HIV, the virus that causes AIDS. The freezing method is also important in screening embryos for identifiable inherited diseases such as cystic fibrosis. Genetic testing in this way allows selection of a disease-free embryo.

Freezing sperm or eggs is an option for men and women undergoing treatment such as chemotherapy which may make them infertile. This isn't offered as a matter of course so make sure that you ask about it if you are interested to know more.

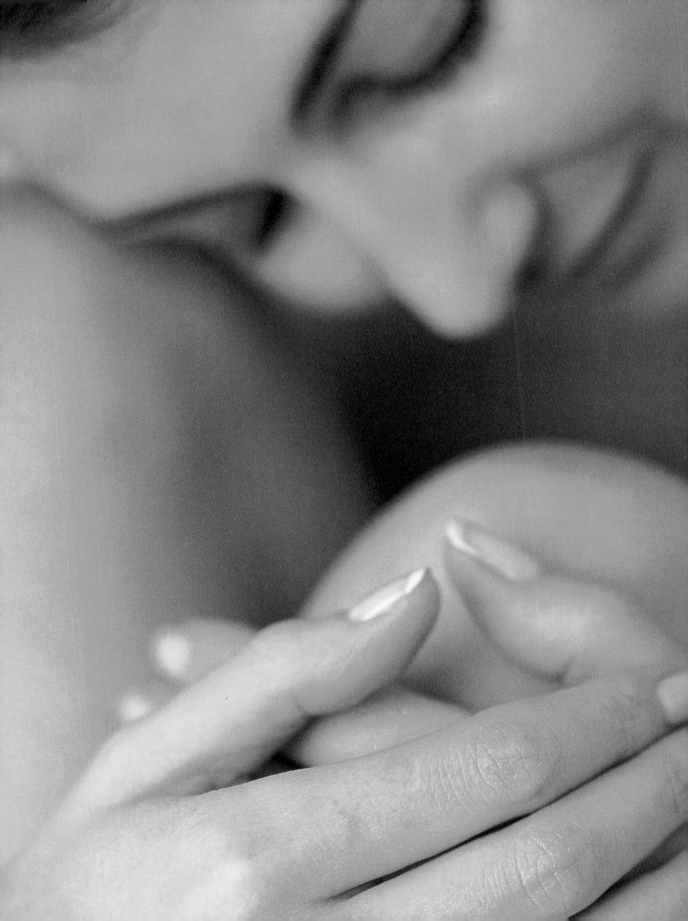

ILLNESSES AND EMERGENCIES

At different times of your life you may experience illnesses that occur because a part of your body malfunctions. It is important that you seek the right help and receive effective treatment as soon as possible so that health is restored. Being aware of how your body works is probably the most significant factor in maintaining good health. Although minor illnesses or infections may be more commonplace than life-threatening ones, if you allow them to come and go without sorting them out you may unwittingly cause a build-up of tension and stress, leading to a general feeling of ill health. If you just accept this, you may forget what is normal for you and even what being well feels like.

URINARY SYSTEM PROBLEMS

Disorders of the urinary tract arise from many causes, often linked to a woman's hormonal changes or as a result of the closely related anatomy of the reproductive and urinary systems. Although these problems can cause discomfort and distress, they can often be ameliorated by taking quick action and simple treatments.

See also:

1/BEING A WELL WOMAN
Healthy body systems p. 37

4/HORMONAL HEALTH
Endocrine system pp. 142–143
Uterine problems pp. 162–166
Pregnancy pp. 172–179

5/ILLNESSES & EMERGENCIES
Acute infections pp. 244–246

See your doctor

Painful urination is not a symptom of incontinence. Nor is urinating several times during the night (nocturia) usual. If you suffer from either of these conditions you should go to your doctor for a check-up.

Incontinence

Urinary incontinence is a condition that is embarrassing and distressing—and far from uncommon in women of all ages. There may be various causes, from childbirth to infection, and from gynaecological surgery to loss of oestrogen at menopause. In too many cases women do not discuss the problem with their doctor early enough for the right help or advice to be given. For many women, incontinence may be more of an annoyance than a serious problem and they can benefit from methods that restore their ability to control urination. Other women may need surgical help (p. 165).

Usually problems can be sorted into three categories: overactive bladder, stress incontinence and mixed symptoms.

HOW IT IS DIAGNOSED

Your doctor will either give you a questionnaire to fill in or ask you a series of questions about your symptoms. These will help determine the bladder-control condition you have. The complete diagnosis will involve a physical examination and a series of simple tests carried out by a urologist, urinary surgeon or gynaecologist, to establish the cause of your problem.

Bladder function is tested by asking the patient to drink large quantities of fluid and seeing how much urine is passed in normal circumstances. A second test, called urodynamics, involves several procedures: the pressure in the bladder and the flow of urine are checked, a sample of urine is taken for analysis to detect any infection or bladder stones, the whole urinary system is examined by ultrasound, and a fibreoptic cystoscope may be inserted into the urethra so that the urinary tract can then be inspected from the inside.

The doctor will want to evaluate all the results, since it is not unusual for a woman to suffer both stress and urge incontinence at the same time. Urinary incontinence may also be a side effect of illnesses such as multiple sclerosis and prolapsed spinal discs in the lower back.

Gynaecological physiotherapy

Kegel and similar exercises are aimed at improving the tone and strength of the muscles of the pelvic floor—the muscles that are used to stop urine from flowing. The exercises involve alternate contraction and release of vaginal and anal muscles to restore the neck of the bladder to its correct position. They are taught in antenatal classes and should be used after childbirth or pelvic surgery as a preventive measure. You can do them standing or sitting, when or where you want (no one will be able to tell that you are doing them).

Keep your legs slightly apart and close your anus as if you are trying to avoid passing gas. At the same time, draw the vagina inward and upward as if trying to stop passing urine. Count to five, relax for a count of five, then repeat.

Start by contracting the muscles three to five times a day; the goal is to hold the passages closed for 15 seconds. After eight weeks' practice you should notice an improvement in bladder control.

BLADDER-CONTROL PROBLEMS

There are different types of incontinence which are brought about by different factors and vary in their symptoms and the discomfort or inconvenience they cause. You need to be able to describe to your doctor what happens to you so that he or she can accurately diagnose the cause and try to help.

Type	Symptoms
Stress incontinence	Small amounts of urine are discharged involuntarily when pressure is put on the bladder by coughing, laughing or sneezing. It is due to weakness in the muscles of the pelvic floor, perhaps caused by a vaginal delivery, obesity, pelvic surgery, a prolapse or a lack of hormones after menopause. It is the most common form of incontinence in women.
Urge incontinence	Larger quantities of urine are discharged by involuntary contractions of the bladder muscles. You may need to urinate several times during the night. The causes include bladder infections, alcohol, diabetes and lack of oestrogen after menopause. Lack of nervous control of the bladder is known as reflex incontinence.
Overflow incontinence	The bladder always feels full, either because of an obstruction caused by a tumour or kidney stones, or some other condition, such as diabetes or a stroke, that affects bladder control. Urine may be forced back up the ureters to the kidneys, carrying serious infection with it.
Functional incontinence	People with this type of incontinence can control urination but are unable, usually because of physical disability, to reach the toilet in time. It is common in older age.
Transient incontinence	Sometimes incontinence is a temporary affliction, the result of an infection of the urinary tract, constipation (faeces press against the urethra, blocking it—common in pregnancy) and certain prescription drugs (such as antidepressants and muscle relaxants).

RANGE OF TREATMENTS

Treatment of incontinence depends on its type. Women suffering from stress incontinence may be referred for gynaecological physiotherapy sessions to learn Kegel and other exercises (see opposite). Postmenopausal women may be asked to consider HRT (p. 144) to restore oestrogen levels. If stress incontinence persists, surgery may be suggested to put the neck of the bladder back in its correct position. The success of this procedure is not guaranteed.

The bladder contractions that cause urge incontinence are treated with anticholinergic and antispasmodic drugs—although these have side effects such as dry mouth and blurred vision—and by treating any underlying condition. With urge incontinence, timed voiding may be suggested. You will be told to go to the toilet at set intervals throughout the day, whether you feel the urge or not. After several days of this, the time between visits is increased. This continues until you can hold urine for three to five hours without leakage. You may be advised to avoid drinking coffee, and to have only a little to drink in the evening.

Bladder retraining for urge incontinence is possible, using devices such as cones, sponges and plugs, which your doctor or physiotherapist may prescribe. The devices have different weights and are held in the vagina, the weight increasing as the muscles strengthen.

WHICH OF THESE APPLY TO YOU?

A number of symptoms are associated with incontinence. You should consult your doctor if you: frequently have a strong, sudden urge to pass urine; go to the toilet eight times or more in 24 hours; get up twice or more in the night to pass urine; are not always able to hold on until you reach the toilet; have a slight loss of urine when you sneeze, cough or laugh; have a loss of urine when exercising or lifting heavy objects; or wear incontinence pads and have to change them two or more times a day.

DIGESTIVE SYSTEM PROBLEMS

When the system is working well every part of the body benefits from the food you eat. In some women, however, for reasons not always known, the efficiency is compromised by a range of problems which in themselves can be a long-term risk to health.

See also:

1/BEING A WELL WOMAN
Essentials of good health
    pp. 16–23

3/GENERAL HEALTH ISSUES
Skeletal system problems
    pp. 78–81
Blood and the circulation
    pp. 118–125
Women and heart disease
    pp. 126–133

4/HORMONAL HEALTH
Endocrine system problems
    pp. 136–137; pp. 142–143
Uterine problems pp. 162–166
Conception problems pp. 180–181

The effects of obesity

When your body weight is much too high in proportion to your age and shape you raise your risk of serious health problems. Between the start and end of the 20th century, due to changes in diet and lifestyle, the shape and weight of men and women changed a great deal, but not for the better. By the millennium, more people were classed as overweight than of normal weight. More important, 27 percent of women and 24 percent of men were clinically obese—their weight was at least 20 percent more than that regarded as desirable for their frame (bones of the skeleton). A worrying number of children were in this category.

WHAT CAUSES OBESITY?

Your natural body weight is influenced by many factors, including your age, sex and shape. You gain weight when what you eat is not used by the body as energy (calories) and is instead stored in adipose (fatty) tissue. In women, this is usually around the hips, thighs and buttocks, the arms and shoulders. In men, fat builds up around the waist and stomach.

Obesity tends to run in families, not only through genetics but because most people acquire their eating habits from their families. Very rarely, obesity is caused by glandular problems, such as an underactive thyroid or overactive adrenals. Getting older can have an effect too—people use less energy, may have joint and mobility problems, lose muscle mass, the metabolic rate slows and more fat is stored.

DANGERS OF BEING OVERWEIGHT

Obesity is not simply a cosmetic problem. Even moderate weight gain as an adult increases your risk of illness later. Many overweight people have high blood pressure and blood fat levels which have been linked to a number of health concerns, including coronary heart disease (CHD), stroke, some cancers (including colorectal and breast cancer), gall stones and adult-onset diabetes.

If you are clinically obese it means your metabolism is putting stress on many organs in your body and the extra load on the bones and joints can make other medical conditions, such as osteoarthritis, worse. Storing weight around the stomach (apple shape) is associated with greater risk of disease than storing fat on the hips and thighs (pear shape). However, if you lose five to 10 percent of this accumulated extra weight and switch to a healthy eating plan with exercise, you can substantially reduce your risk.

FAT DISTRIBUTION
Near right: a certain amount of fat is natural on a woman's body. Centre: if through her life a woman's weight comes more from muscle or bone than fat, her outline is pear-shaped. Far right: if a woman aged between 40 and 60 builds up fat around waist and stomach, and becomes apple-shaped, she runs the risk of heart disease, stroke, diabetes and gall bladder problems.

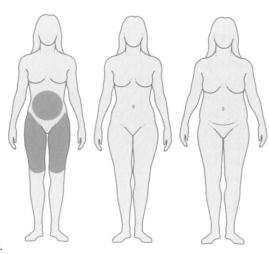

General fat distribution   Pear shape   Apple shape

ASSESSING YOUR HEALTH RISK

To calculate your body fat in relation to your frame, doctors use the Body Mass Index (BMI). This figure is reached by dividing your weight (without shoes) in kilograms by your height in metres squared (rounded off to nearest decimal point). A woman who is 1.6 m tall and weighs 60 kg can work out her BMI as: 1. 6 multiplied by 1.6 = 2.6; then 60 divided by 2.6 = 23.1.

For women, the desirable BMI is between 19 and 24. If it is under 19, you are underweight. If it is 25 to 27, you are overweight. If it is between 27 and 30, you are considered obese. Over 30 is described as clinically obese.

Doctors may do another assessment, the waist-to-hip ratio: your waist measurement is divided by your hip measurement. If your waist is 75 cm (30 in) and your hips 92.5 cm (37 in), your ratio is 0.8. Women should ideally have a ratio of less than 0.8 (the waist is not greater than 80 percent of the hips); if 0.9 or higher, they have more than three times the risk of heart disease as women with a ratio of less than 0.7, even if their weight is normal.

A third measurement, often taken at a gym, determines your lean body mass (which reflects your bones and muscle) and fat mass. Exercise programmes aim to turn body fat to muscle.

Your metabolism

Your metabolic rate is the speed at which your body turns food into the energy it needs to keep all parts functioning well. Regular aerobic exercise that makes you out of breath, such as brisk walking, tennis or cycling, increases your muscle mass which leads to a higher metabolic rate.

The effect of the increase goes on for longer than you spent exercising so you go on using up body fat even at rest. If you are fit and exercise regularly, extra calories you eat will burn up rather than be stored. If you stop regular exercise your metabolic rate slows, muscle mass breaks down and your weight may return to what it was.

If you crash diet (eat very few calories), your body responds by decreasing its metabolic rate. When you return to your normal eating pattern your body can no longer burn extra calories as efficiently, so excess energy is stored as fat and you put on weight. Recurrent crash diets also adversely affect protective HDL cholesterol levels.

ACID REFLUX AND HIATUS HERNIA

Doctors call it gastro-oesophageal reflux disease and it occurs when stomach acid comes up the food pipe into the mouth. It affects about 30 percent of adults and most pregnant women although it stops after the baby is born.

The common symptoms are heartburn (burning sensation) and regurgitation of food or acid, both of which happen after meals, when bending over or lying down. Some people may also have chest pain, which can be mistaken for a heart attack, and wheezing and coughing. The cause usually lies either with the muscular valve or a hiatus hernia, where part of the stomach rises through a hole in the diaphragm (the hiatus) into the chest. Hiatus hernia is common in middle-aged women, and in smokers and people who are overweight. Heavy lifting, sneezing or coughing can also cause this type of hernia.

Tests such as a gastroscopy or barium swallow may be done to confirm the diagnosis and you will be advised to change your lifestyle: cut down on alcohol, stop smoking, lose weight, exercise daily and raise the head of your bed about 10 cm (4 in). Eat small. frequent meals slowly, chew food well and reduce fat intake.

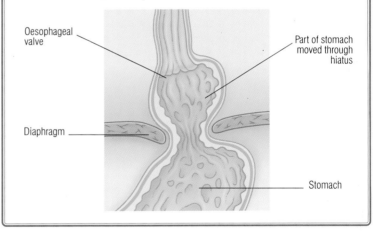

Oesophageal valve

Part of stomach moved through hiatus

Diaphragm

Stomach

FAT AND THE MENOPAUSE

Most women tend to put on weight between the ages of 40 and 60. Though overall oestrogen levels drop, if at this time there is a substantial proportion of fat on the body, oestrogen is still produced by the fat. Some women attribute weight gain to the combination pill, progestogen-only contraception and HRT, but reduced activity resulting in loss of muscle mass may be more pertinent. Walking for at least 30 minutes daily, three hours a week, reduces the risk of CHD and stroke by 40 percent. Walking strengthens muscles and bones by placing one and a half times the body weight on them.

Hepatitis

! Caution

If you have hepatitis A you must avoid spreading it to other people in your household. Use separate eating utensils and be extra vigilant about hygiene. People who have contracted hepatitis B or C can be carriers; for example, a mother can pass hepatitis B to her child by breastfeeding.

Hepatitis (inflammation of the liver) is usually caused by one of three viruses. It can also stem from lifestyle and overindulgence. In some cases it is life threatening.

The viruses that cause hepatitis are known as A, B and C; D and E also exist, but are much rarer. Non-infectious hepatitis can occur as a result of alcohol abuse, industrial chemicals, some autoimmune disorders (in which your immune system attacks your own liver cells) or overdosing on drugs, such as paracetamol. Other viruses, such as glandular fever or cytomegalovirus, can also cause hepatitis.

Hepatitis can be acute or chronic, and will need medical attention. The acute illness lasts for a few months, has no long-term effects and gradually you feel better. The chronic illness is more serious, since it can destroy the liver.

? Did you know?

There is no cure for hepatitis. Sometimes a doctor will prescribe medication such as interferons (which have a nonspecific antiviral action) or a drug to treat specific symptoms such as nausea.

TREATMENT

Many hepatitis patients recover without any specific treatment; the doctor usually recommends rest for a few weeks until the jaundice disappears.

Because of the role the liver plays in the digestive process, you may be advised not to take certain medicines (such as birth control pills) or alcohol. Jaundice can last many months, leaving you feeling very tired, even after the infection has passed. You should give the liver time to recover by avoiding alcohol for the time recommended by your doctor.

PREVENTION

Noninfectious hepatitis can be prevented by avoiding excesses of alcohol. Viral hepatitis is spread in contaminated blood, water and food and is most likely to be caught in developing countries. Vaccines are available against hepatitis A and B and are usually recommended for people at high risk, including healthcare workers and travellers to these countries.

Good hygiene is essential while travelling. Drink only boiled or bottled water, avoid ice in drinks and don't eat food stored or prepared in unhygienic conditions. You should also avoid unprotected sex (p. 72) or sharing needles.

TYPES AND SYMPTOMS

There is more than one type of hepatitis and the symptoms depends on the virus involved. A diagnosis is made by a physical examination, urine and blood tests.

Approximately 10 percent of patients with hepatitis B later acquire chronic hepatitis; this is extremely rare for people with hepatitis A.

Disease	Symptoms
Hepatitis A (HAV)	Causes an acute flu-like illness, with headaches and fever, aching joints or muscles, nausea, diarrhoea and vomiting, loss of appetite and abdominal pain. If the condition is severe, within a few days there may be jaundice—yellowing of the skin and whites of the eyes caused by a build-up of bile pigments in the blood. You may also pass pale-coloured stools and dark urine.
Hepatitis B (HBV)	Has similar symptoms to those above, but is a greater problem since it can lead to a chronic illness, with severe, persistent liver inflammation that can result in cirrhosis and liver failure. It may also cause cancer of the liver.
Hepatitis C (HCV)	Mainly chronic, but symptoms may be no worse than generally feeling unwell. It, too, can lead to cirrhosis. It is most usually the result of blood transfusion, which is less likely now that donated blood is screened. Both hepatitis B and C can be sexually transmitted.

Cirrhosis

This life-threatening disease of the liver is characterized by the progressive destruction of cells within an organ that is central to your body's health. Chronic alcoholism over a number of years is the most common cause of cirrhosis, although chronic viral hepatitis and, in some rare cases, inherited diseases can also be the culprits. Although a woman may drink less than a man, she may be at an equal risk of cirrhosis, because of her smaller body size and slower metabolism of alcohol.

The most common form of cirrhosis, called primary biliary cirrhosis, mainly affects women aged 30 to 60. It occurs when small bile ducts, which deliver bile to the intestines for the digestion of fats, become inflamed and blocked. It is an autoimmune disorder.

SIGNS AND SYMPTOMS

The onset of cirrhosis may be fairly gradual and no specific symptoms may be noticed at first. Signs to be aware of include tiredness and sleep disturbance, generalized itching, swollen feet and legs, menstrual disturbances, nausea, loss of muscle bulk and slight jaundice.

In more advanced cirrhosis, the cells are replaced with fibrous scar tissue and the liver becomes less effective. There may be malabsorption of vitamins, such as vitamin D, leading to loss of bone mass. A build-up of female hormones causes spidery small red marks on the chest and upper body, while an accumulation of waste products can affect the brain, causing confusion and coma.

Once the liver begins to harden, blood pressure in internal organs may increase, leading to sudden internal bleeding. The cell death and scarring can be serious enough to cause liver failure.

TREATING CIRRHOSIS

The liver has a remarkable ability to repair itself. If the early signs of cirrhosis are recognized, most people have a good chance of recovery. Since the liver cell damage is most commonly caused by heavy alcohol consumption, alcoholics must stop drinking alcohol. They may be helped to stop by drug treatment that disrupts alcohol metabolism in the liver leading to nausea and vomiting if alcohol is ingested.

Steroids or antiviral drugs may be given to treat chronic hepatitis and other drugs can be used to control symptoms such as itching.

If no action is taken or the cirrhosis is far advanced, permanent damage may occur and the only chance of a long-term cure will be a liver transplant.

See also:

1/BEING A WELL WOMAN
Essentials of good health
pp. 20–21
Healthy body systems
p. 34; p. 36

3/GENERAL HEALTH ISSUES
Problems of the mind pp. 95–97

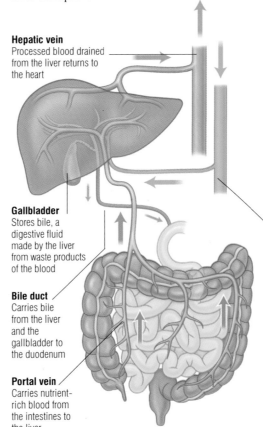

Hepatic vein
Processed blood drained from the liver returns to the heart

Gallbladder
Stores bile, a digestive fluid made by the liver from waste products of the blood

Bile duct
Carries bile from the liver and the gallbladder to the duodenum

Portal vein
Carries nutrient-rich blood from the intestines to the liver

THE LIVER
The liver has a vital role in the control of chemicals in the body. It absorbs oxygen and nutrients from the blood, regulates levels of glucose and amino-acids, manufactures proteins and removes toxic substances.

Hepatic artery
Carries oxygenated blood from the heart to the liver

> **! Caution**
>
> As well as damaging the liver, excessive alcohol intake, especially on a regular basis and without food, can damage other parts of the body, such as the stomach lining. Damage can cause ulcers, stomach and bowel cancers and disorders of the pancreas (such as diabetes). The short-term effects of drinking too much alcohol include an upset stomach and dehydration. Alcohol also interacts with many medicines.
>
> Even light drinkers who drink an unusual amount over a short period may be at risk of developing fatty liver—a condition that produces pain and tenderness, caused when the liver becomes swollen with fat and water, which it is unable to process in the normal way.

Alcoholic neuropathy

Excess intake of alcohol can cause alcoholic neuropathy, a condition causing permanent nerve damage. It is usually associated with vitamin deficiencies, usually of the B vitamins. The symptoms include numbness, abnormal sensations, muscle weakness, incontinence, constipation and diarrhoea. The symptoms may develop gradually and progressively worsen over weeks or even years. It is possible to control the condition with medication and replace the missing nutrients with dietary supplements.

Gallbladder disorders

The gallbladder is a small pear-shaped sac lying directly beneath, and connected to, your liver. It has a profound effect on digestion.

Every time you eat, the gallbladder responds by releasing bile, a yellow fluid produced in your liver that breaks up fats from food and blood. The gallbladder is also involved in removing waste products to the small intestine through a tube-shaped duct.

Inflammation of the gallbladder, called cholecystitis, is common in women. The most usual cause is gallstones, which develop if the bile becomes too concentrated and hardens.

SIGNS AND RISK FACTORS

No one knows why some people get gallstones and others don't. However, there is increasing evidence that oestrogen influences the making of cholesterol, which in turn combines with bile pigments to form crystals—gallstones—which vary in size from a tiny bead to a pigeon's egg. Stones may take years to form with no symptoms if they remain in the gallbladder. It's when they leave and get caught in the ducts that pain occurs.

Gallstones affect one in 10 people and are two to three times more common in women than in men. You are at greater risk if you are over 50, overweight or diabetic, have high triglyceride levels in the blood, have had several children or take contraceptives or HRT in pill form (these are metabolized by the liver). Also at risk are women with a history of rapid weight-loss diets with low calorie intake: not enough bile acids to dissolve the cholesterol may allow crystals to form.

The cholesterol link

Gallstones may contain cholesterol, bile pigments or a mixture of the two. Cholesterol stones can grow very large—big enough to block the common bile duct— whereas pigment stones are generally much smaller. Cholesterol stones are formed if bile contains too much cholesterol, which is made from the breakdown of saturated fats. Therefore, eating a diet that has little saturated fat (from meat and dairy products) is a good preventive measure. If you already have gallstones, fatty foods can make your symptoms worse.

SYMPTOMS

Although you can have gallstones without being aware of it, if a large stone does get stuck in the common bile duct you will certainly feel it. Typically, it causes intense pain on the right hand side of the body under the ribs (called biliary colic). The pain may be very brief or may last for up to several hours and can spread towards the shoulder blades. Accompanying symptoms may include bloating of the stomach, nausea and vomiting.

If the gallstone prevents bile from reaching the intestines, the stools may turn putty-coloured and, if the liver can't get rid of bile, this can lead to jaundice. Occasionally the gallstone blocks the bile flow in the common bile duct, leading to pancreatitis (an inflammation of the pancreas).

TREATING GALLSTONES

If you are not in any pain, gallstones can be left to their own devices. If the stones are causing discomfort, however, bile salts may be prescribed to try and dissolve them, although these can take up to two years to work and the stones can often recur.

Lithotripsy (shock-wave therapy), which uses high-frequency sound waves, may be performed to break up the stones. Alternatively, the gallbladder may be removed by surgery. This is called a cholecystectomy. You can function perfectly well without a gallbladder, because your body is able to create a reservoir of bile within the liver.

GALLSTONES
Gallstones vary in size and can occur singly or in groups of up to 10. Increasingly surgeons locate and remove them laparoscopically, using a flexible endoscope—a fibreoptic viewing instrument.

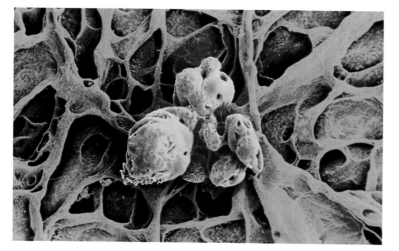

Digestive tract ulcers

Ulcers are sensitive raw patches that occur in the lining of the digestive tract from the oesophagus to the stomach and duodenum (the first part of the intestines). Collectively, stomach (gastric) and duodenal ulcers are called peptic ulcers.

Digestion is a carefully balanced process. Your stomach produces hydrochloric acid and the enzyme called pepsin so food can be broken down and its nutrients absorbed. These gastric juices are kept from attacking the smooth, muscular walls of your stomach and duodenum by a protective mucus membrane. It is when this breaks down that an ulcer forms.

A peptic ulcer can cause severe, burning abdominal pain that may be temporarily relieved by eating. It is often worse at night. Other symptoms include nausea, vomiting, belching, bloating and weight loss. In severe cases the ulcer may cause bleeding, triggering anaemia. Severe ulcers may, in rare cases, perforate the stomach lining, leading to peritonitis—inflammation of the abdominal lining.

If there is any doubt about where the ulcer is, diagnosis will be by endoscopic examination (gastroscopy) under short-term general anaesthetic. A flexible fibreoptic tube is passed from the oesophagus to the stomach and duodenum while the doctor views the area on a screen. A piece of tissue will be taken (a biopsy) to check for the presence of bacteria or cancer.

WHO IS AT RISK?

Peptic ulcers affect one woman in 15, particularly those over the age of 50. Ulcers tend to occur in families, possibly passed through close contact. The primary culprit is a bacterium called Helicobacter pylori (see box). Ulcers are also common in heavy drinkers, smokers and people who regularly take nonsteroidal anti-inflammatory drugs (NSAIDs), which are used in the treatment of arthritis.

The symptoms can often be relieved by avoiding any foods that make them worse—milk and too hot spices, for instance—by eating regular meals, giving up smoking and drinking less alcohol. The doctor may prescribe drugs to prevent acid secretion, and liquid antacids to neutralize the acid and protect the stomach lining. Surgery is a last resort.

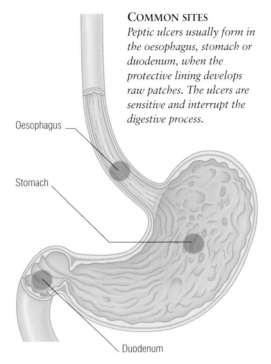

COMMON SITES
Peptic ulcers usually form in the oesophagus, stomach or duodenum, when the protective lining develops raw patches. The ulcers are sensitive and interrupt the digestive process.

Oesophagus

Stomach

Duodenum

See also:

1/BEING A WELL WOMAN
Essentials of good health pp. 16–19
Healthy body systems p. 36

3/GENERAL HEALTH ISSUES
Problems of the mind pp. 95–103
Blood and the circulation p. 116

6/TREATMENTS & THERAPIES
Conventional treatments pp. 272–277

See your doctor

Ulcers that are left untreated may bleed, which in turn can cause anaemia (p. 116). A prime symptom of this is tiredness, as well as dark red, bloody or black stools which indicate internal bleeding. See your doctor immediately.

The bacterial breakthrough

For many years it was thought that stress and diet caused stomach ulcers. However, since the mid-1980s, it has been known that bacteria called *Helicobacter pylori* (*H. pylori*) are involved in the formation of 95 percent of duodenal ulcers and 70 percent of gastric ulcers. The bacteria live in the stomach lining, making it more sensitive to acid and causing inflammation. Most people are infected in childhood, although not everyone will have symptoms. Once symptoms appear—the most usual being indigestion, reflux (backflow) and stomach pain—your doctor can arrange a blood or breath test for *H. pylori*.

If the bacteria are found, a multi-layer regime will be prescribed, consisting of powerful antibiotics and histamine blocker drugs to reduce acid production. These drugs will be taken over one to three weeks. It is essential to complete the course of therapy for the length of time advised. Side effects that may occur are explained in leaflets accompanying the prescriptions. If in doubt, ask your doctor or pharmacist.

! Caution

Over-the-counter pain relievers (such as aspirin) and NSAIDs (such as ibuprofen) can make an ulcer worse. While paracetamol does not affect the stomach lining, it can relieve pain. If you have an ulcer and develop anaemia, ensure you do not take too much iron as a supplement, since this can irritate the stomach lining. Discuss with your doctor the amount you need to counteract one problem without exacerbating the other.

Constipation

See also:

1/BEING A WELL WOMAN
Essentials of good health
pp. 16–21
Healthy body systems p. 36

3/GENERAL HEALTH ISSUES
Problems of the mind pp. 102–103

4/HORMONAL HEALTH
Reproductive problems
pp. 146–149
Pregnancy and motherhood
pp. 170–175

? Did you know?
Lack of fibre is the most common cause of constipation—you should eat high-fibre foods daily. However, you can also be at risk if you drink too much caffeine and not enough water, eat too much chocolate and do not take enough physical exercise.

Normal bowel habits vary from person to person, ranging from three times a day to four times a week. Medically speaking, however, you are usually considered constipated if three or more days go by without a bowel movement and if your stools are hard, dry and difficult to pass. Chronic constipation occurs most often in women, children and in people over the age of 65.

Constipation usually occurs when the bowel lacks water and works too slowly, causing stools to harden. As food and waste pass through the intestines, the body absorbs water in order to maintain blood pressure at the right level. Other reasons for constipation include eating foods that contain too little fibre or fibrous material, bowel diseases and chronic medical conditions such as multiple sclerosis (p. 210). It can also be a side effect of some drugs and may occur during the menstrual cycle and pregnancy.

Constantly straining to empty your bowels can lead to haemorrhoids (piles), which are swollen veins in the rectal area. The skin in the area is thin and veins may rupture, causing bleeding. Chronic constipation in people who are elderly or immobile can lead to impacted faeces, when the hard stools are so tightly wedged that they cannot be removed with normal pushing. A doctor may consider it necessary to soften these with arachis oil or phosphate enemas. In particularly difficult cases the doctor may remove part of the hardened stool by inserting one or two (gloved and lubricated) fingers into the anus.

LIFESTYLE CHANGES CAN HELP

You can prevent constipation by eating at least 15 g ($^1/_2$ oz) of fibre a day (beans and pulses, wholemeal bread, bran cereals, fresh or dried fruit such as prunes, and fresh vegetables). The fibre adds water-retaining bulk to stools so they don't become hard. The general recommendation of daily fibre intake is 30g (1 oz).

You can make bowel movements easier by drinking at least eight glasses of water a day. Avoid alcohol and caffeine, since drinks containing these cause dehydration.

Muscles play an important part in the peristaltic action of your bowels, which propels the waste along. Regular daily exercise will tone your muscles and improve digestion.

THE ROLE OF LAXATIVES

Laxatives treat acute constipation by stimulating the large intestine to contract. There are different types of laxatives. Stool softeners and some gentle laxatives make the stools bulkier, just as food fibre does, while others make them greasier. Pills or liquid are taken by mouth; suppositories are inserted in the rectum.

Laxatives should only be taken for a short period of time and only if a change to a high-fibre diet doesn't work. They should not be taken regularly as the colon begins to rely on them to bring on faecal movements. Over a period of time, this can affect the colon's ability to contract. This may cause diarrhoea and interfere with the body's absorption of nutrients. Laxatives also interact with various medicines. For these reasons, a self-help routine without laxatives is the preferred treatment.

CONSTIPATION IN PREGNANCY

Constipation is common during pregnancy because hormones relax the bowels and slow the action of the muscles, causing the heavy uterus to press against the intestines. Iron pills, which may be prescribed for anaemia, can make matters worse. The best advice is to drink plenty of water every day, eat lots of fresh fruit and vegetables and walk regularly. Sitting on the toilet with your feet raised on a pile of books may make passing stools easier. Laxatives should only be taken during pregnancy on medical advice, because they can cause the uterus to contract.

Constipation usually disappears after giving birth.

HELPING YOURSELF
Gentle exercise will improve muscle tone during pregnancy. Combine stretching exercises with swimming or walking.

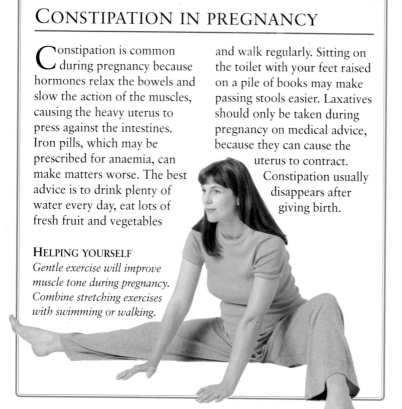

Diarrhoea

Diarrhoea occurs when the bowels contract too quickly or too much fluid passes into the gut, causing more frequent or runnier stools than usual. It may be an acute attack or an on-going problem related to a medical condition.

An attack of acute diarrhoea comes on suddenly and can last for three to four days, but tends to clear after 48 hours. The first sign is an urgent need to empty your bowels frequently. You may feel nauseous. If the bouts are accompanied by vomiting and abdominal pain, you can suspect food poisoning (see box below).

In general, diarrhoea is caused by a change in routine, anxiety, rich or spicy foods, a reaction to monosodium glutamate (the food additive MSG) and some antibiotics. Traveller's diarrhoea occurs through exposure to foreign viruses and bacteria in contaminated food and water.

What appears to be diarrhoea may also occur after prolonged constipation or use of laxatives, when the colon loses its ability to function. Any involuntary leakage from the rectum needs medical help. A drug will be prescribed to encourage the nerves and muscles to return to normal.

Gastroenteritis

Gastroenteritis is the medical term for infection of the digestive system. If it is caused by a virus, it is usually part of flu. If it is caused by bacterial contamination of food, it is known as food poisoning.

The symptoms of food poisoning are sudden fever, vomiting, abdominal pain and diarrhoea. The most common culprits are Campylobacter, *E. coli* and Salmonella from poorly cooked meat and poultry, unpasteurized milk or dairy products. You may be asked for a stool sample that will be analysed in the laboratory so the doctor can identify the bacteria. If several people are infected, public health inspectors try to find the source to limit the spread of the infection.

Most cases resolve without treatment other than the prevention of dehydration, although antibiotics may sometimes be prescribed. Young children and the aged and frail are most at risk from gastroenteritis and may require hospital treatment. Food poisoning can be prevented by strict hygiene in food preparation.

HOW TO HELP YOURSELF

After a bout of diarrhoea you should avoid food for the first 24 hours, but sip plenty of boiled or bottled water. You can try weak black tea with lemon or herb tea, but avoid milk or dairy products or fruit juices since these make diarrhoea worse. Light, bland food can be gradually introduced into your diet as the bouts of diarrhoea become less frequent.

You can take antidiarrhoeal medicines to slow down the activity of the bowels (though one school of thought suggests it is better to let whatever caused the diarrhoea leave the body). Severe dehydration can damage the kidneys, especially in children and the elderly. If you have severe symptoms, you should see your doctor. Oral rehydration solutions to replace fluids and mineral salts will probably be recommended. These can be bought from pharmacies or you can make your own by dissolving a generous pinch of salt and 5 ml (1 teaspoon) of sugar in 275 ml ($^1/_2$ pint) of water.

Observe strict hygiene, making sure to wash your hands after a visit to the toilet, in case the diarrhoea is infectious.

CHRONIC DIARRHOEA

Persistent diarrhoea should be investigated. It may occur in conditions such as inflammatory bowel disease, irritable bowel syndrome and diverticulitis and may also stem from intolerance to foods, including gluten (in coeliac disease) and lactose. A reduced ability to absorb foodstuffs in the intestine—the result of hormonal changes—will also cause diarrhoea.

FOOD INTOLERANCE
Wheat and dairy foods may trigger an allergic reaction in some people, causing diarrhoea.

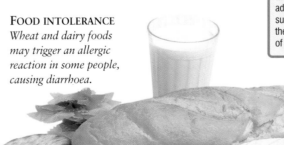

See also:

1/BEING A WELL WOMAN
Essentials of good health
pp. 16–23

5/ILLNESSES & EMERGENCIES
Digestive system problems
pp. 198–203

6/TREATMENTS & THERAPIES
Conventional treatments
pp. 272–277

● See your doctor

Consult your doctor if you have severe abdominal pain, vomiting, fever or blood or mucus in the stools. You should also see your doctor if the diarrhoea wakens you from your sleep, if it continues for more than two days, if you are severely dehydrated or if you have recently travelled abroad. If a bacterial or amoebic infection, such as dysentery, is diagnosed or suspected, a doctor will prescribe antibiotics or an amoebicide to kill the parasites.

! Caution

Oral contraceptives are less reliable if you have diarrhoea for more than 24 hours—continue taking the pill, but use additional precautions such as condoms during the illness and for the rest of the cycle.

Appendicitis

See also:

1/BEING A WELL WOMAN
Essentials of good health
pp. 16–19
Healthy body systems
p. 36; p. 40

6/TREATMENTS & THERAPIES
Treatment plans pp. 262–269

The appendix is situated at the beginning of the large intestine and is a narrow, tube-like sac that resembles a tail. It contains lymph nodes and may be part of the immune system, although it is thought the body can survive without it.

In appendicitis, the appendix becomes infected, although the cause cannot always be found. The appendix may become inflamed if its opening is blocked by faecal matter. The blockage may be triggered by a lack of fibre, which causes food to pass through the intestines slowly.

Most cases of appendicitis occur in people before the age of 30. It is rare in babies younger than two. The condition can be difficult to diagnose in women because the pain can be mimicked by gynaecological discomfort from the ovaries or uterus.

During pregnancy, because of the growing uterus, appendicitis may often be overlooked. The tube-like sac is pushed out of position and moves from near the right groin area in the right lower quadrant of the abdomen to just under the liver. If the appendix ruptures, the resultant scarring can cause a blockage of the Fallopian tubes as the scar tissue builds up, and this in turn can lead to infertility. A high-fibre diet in pregnancy is the best preventive measure.

> **! Caution**
>
> If you do have the symptoms, especially the pain as described, it is important not to eat, drink or take painkillers or antacids, because these may cause the appendix to rupture. Seek medical help as soon as possible.

SYMPTOMS AND DIAGNOSIS

The early symptoms of appendicitis are indistinguishable from many other abdominal disorders. There may be some discomfort in the abdomen, with a dull pain near the navel, loss of appetite, nausea, constipation or diarrhoea and slight fever. After six to 12 hours, however, the symptoms become more recognizable. Typically, a sharp pain shifts from the lower mid-abdomen to the lower right-hand side and is aggravated by movement, particularly if the right leg is flexed up. Pain may also be felt in the back or around the rectum. The pain usually becomes progressively worse, although in some people it may come and go.

A doctor will press the stomach area to establish where the pain hurts the most. If there is tenderness in the right lower abdomen, just under the pelvic bone, the doctor may perform an internal physical examination to establish the cause. The doctor may also examine the rectum with a gloved and lubricated finger.

TREATMENT AND COMPLICATIONS

Acute appendicitis is a medical emergency. Most doctors operate immediately to remove the appendix, since complications may occur if it is neglected. An appendicectomy is a simple, hour-long, laparoscopic operation, usually done under general anaesthetic through a keyhole incision. In women it may be done as part of a hysterectomy. Antibiotics are given routinely to treat any possible infection.

If appendicitis is not recognized and treated early enough, the appendix can rupture, releasing its contents into the abdomen. At this point the local pain stops, but urgent help is needed. The escape of the bacteria from the appendix into the abdominal cavity leads to peritonitis—a serious infection and inflammation of the walls of the abdomen. The symptoms of this are pain and tenderness in the abdomen and a fever. Peristalsis (the muscular contraction in the gut) ceases and severe dehydration can result.

If the appendix has ruptured, the abdominal cavity will have to be drained of pus and rinsed with a saline solution.

THE APPENDIX IN WOMEN
Because of where the appendix lies—at the end of the small intestine—discomfort or pain in women may be mistakenly attributed to the ovaries or uterus, which lie to the front of the pelvic area.

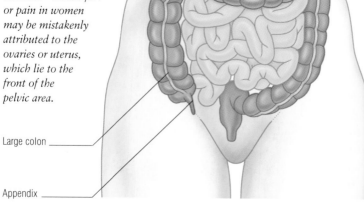

Large colon

Appendix

Diverticular disease

The walls of the lower part of the colon can develop small pouches, known as diverticula, which may be caused by pressure build-up in the bowel as it contracts. The pouches tend to form at weak spots, usually where blood vessels enter the intestinal tract. If hard faecal matter gets caught in them, interfering with their blood supply, inflammation occurs, causing a condition called diverticulitis. If it continually recurs it is known as diverticular disease.

Symptoms include pain and severe cramping, nausea, abdominal tenderness, alternating diarrhoea and constipation and, in rare cases, rectal bleeding. If the diverticula become infected, they may bleed profusely or perforate the intestinal wall, leading to peritonitis, which needs emergency treatment.

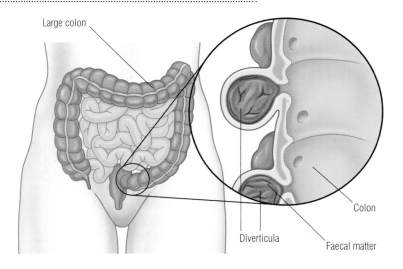

Large colon

Colon

Diverticula

Faecal matter

WHO IS AT RISK?

It is thought that the tendency to have diverticula can be inherited. However, since diverticular disease mainly occurs in countries in which low-fibre diets are not uncommon it is also linked with lifestyle and eating habits. It mostly affects people over the age of 50. It is most common after the age of 70, particularly in those with chronic constipation—which is both a symptom and cause, since diverticular disease increases the pressure in the colon. Others at risk include those with coronary artery disease, gallbladder disease and obesity.

DIAGNOSIS AND TREATMENT

As diverticula do not always cause symptoms, they are often found by chance. If there is local tenderness, doctors have three options for diagnosis: ultrasound to look for an abscess; a barium enema to outline the bowel; or a colonoscopy or sigmoidoscopy for an internal examination of the intestines. A CAT scan may also be done so that other diseases with similar symptoms, such as irritable bowel syndrome and digestive tract ulcers, can be ruled out.

Diverticula are not generally treated, but the symptoms can be. Constipation may be eased by eating a high-fibre diet or taking bulk laxatives for a short period of time. Some doctors also recommend avoiding foods with small seeds, such as tomatoes, grapes or strawberries, because the seeds can get caught in the

pouches. If diverticulitis develops, you will need antibiotics, painkillers, drugs to stop abdominal spasms, and bed rest until the pain and inflammation subside. Severe cases may require a liquid diet or intravenous feeding to give the colon a complete rest. If attacks are frequent or very severe, a doctor may recommend surgery to remove the affected area.

Why your stomach rumbles

Stomach rumbling may not be regarded as a medical problem, but it can be a social embarrassment. The noises, which are known medically as borborygmi, are produced when liquid and gas in the stomach are shuffled to and fro by vigorous muscular contractions. This action may be triggered by hunger, anxiety or a fright, or it may be the result of eating high-gas foods such as beans. A noisy stomach can be common in some diseases, such as irritable bowel syndrome, for which antispasmodic drugs may be given. Swallowing air when eating or talking rapidly and drinking too many carbonated drinks are other culprits.

The noises may diminish if you eat regularly and slowly. Having five small meals a day instead of three large ones may help. Loud rumblings with severe abdominal pain should be reported to a doctor. They may be caused by a variety of digestive or other disorders, including gynaecological ones.

? Did you know?

Not all laxatives are the same. Bulk-forming laxatives, taken orally, help to retain water and soften faeces, and encourage peristalsis (the muscular contraction of the gut, moving food and waste). People who suffer constipation with diverticular disease, but who find it difficult to eat or even increase their intake of high-fibre foods, can benefit from these laxatives. It is important to drink plenty of water every day you take them.

Irritable bowel syndrome

Women are twice as likely as men to report symptoms of irritable bowel syndrome, which is also known as IBS, spastic colon or nervous diarrhoea. Many people never seek medical help, yet it is thought to affect one in five people at some time in their lives, usually at a time of significant change or stress.

There is no established cause and the condition is not hereditary. With IBS, either the bowel is not functioning properly—the muscles work too quickly, too slowly or are out of synchronization—or the bowel is hypersensitive to the normal muscular activity within it. IBS may often occur after a bout of food poisoning (gastroenteritis) or a stressful life event such as pregnancy or childbirth, marriage or bereavement. The symptoms may disappear for long periods of time, but the condition usually recurs.

HOW IBS IS DIAGNOSED

Irritable bowel syndrome is difficult to diagnose because it does not cause any physical changes in the bowel, such as inflammation. No test can give a definitive diagnosis, but a doctor needs to rule out more serious illnesses, such as inflammatory bowel disease, which can have similar symptoms (p. 202). Women over the age of 50 need to have a thorough investigation, especially if symptoms include weight loss or blood in the stools, which are not typical of IBS.

Your doctor may perform some or all of the following tests: a sigmoidoscopy or colonoscopy to examine the intestine wall; an ultrasound to check the intestine wall; a barium enema—an X-ray procedure to make sure there are no blockages; lab testing of a stool culture to check for parasites or rule out other causes; and a full blood count and blood test to reveal any infection or inflammation.

Signs and symptoms

Symptoms vary from person to person, may be mild or severe and can come and go at different times. They may include:

Abdominal cramping, especially on the left side of the body or across the lower right abdomen. The pain is often relieved on passing wind or after a bowel movement.

♀ A feeling of bloating and fullness, which may make clothes feel tight and uncomfortable.

♀ Excessive flatulence.

♀ Constipation and/or diarrhoea.

♀ A sudden urge to rush to the toilet.

♀ A sensation of incomplete emptying of the bowel.

Nausea.

Pellet-like stools, often containing mucus.

Stomach-rumbling sounds.

Some people with IBS find that stress and certain foods make their symptoms worse. Women often find their symptoms are worse around the time of menstruation and they may also experience occasional urinary incontinence, painful periods, discomfort during sex and cystitis-like pain.

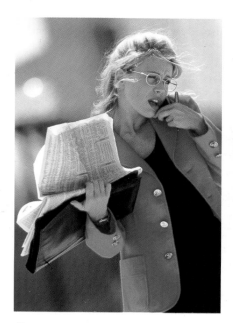

CAREER WOMAN
The constant stress of a high-powered job can be exciting but it can also be debilitating. When the "fight or flight" response is a regular event in a day's work, physiological changes occur in the body. These are made worse when personal habits such as eating and going to the toilet are irregular.

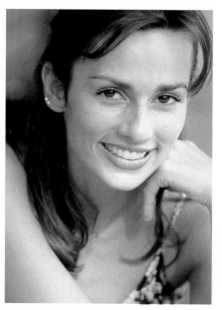

SUPER WOMAN
Trying to do too much—as wife, mother, working woman—can cause the body systems to react. Digestion is particularly susceptible, since little time is available to sit down and enjoy food and to relax. To coax the digestive tract back into working order may require some self-nurturing.

RANGE OF TREATMENTS

IBS cannot lead to complications or cancer. However, the symptoms are highly distressing and should be brought to the attention of your doctor. They can normally be kept under control with medication, although there is no single solution and several drugs may be tried. The most commonly used include antispasmodics to reduce intestinal muscle contraction causing diarrhoea and abdominal pain, laxatives to reduce constipation and peppermint oil for bloating and gas problems.

When none of these succeed, a doctor may sometimes prescribe a tricyclic antidepressant to calm the nervous system and so the intestines. If stress is a contributory factor, your doctor may suggest psychotherapy, hypnotherapy or mind/body therapy. Self-nurturing through relaxation techniques and regular exercise can also have beneficial effects.

DIETARY CHANGES

People with IBS are advised to eat a well-balanced diet with meals at set times, since this can reduce the symptoms. Knowing what provokes your symptoms is also important, so your doctor may suggest you try an exclusion diet for a few weeks. Common culprits include wheat, dairy products, fatty or spicy foods, beans and pulses, soft drinks, caffeine and some fruits and vegetables such as the brassicas—cabbage, cauliflower and Brussels sprouts. Eating more fibrous foods helps some people, but makes others feel worse because of the gas problem. You can also try a soluble fibre dietary product such as psyllium husks, to encourage bulk-forming in your stools.

Tests may be carried out to find out if you are lactose intolerant (meaning you lack the enzyme lactase that metabolizes lactose, a sugar found in milk and other dairy products); or have an intolerance to gluten, a protein in wheat and other grains; or have too much of the yeast *Candida albicans* in the gut. All conditions have symptoms that are similar to IBS.

> **! Caution**
> The most common medicines to relieve symptoms of IBS are available over the counter from pharmacies or health-food stores. However, you should not try to treat yourself before you are sure that you have IBS. It is important that the condition is diagnosed first, to rule out anything more serious.

CHANGES IN BOWEL MOVEMENTS

If your stools change colour, odour or consistency for longer than two weeks, you should consult a doctor. Your doctor may ask you to provide a stool sample, which will be sent to a lab for analysis, and may perform a rectal examination (with a gloved and lubricated finger) to discover the source of the problem.

In most cases the changes in stools are harmless, but in some people they may relate to a disorder of the digestive system. Pale, smelly or bulky stools can be a sign of coeliac disease (gluten intolerance), caused by the malabsorption of food. Loose stools with mucus may be associated with constipation or IBS; if blood is also present it may be a sign of inflammatory bowel disease (IBD) or cancer. Dark stools can be caused by eating too much of a food such as beetroot. But if they contain blood, it can be a sign of haemorrhoids, diverticulitis or, rarely, colorectal cancer.

Symptoms	What it may indicate
Hard, infrequent stools, much straining needed	Constipation
Runny, frequent stools	Diarrhoea
Alternating hard/infrequent and runny/frequent stools	Irritable bowel syndrome, diabetes, misuse of laxatives
Visible blood, blood in stools	Haemorrhoids, irritable bowel syndrome, IBD, colorectal cancer
Thin ribbon-like stools, anal blood	Possible cancer
Pale clay-like stools	Liver disease
Dark metallic-smelling stools	Bleeding in gastrointestinal tract, possibly certain medicines
Foul-smelling large stools, abdominal pain	Pancreatic problems, coeliac disease
Light-coloured threads in stools, anal itching	Worm infection
Pale chalky stools, dark urine	Gallbladder-related problems, disorders of the liver

Inflammatory bowel disease

See also:

1/BEING A WELL WOMAN
Essentials of good health p. 16
Healthy body systems p. 36

3/GENERAL HEALTH ISSUES
Blood and the circulation p. 116

4/HORMONAL HEALTH
Pregnancy and motherhood p. 170

6/TREATMENTS & THERAPIES
Treatment plans pp. 262– 269

Crohn's disease and ulcerative colitis are two related diseases that cause inflammation of the intestines. Together they are called inflammatory bowel disease (IBD). Crohn's disease can affect any part of the digestive tract, with parts becoming red and inflamed; in ulcerative colitis there is inflammation and ulceration only of the colon and lining of the rectum.

IBD is more common in women than in men. The cause is unknown, although the condition has been linked to a long-term reaction to bacteria or viruses, such as measles. It is not caused by anxiety, stress or psychological disorders. IBD can run in families.

SIGNS AND SYMPTOMS

Crohn's disease causes abdominal pain, diarrhoea (with occasional bleeding), vomiting and inflammation around the anus. Children with Crohn's disease may have poor growth. Sometimes leaks, called fistula, break through the inflamed gut, leading to infections, or scar tissue builds up that narrows and obstructs the bowel. In severe ulcerative colitis, there is frequent diarrhoea with blood and mucus, and abdominal pain. It can also cause skin and mouth ulcers, eye inflammation and joint pain. Both Crohn's disease and ulcerative colitis can lead to fatigue, weight loss and anaemia.

Flare-ups can occur at any time of life. Active disease can reduce fertility in women, who may be advised to try to get pregnant while in remission. Active IBD can also complicate a pregnancy.

People with widespread and severe ulcerative colitis have a high risk of developing bowel cancer and need regular colonoscopies.

METHODS OF DIAGNOSIS

It can take time for a diagnosis to be finally made, as most people feel fine between flare-ups. In addition, the two conditions are alike and they share symptoms with other, more minor, digestive tract problems.

A doctor may choose a range of tests, which can include: a barium enema to show up any intestinal thickening and identify the parts affected; an internal examination by sigmoidoscopy or colonoscopy to assess the disease's severity; biopsies to analyse the intestinal lining; analysis of stool samples; and blood tests to detect anaemia and nutritional deficiencies.

TREATMENTS

Acute mild to moderate IBD affecting the rectum or distal colon is treated initially with local application of steroids (liquids or foams) and aminosalicylates, such as mesalazine. More severe or widespread disease that does not respond to local treatment requires oral aminosalicylates (mesalazine or olsalazine) and corticosteroids (prednisolone or budesonide).

Severe disease calls for hospital admission and intravenous corticosteroids and nutrition, because there is a risk of dehydration and the colon bursting. Antidiarrhoeal agents are used in Crohn's disease. Badly diseased sections of the colon can be surgically removed, but the inflammation often returns elsewhere along the digestive tract. Surgery may repair leaks or widen badly scarred areas. Sometimes surgery can cure the disease by taking away all or part of the colon—a procedure called a colectomy.

DURING PREGNANCY
Patients with IBD who are pregnant should be monitored carefully for flare-ups.

Questions to ask your doctor

♀ If I'm on steroids for IBD, am I at risk of osteoporosis?
♀ How can I avoid osteoporosis?
♀ What are the side effects of my medicines?
♀ Are there any foods that I should avoid?
♀ Will I need surgery?
♀ Am I at risk of contracting bowel cancer?

Colorectal cancer

Colorectal (bowel) cancer is the second most common cancer. It often develops when cells in the lining of the colon (the large intestine or bowel) or rectum become abnormal and form small growths called polyps. Although most polyps are harmless, they may sometimes become cancerous.

WHO IS AT RISK?

Colorectal cancer is primarily a disease of the Western world, linked to a diet rich in saturated fats and sugar and low in fibre. Excessive alcohol intake, a sedentary lifestyle and obesity also increase the risk. Colorectal cancer can occur at any age but is rare in people under the age of 40 and is common in the elderly. People with IBD (see opposite) have a slightly increased risk.

The risk of developing colorectal cancer can be reduced by eating a balanced diet. You should eat at least 15g (¹/₂ oz) of fibre (a minimum of five portions of fruit and vegetables) a day, which aids the passage of food through the body and ensures the elimination of waste. Water also flushes the intestine and helps waste to pass through. Antioxidant vitamins, such as beta carotene and vitamin C, may have a protective effect. Avoid high-salt and smoked foods, which are thought to increase the levels of carcinogens in the body.

As many as 10 percent of those diagnosed have a family history of colorectal cancer. In these families the disease often appears before the age of 45 and may affect two or more close relatives. Hereditary colorectal cancer has also been linked to other forms of cancer.

WARNING SIGNS

Colorectal cancer often has no symptoms in the early stages. Many of the advanced symptoms are also found in other bowel disorders, such as inflammatory bowel disease. They include a persistent change in bowel habit for three or more weeks (for example, constipation or diarrhoea); rectal bleeding; anaemia with or without tiredness; and sudden unexplained weight loss. The cancer can also partially or completely block the bowel, with abdominal pain, bloating and vomiting.

METHODS OF DIAGNOSIS

Colorectal cancer can be difficult to diagnose. Many people are only diagnosed in advanced stages because of a delay in seeking help. If you have symptoms that could indicate colorectal cancer, note down the time and type of your bowel movements or bleeding and consult your doctor, who may refer you to a specialist.

The tests for colorectal cancer include: a rectal examination to check for polyps; a stool analysis to check for blood; a barium enema to check for blockages; an internal examination by sigmoidoscopy to look for changes in the bowel lining; a biopsy (cell sample); an ultrasound scan; and a colonoscopy (examining the inside of the colon).

TREATMENTS

If the cancer is caught in its early stages, the chance of surviving five years after diagnosis is high. When polyps are found, they are removed and examined to see whether they are cancerous and if the cancer has spread further. If the cancer has spread, a second operation may be performed to cut out part of the bowel. In advanced cases, the whole bowel may be removed and replaced with an external pouch. Some people may benefit from chemotherapy or radiotherapy to shrink the tumour before surgery, kill cancer cells at other sites or reduce the risk of recurrence.

In advanced colorectal cancer, tumour cells break away to form a secondary tumour elsewhere in the body (called a metastasis), usually in the liver. Treatments may include chemotherapy or surgery to remove the secondary tumours.

See also:

1/BEING A WELL WOMAN
Essentials of good health p. 16
Healthy body systems p. 36

6/TREATMENTS & THERAPIES
Treatment plans
pp. 262–269
Conventional treatments
pp. 278–281

> **! Caution**
> It is important to be familiar with your own bowel habits so that you can recognize anything out of the ordinary. With colorectal cancer early diagnosis is vital, significantly increasing the chance of survival.

> **● See your doctor**
> It is recommended that everyone over the age of 50 (with or without a family history of colorectal cancer) should be screened yearly. The screening involves a rectal examination and a physical check of your lymph nodes and abdomen for signs of swelling or a mass. A stool or blood sample should be provided for analysis.

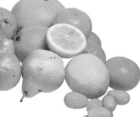

DIET HELPS
A high-fibre diet helps to clear out the intestine and keep it healthy.

IMMUNE SYSTEM PROBLEMS

Your body's ability to protect itself relies on the healthy and efficient operation of the blood and lymphatic systems. In some instances the various white cells that tackle infection are affected by an allergic reaction that makes them unable to cope. The most common problems are caused by substances and organisms in the world around us.

See also:

1/BEING A WELL WOMAN
Healthy body systems pp. 40–43

5/ILLNESSES & EMERGENCIES
Respiratory problems pp. 213–221

6/TREATMENTS & THERAPIES
Alternative medicine pp. 298–311

Maintaining your defences

Your body has a complex and usually effective system of defending itself against attack from organisms such as bacteria, viruses and parasites. However, the system can malfunction in a number of ways.

It may mistakenly attack certain of its own cells or tissues, as in so-called autoimmune disease. It can also respond to substances that are in fact harmless, such as dust or pollen, causing an allergic reaction. This kind of response, known as atopy, often runs in families. The system can also fail partially or completely, as in AIDS (p. 208), or in response to drugs designed to prevent the destruction of transplanted tissue, such as a new kidney.

Allergies come in many forms and most appear before the age of 40. One sensitivity may make you susceptible to another. For example,

if you suffer from asthma, you are also more likely to have a skin allergy. In rare instances, people develop "total allergy syndrome" in which they react adversely to almost everything in their surroundings.

PROBLEM FOODS
Allergies may relate to anything from perfume to food. The most common foods known to provoke an allergic response are cow's milk, wheat (in bread and pasta), soya beans, egg white, citrus fruits, strawberries and shellfish such as shrimps, mussels and clams.

Sensitization and triggers

From a medical viewpoint, sensitivity and intolerance are controversial areas. Even if someone does not suffer a full immune system response, as with allergies, she may become physically ill or weak from contact with certain foods or ingredients. Headaches, flushing and numbness occur, for example, in response to the flavour enhancer monosodium glutamate (MSG). Certain preservatives such as sugar, and additives such as sulphites (found in a range of dried fruit and vegetables, wine, beer, dehydrated soups and baking mixes) may cause reactions in individuals with an allergic susceptibility.

Various diagnostic techniques are used to pinpoint suspected triggers. Your doctor may advise you to undergo sensitivity tests in which a tiny amount of one allergen at a time is placed under the skin and your reaction is noted. One recommended treatment may be immunotherapy—also called desensitization—which gradually introduces by injection small but increasing amounts of an offending allergen to try to encourage your immune system to learn tolerance.

THE MOST COMMON ALLERGIES

Allergy	Self-help

Hay fever

Inhaling pollens from a vast assortment of trees, grasses and other plants can set off the misery of hay fever symptoms for millions of people every spring and summer. Watery, sore eyes, a running nose and itchy throat are the result of the immune system reacting to the pollen and triggering an immune response. Nasal steroid sprays can help to suppress the immune response, supplemented with over-the-counter antihistamines (though these may cause drowsiness), eye drops and nasal decongestants as required.

Wear sunglasses, keep car and bedroom windows closed and stay inside as much as possible when pollen counts peak in the early morning and evening. Take early evening showers to remove pollen.

Eczema

An immune response to allergens in the environment can cause this skin condition in susceptible people. The droppings of dust mites, animal skin scales and pollens are common triggers, causing the skin to erupt in scaly patches and watery blisters which become crusty and may ooze. Emollients moisturize the skin and help soothe itching, and steroid creams help to get rid of inflammation and encourage healing.

Keep the skin cool and wear natural fibres such as cotton, rather than synthetics, next to the skin. (For more on eczema, see p. 224.)

Asthma

People with allergic asthma become wheezy and breathless when an allergen such as pollen or animal skin scales enters the tiny airways in their lungs, causing the bronchioles (airways) to narrow and fill up with mucus. The bronchioles are hyper-responsive to irritants that would not affect other people. Because the flow of oxygen through the lungs is also restricted, an asthma attack is potentially serious.

Keep your environment as free as possible of known allergens. Help to prevent attacks by avoiding cigarette smoke, fuel fumes and other environmental pollutants.

Stings

Some people develop an allergic response to insect stings, especially those from bees. This response may range from highly unpleasant, with severe itching, dizziness, faintness or vomiting, to potentially fatal if the person goes into anaphylactic shock. This can happen within minutes, and is caused by a massive release of histamine which restricts breathing and causes blood pressure to drop disastrously if urgent action is not taken (p. 254).

Prompt treatment with an injection of adrenaline is essential. Carry a kit (an Epipen) with you at all times.

Food

A genuine food allergy, rather than a food sensitivity, causes a release of histamine that produces serious symptoms such as hives on the skin, nausea and vomiting, and sometimes asthma. In severe cases it can cause anaphylactic shock (p. 254). Common triggers are peanuts, peanut oil and other protein foods.

If the trigger is known, always read labels on prepared foods and ask in restaurants if the ingredient is included. Carry an adrenaline injection kit with you at all times.

Chronic fatigue syndrome

No one knows exactly what chronic fatigue syndrome (CFS) is or what causes it. Some doctors dispute that it exists at all, believing that it is simply a form of depression or other psychological disorder.

The confusion is reflected in the various names by which it is known: post-viral syndrome or myalgic encephalomyelitis (ME), chronic Epstein-Barr virus (CEBV) and immune dysfunction syndrome. Although it was once thought to be a type of influenza, it is now considered to be a type of immune system weakness or malfunction that is sparked by a viral infection, major stress or environmental pollution—any or all of which may combine with a genetic predisposition to trigger the illness in susceptible people. Women are much more likely to contract CFS than men; 80 percent of those with CFS are women under the age of 45.

Symptoms may come and go and vary both in severity and from one person to another, but some are common to all. They are long-lasting (up to two years or more) and have a significant impact on the sufferer's normal lifestyle.

COMMON SYMPTOMS

The predominant symptom is fatigue, often to the point of exhaustion, and an overall lack of energy. You may have pain or aches in joints and muscles, usually in your arms, but without any swelling or tenderness. The lymph glands under your jaw and ears may feel swollen. Your throat

THE ONGOING PROBLEM OF LUPUS

Systemic lupus erythematosus (SLE or lupus) is a condition affecting the joints, connective tissues and small blood vessels as a result of an immune system malfunction (p. 83). As with other autoimmune diseases, it is not clear why the body's defence system turns against itself, but external factors that may trigger it in a person who has inherited a genetic susceptibility include childbirth, exposure to sunlight, arrival of the menopause and viral infections.

Women between the ages of 15 and 40 make up 90 percent of cases of lupus. Some women are more severely affected than others and many only have relatively mild symptoms. The disease tends to flare up then subside periodically, with the symptoms often rising and subsiding with the menstrual cycle.

In an active phase, you may feel as though you have flu, with a raised temperature, achiness and weakness. Inflammation makes joints in the hands, elbows, knees and ankles swollen and painful, and

some people get a red rash, known as a butterfly rash from its shape, across their nose and face.

A common and serious consequence of lupus is some form of kidney disorder. More than half of lupus sufferers will develop some degree of renal failure.

Steroids keep the condition under control for many people, although they may need increased doses during a flare-up. Drugs more familiar as malaria preventives, such as hydroxychloroquine, are also effective, while NSAIDs (nonsteroidal anti-inflammatory drugs) can reduce pain and inflammation. Immunosuppressive drugs may weaken the immune system's attack on the body. Mild steroid creams can help with rashes, and sun protection should be used in all seasons. Physical therapy can help prevent loss of mobility.

Women with lupus would at one time have been advised not to have children. Now, with close monitoring by their doctors, many have healthy, normal pregnancies.

There is, however, an increased risk of miscarriage and preeclampsia, and babies are commonly born small and prematurely.

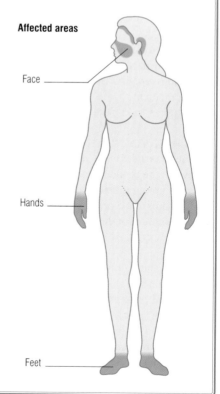

Affected areas

Face

Hands

Feet

may be constantly sore, and headaches will be frequent. You may be aware that you always seem to have a slight temperature and you find yourself responding to a new allergy, or an old one flares up. You may have difficulty with short-term memory and you may have problems concentrating for any length of time.

In addition, your sleep pattern can go awry. First there may be insomnia, then waking in the early hours of the morning filled with anxiety. After this, there may be a period of oversleeping—being so tired that you can't wake up at the normal time. You may have dramatic mood swings and generally not feel well.

CAN YOUR DOCTOR HELP?

Your doctor will want to rule out other causes for your symptoms, such as depression, thyroid malfunction, glandular fever, arthritis and cancer, and will arrange tests. If these prove clear, your doctor may conclude from your medical history and your symptoms that you are suffering from CFS. Although researchers are developing possible diagnostic tests, there are no reliable ones in use as yet.

Your doctor can prescribe treatment to alleviate symptoms. Since people with FS can be ultra-sensitive to drugs, any medication will be prescribed in minimum doses at first and can be increased later if it is thought necessary.

Alternative medicine may be helpful in alleviating symptoms. Qualified practitioners of herbal, homeopathic, Ayurvedic and traditional Chinese medicine have a holistic approach that looks at the whole person.

HELPING YOURSELF

You may be told to rest, and when symptoms are severe you will have no alternative. When you have the time and energy available, consider some of these other suggestions.

Exercise An individually tailored programme of gentle, slow-building aerobic exercise may improve low-energy levels. Find a gym or personal trainer who understands your needs.

Mind and body Meditation, progressive relaxation, breathing techniques, guided imagery, qigong and yoga all reduce stress and may boost your energy levels. Investigate the various Chinese exercise systems that involve little physical movement but stimulate the flow of chi (energy) in the body.

Find a class and learn autogenic training, which aims to promote the body's self-healing powers. There are six main exercises using the power of visualization to switch off stress. You learn in a class until you are self reliant, but it does require you to have enough discipline to practise for 15 minutes, once or twice a day.

Therapeutic body massage and reflexology both focus on achieving a state of relaxation. Acumassage is more rigorous: it combines lymphatic drainage massage with acupressure to remove toxins and pep up the immune system.

Nutrition Pay attention to the food you eat. Increase the garlic content of your diet and take antioxidant supplements, which help the body's defence system. Fresh fruit, vegetables and green tea are good daily sources of antioxidants. You could also try herbal supplements—*Echinacea* to stimulate the immune system and St John's wort, a natural antidepressant and remedy for anxiety, insomnia and poor concentration. Check with your doctor before taking supplements in case they clash with whatever conventional medication has been prescribed.

A cycle of stress

CFS is probably associated with chronic stress that builds up slowly, from pressures at work, problems in relationships, looking after a sick parent or child or dealing with an illness. Stress takes a gradual toll, straining the nervous system so the body is in a constant state of mental and physical readiness for what might happen next.

The ever-present low-level anxiety that accompanies this adds to the stress, which may then affect the immune system and upset its normal protective role.

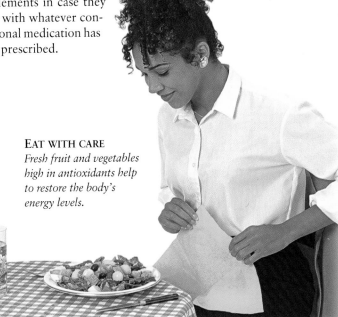

EAT WITH CARE
Fresh fruit and vegetables high in antioxidants help to restore the body's energy levels.

HIV and AIDS

See also:

2/SEX & SEXUALITY
Contraception pp. 60–65
Sexual infections pp. 72–75

3/GENERAL HEALTH ISSUES
Problems of the mind
pp. 100–101

HIV, the human immunodeficiency virus, is passed on when an infected person's body fluids—such as blood or semen—enter another person's bloodstream. This is most likely to happen during sexual intercourse, both heterosexual and homosexual. Women generally acquire the virus from men rather than passing the virus to their male partners.

Other methods of transmission are through the use of a hypodermic needle shared with someone who is HIV-positive, or when the infection is passed on by a woman in childbirth or to a baby from its mother's breast milk. In the past, some people were infected through treatment with blood or blood constituents contaminated with the virus, but these substances are now screened before use. Although the virus is present in the saliva of infected people, there is no evidence that it can be passed on by activities such as kissing or sharing a drinking glass. Bleeding gums, however, can be an entry point. Anal intercourse is risky because the tissues in the rectum tear easily. Women who have open sores on their genitals from herpes, for example, are also at risk during sexual intercourse.

Once in the bloodstream, the HIV virus attacks T-cells in the immune system called CD4 lymphocytes, which are taken over and begin reproducing the virus instead of performing their normal task of defending the body against infection. If these T-cells are destroyed in sufficient numbers, the infected person develops acquired immunodeficiency syndrome (AIDS), although it may take many years, even a decade, before this stage is reached.

HOW HIV IS DIAGNOSED

Blood is tested for antibodies that the body produces against the HIV virus. However, the antibodies may not appear in measurable quantities until at least three months after infection and in some cases up to a year.

A positive result has profound implications for the person concerned, as well as for those close to him or her and for anyone with whom they have had unprotected sex. It is therefore important to prepare for the test by discussing the possible outcome with a counsellor; this will normally be offered at clinics specializing in HIV concerns as well as through national support organizations. A counsellor will also be able to discuss the various treatment options that are now available and advise who should be told about the diagnosis. In addition, decisions about employment and insurance may have to be made. The counsellor may have advice on making lifestyle changes, including practising safe sex.

LIMITING DAMAGE

There is as yet no cure for HIV or AIDS, but modern treatments can often temporarily halt or retard the progression from HIV infection to the development of the syndrome. Since a person who is HIV-positive may continue to feel well, the CD4 cell count and viral load are

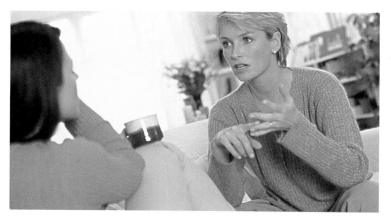

COUNSELLING
One of the chief problems if you have HIV is that you feel you can't talk about your condition. The help of a trained counsellor can guide you through the everyday problems of living with the virus.

HIV and pregnancy

Most children with HIV acquire it from their mothers. The infection is passed on either in the uterus or during breastfeeding. If a woman who is HIV-positive has a baby and breastfeeds it, there is a 25–35 percent risk of the baby becoming infected, unless preventive measures are taken.

Antiviral drugs are now available that can reduce this factor to as little as 2 percent. In developed countries, antiviral drugs such as zidovudine can be given in cocktails to pregnant women and can reduce their viral load so that the risk of transmission is much reduced. If the mother has not been treated, small amounts of antiviral drugs can also be given to infants, which significantly reduces their risk of infection.

monitored closely. When the CD4 cell level goes down and the viral load up, treatment is started. Doctors usually recommend prophylactic medication before the immune system is irreversibly damaged. Issues that need to be considered include the fact that the drug therapy for HIV is costly, complex, disruptive and has psychological as well as physical side effects.

TREATMENT

The first objective of treatment is to stem the proliferation of the virus in the body, the second is to prevent and treat so-called opportunistic infections (box, right) and the third is to boost and maintain immune system function.

Anti-HIV drugs are usually taken in combination. While they cannot eradicate HIV infection, they can often slow viral replication and maintain the protective T-cells at near-normal levels. It is essential to take such medications exactly as prescribed (which may involve waking up to do so at night), despite experiencing unpleasant side effects. A powerful drug called interleukin–2 has been shown to boost the immune system by stimulating T-cells and may help to slow the progress of HIV to AIDS.

Although early symptoms such as aches and pains, fever, diarrhoea, breathing difficulties, swollen glands, weight loss and persistent dry cough will be the same in women as in men, women may also have menstrual problems. Abnormal cervical smear results may occur and recurrent yeast infections may not clear up.

LIVING WITH HIV

The advice usually given when someone has been found to be HIV-positive is to pay careful attention to a healthy diet and food hygiene.

With a weakened immune system, you should be scrupulous when handling uncooked meat that may harbour infectious organisms such as Campylobacter and Salmonella. You should avoid raw or lightly cooked eggs for the same reason and drink boiled tap water or bottled mineral water because of the risk of cryptosporidium infection (box, above right). A consultation with a nutritionist or dietician can be useful to devise a healthy and affordable diet.

Keeping up to date with information on the constant new developments in treatment is important. Counselling and support from various organizations offer help to HIV-positive people, their partners, friends and families.

Threats from infections

When the immune system is not functioning properly, the individual is vulnerable to infections that would be easily controlled by a healthy person. These are called opportunistic infections and affect the susceptible—the very young, old, frail and people who are HIV-positive. Common infections for HIV-positive men are a type of pneumonia called PCP (pneumocystis carinii) and infection from an organism called cryptosporidium, which is found in water. These infections can be treated, and prophylactic medication to prevent them may be recommended for people when blood tests show their immune system is weak. For women, the most dangerous infection is bacterial pneumonia.

The diagnosis of AIDS is usually made after a person has contracted one or more life-threatening infections. For a woman these may be invasive cervical cancer and serious ulcerative genital lesions, both of which are difficult to treat. A CD4 count of less than 200 is another sign—CD4 cells are the most important white blood cells involved in immunity. Women and men with AIDS can develop tuberculosis, non-Hodgkin's lymphoma, and a herpes infection called CMV (cytomegalovirus) that leads to blindness, colitis and oesophagitis (inflammation of the oesophagus).

TREATING AIDS

Controlling the infections—which are inevitable with AIDS—with antibiotics or blocking the reproduction of the virus with a drug such as zidovudine (AZT) can improve the survival rates for AIDs sufferers. AZT may be given while a woman is pregnant as it appears not to affect the mother or child adversely and reduces the chances of transmitting the virus to the child. Combination therapy has proved more effective than monotherapy.

Immunizations against contagious and life-threatening illnesses such as diphtheria, mumps, measles, rubella, tetanus, hepatitis B and influenza should be administered. Women should have a cervical smear every six months. Blood tests should be performed every three to six months so that the levels of CD4 cells and viral load can be measured. There is no vaccine to prevent AIDS although there continues to be extensive research.

> **! Caution**
> Male or female condoms can substantially reduce the risk of infecting the partners of HIV-positive people. HIV-positive people who have sexual intercourse with a person who is also HIV-positive should take precautions as well, because there may be a potential risk of infection from a different or drug-resistant strain of the virus.

NERVOUS SYSTEM PROBLEMS

An extensive nerve network reaches every part of your body, operating by a system of signals and impulses that process information at high speed and initiate action. The nerves themselves are composed of a chain of nerve cells, and they rely on chemical messengers. Problems arise if nerves lose the ability to carry messages from the brain.

See also:

1/BEING A WELL WOMAN
Healthy body systems p. 32

Nerve and muscle diseases

More women than men get multiple sclerosis (MS), a disease of the central nervous system. Some symptoms are more likely to appear in your 20s or 30s, although the disease can strike earlier or later in life, and is more common in people who live in temperate climates. Probably an autoimmune disorder, the cause of MS remains unsolved. Evidence suggests that an environmental, probably viral agent operates in a genetically susceptible individual. Herpes virus 6 and chlamydia pneumoniae are possible triggers.

The symptoms of MS are the result of damage to the myelin sheath—the fatty insulating layer that surrounds the nerves controlling movement and sensation throughout the body. The form that symptoms take and their severity depends on which part of the central nervous system is affected and how badly. This, together with the fact that there is no definitive test for MS, can make the condition difficult to diagnose and it may only be confirmed once a person has had several attacks.

INDIVIDUAL SYMPTOMS

The course that MS takes varies, ranging from mild, occasional symptoms to a more progressive deterioration. Many people have periods of active disease interspersed with periods of remission when symptoms disappear partially or even completely.

Doctors distinguish between relapsing-remitting and progressive MS, but the difference is not always clear. Some people whose MS begins as relapsing-remitting eventually develop the progressive form, while about 15 percent do not experience remissions at all. At the other extreme, some people have relatively mild symptoms with long periods of remission.

DIAGNOSIS AND TREATMENT

Your medical history and the results of a neurological examination, plus other tests including, ideally, a scan called an MRI, can usually confirm a diagnosis of MS. No one can tell you, however, what course the illness may take in the future and there is as yet no treatment that can cure it. However, this does not mean that nothing can be done.

The past few years have seen the launch of a new treatment with antiviral drugs known as interferons, which inhibit the multiplication of viruses and may slow the progress of MS in some people. Although the drugs cannot stop MS altogether, they are effective for relapsing-remitting MS. Glatiramer acetate may be prescribed. This mixture of polypeptides may act by blocking immune responses to one of the myelin proteins. It can reduce relapse rate and so significantly affect disability. Other drug treatments can help ease specific symptoms, such as muscle spasm, and courses of steroids

Symptoms of MS

The fact that symptoms of MS come and go and are often vague and ill-defined means that many people may dismiss them at first. No one with MS is likely to experience all the symptoms at the same time. The following symptoms can be the result of the disease, but may also have other causes:

♀ Visual problems such as blurring, double vision and blind spots.
♀ Loss of coordination, with clumsy or jerky movements.
♀ Loss of balance and feelings of dizziness.
♀ Physical weakness.
♀ Strange sensations in the hands and feet, such as pins and needles and tingling, and heaviness of the limbs.
♀ Fatigue.
♀ Muscle stiffness and spasms.
♀ Having to empty your bladder often and urgently.
♀ Psychological difficulties, including poor concentration, memory loss and mood swings.

can be effective in relieving or shortening an attack, especially when the eyes are affected. Nonmedical approaches, including physical therapy, nutritional and occupational therapy and counselling from specialist neurorehabilitation professionals, may also be beneficial.

ADVICE AND SUPPORT

The amount of support offered by doctors to people with MS varies and may depend on where you live. You may need to find out what is available for yourself. Specialized MS nurses are particularly helpful. The MS Society (p. 314) can provide information and advice on treatment and suggest other types of help and support available to people with the condition and also to their families.

Many people with MS say that one of the worst things about it is its unpredictability and the feeling that they have no control over how it will affect them. This can lead to stress in relationships and at work as well as anxiety about the future. It can be almost impossible for other people to understand how you feel, but meeting those who are going through similar experiences can be therapeutic. A number of organizations run local support groups; contact the MS Society for details.

Because of the lack of any effective medical treatment for MS, many people look instead to alternative medicine and complementary therapies. While none has been shown to have any long-term effect on slowing the progress of the disease, many people nevertheless feel that they have benefited both physically and psychologically. Some therapies that people have tried, which can help them live with their condition, include aromatherapy, acupuncture, reflexology, homeopathy, osteopathy, chiropractic, massage and healing.

It is difficult to assess whether any type of treatment—conventional or complementary— is working because of the way symptoms tend to come and go on their own. Claims for a range of treatments, from pressurized oxygen to gluten-free diets and many others, have been made, but none has so far been substantiated.

MOTOR NEURONE DISEASE

The clinical name for this incurable, degenerative neurological disorder is amyotrophic lateral sclerosis (ALS). It is not known what causes the motor neuron cells of the brain and spinal

HOW NERVES ARE AFFECTED

Nerves consist of a chain of neurons along which messages from the brain to all parts of the body travel. Nerves are covered in a myelin sheath that acts as an insulator. When this protective covering is damaged in some way, the messages can no longer travel along the nerve. In multiple sclerosis, this can mean a loss of response in sensitive areas.

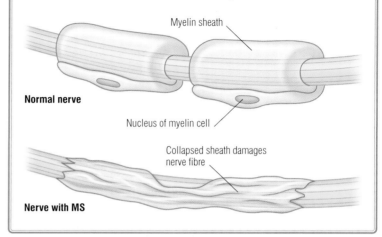

Myelin sheath

Normal nerve

Nucleus of myelin cell

Collapsed sheath damages nerve fibre

Nerve with MS

cord (which control voluntary muscle movement) to die gradually, nor why they should be the only nerve cells affected. During the deterioration, which usually takes between two and five years, the muscles waste away, causing paralysis of the head, lungs and limbs. The mind continues to act as normal and no pain is felt.

Motor neurone disease is a rare and distressing disease. It affects more men than women. It is believed that between 5 and 10 percent of cases are inherited ALS, which is the result of a defective gene that normally prevents oxygen molecules called free radicals from damaging body tissue. In noninherited ALS (the more common form) environmental toxins as well as defects in protective enzymes are thought to play a role. The inherited form normally appears at the age of 50; 60 is the average age for the onset of noninherited ALS.

When symptoms appear, a neurologist will carry out tests to rule out MS and spinal cord diseases, then perform an electromyogram (EMG) to test electrical activity in the muscles and assess nerve damage. Electronic and other equipment is available to enable people with ALS to eat, talk, breathe and move, but physical assistance from a caregiver may become necessary as the disease progresses.

Brain disorders

? Did you know?

♀ There is no established link between high blood pressure and a decline in cognitive or mental function.
♀ Memory can be impaired at any age—it is not always the first sign of dementia. Other causes include fatigue, stress, grief, vision or hearing loss, excessive alcohol consumption and working too hard.

Some mental disorders are more often found in older people and are sometimes linked to ageing, although not everyone who lives longer will necessarily be affected.

DEMENTIA

There are various specific disorders called dementia, which display symptoms showing a decline in a person's mental ability severe enough to interfere with everyday life. Although once known as senility or senile dementia, dementia need not inevitably be a part of ageing. Some illnesses, like thyroid disease, vitamin B deficiency and depression, cause dementia-like symptoms that can be reversed when the underlying disease is treated. Other causes of dementia, including vascular disease, multiple strokes and Alzheimer's disease, are not curable. But intervention and new medication may slow the progress of the disease.

Advanced symptoms may include short-term loss of memory, confusion and non-recognition of people. There may be emotional outbursts, such as anger and irritability, or embarrassing behaviour. Eventually this subsides into a state of non-emotion in which personal habits deteriorate and 24-hour care is needed.

ALZHEIMER'S DISEASE

This is the most common form of dementia. Scientists do not yet know the cause of the disease, which affects about 10 percent of elderly people and causes brain cells to die.

One of the hallmarks of Alzheimer's is the deterioration of nerve cells releasing the neurotransmitter acetylcholine that carries messages between brain cells. At the same time, the enzyme acetycholinesterase (AChE) breaks down acetylcholine in the body at an incredible rate. Several drugs (Aricept, HupA and Cognex) are used to try and restore these acetylcholine levels by inhibiting AChE activity.

Brain "plaques" are another hallmark of the disease. Protein, called amyloid-beta (A-beta), is naturally made in the brain, but when it clumps and forms plaques it causes inflammation and other changes in brain tissue that eventually rob sufferers of the ability to think and function. Researchers aim to develop a drug that lowers A-beta levels. Research is also being done on genetic disposition, and on calcium usage, which is essential for neurotransmission but is affected by Alzheimer's.

People with Down's syndrome (caused by an extra copy of chromosome 21) are at high risk of developing Alzheimer's. Problems with reasoning and judgement, changes in mood and behaviour patterns and an inability to manage work and social life are all characteristic of the disease. Medications may be given for depression, insomnia and behaviour problems.

PARKINSON'S DISEASE

The characteristic symptoms of Parkinson's are muscle tremor or stiffness, slow movements, shuffling walk, stooped posture, loss of balance and a fixed expression. It is a progressive degenerative disease of the nerves that generally appears in people aged 50 to 65. If it is treated, it may not be directly life threatening and its course may be mild or severely debilitating. Dementia also occurs in about a third of cases.

There is no cure, but several drugs are available which improve quality of life. Treatment focuses on improving morale and mobility, social activities and reassurance. Links with a support group are essential for the caregiver as well as the patient.

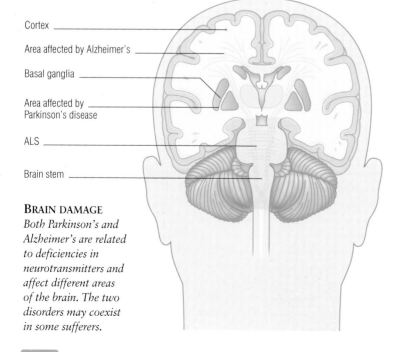

Cortex

Area affected by Alzheimer's

Basal ganglia

Area affected by
Parkinson's disease

ALS

Brain stem

BRAIN DAMAGE

Both Parkinson's and Alzheimer's are related to deficiencies in neurotransmitters and affect different areas of the brain. The two disorders may coexist in some sufferers.

RESPIRATORY PROBLEMS

Women are susceptible to a wide range of diseases that affect the nasal passage, airways and lungs. Problems range from contagious illnesses that are spread by viruses and bacteria to occupational hazards that may have long-lasting effects.

Pneumonia

Inflammation of the tissues and airways of the lungs is termed pneumonia. Depending on its cause and the vulnerability of the sufferer, pneumonia can range from mild to life threatening. Those particularly at risk include the elderly, the very young, those suffering from immune-related disorders, heart or lung disorders, diabetes and alcoholism, and smokers. These people should be vaccinated against influenza and pneumococcus. Pneumonia is a common cause of death in post-operative patients.

BACTERIAL PNEUMONIA

This type can arise spontaneously, but usually results from an infection following some other disorder, such as influenza or chronic bronchitis. Generally, the bacteria responsible are *Streptococcus pneumoniae* (also known as *pneumococci*) though *Staphylococcus aureus* is often implicated when pneumonia follows influenza. There is a high fever, with chills and the production of coloured sputum, which may be flecked with blood, and, especially in the elderly, there may be confusion. Pleurisy (inflammation of the lining of the lungs) is also a common complication. The usual treatment is antibiotics.

VIRAL PNEUMONIA

Many viruses responsible for other lung infections, including the influenza virus, can cause viral pneumonia. Its onset is often slower than that of bacterial pneumonia. Initially there is a dry cough with a headache, aching muscles, fever and lethargy. Symptoms progress to a productive cough, often with blood-flecked sputum and breathlessness. An attack may be followed by bacterial pneumonia.

MYCOPLASMA PNEUMONIA

This type of pneumonia is caused by a microorganism called *Mycoplasma pneumoniae*. The symptoms of the condition are similar to those of bacterial and viral pneumonia, although they are usually milder and the condition tends to progress slowly. The most common treatment is antibiotics.

See also:

1/BEING A WELL WOMAN
Healthy body systems p. 35

3/GENERAL HEALTH ISSUES
Problems of the mind pp. 98–99

6/TREATMENTS & THERAPIES
Conventional treatments pp. 272–277
Alternative medicine pp. 298–311

LUNG DISEASES

Different parts of the lungs are affected by different diseases. Bronchitis affects the main respiratory tubes and pneumonia the lesser tubes and alveoli. In emphysema, these alveoli break down, reducing the area for oxygen exchange.

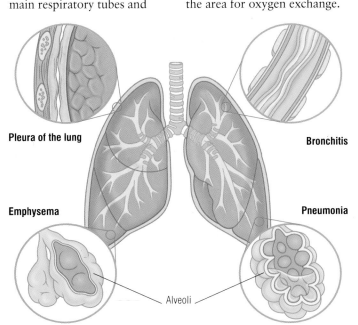

Pleura of the lung

Bronchitis

Emphysema

Pneumonia

Alveoli

See also:

1/BEING A WELL WOMAN
Healthy body systems p. 35

3/GENERAL HEALTH ISSUES
Problems of the mind pp 98–99

6/TREATMENTS & THERAPIES
Treatment plans pp. 262–265
Conventional treatments
pp. 270–277

Influenza

An acute respiratory illness, influenza—flu, as it is popularly known—attacks both the upper and lower respiratory tract. It also causes fever, aching limbs, headache, sore throat, weakness and lethargy. These symptoms may be less apparent in milder forms of influenza, but coughs and a runny nose are common. The cause is a virus: either of the influenza A or B type. A third influenza virus, C, causes symptoms that are almost indistinguishable from those of the common cold—there are no aching muscles or fever and the onset is usually slow.

Influenza strikes nearly every winter, though there can be an outbreak at any time of year. It is defined as epidemic when it affects 400 or more in every 100,000 people. The severity of symptoms varies according to the precise strain of the virus, which mutates frequently, and the constitution of the sufferer. The most severe form of influenza is caused by A-type viruses. The virus is spread in minute droplets exhaled in coughs and sneezes. Symptoms generally appear suddenly, between one and three days after infection, and last for six to 10 days.

The best treatment is to rest in bed for three to four days, drink plenty of fluids and take NSAIDs (nonsteroidal anti-inflammatory drugs) to reduce body temperature and ease aches. The biggest danger for influenza sufferers is secondary, opportunistic bacterial infections of the lungs. These can range from acute bronchitis to severe bacterial pneumonia, and the young, the elderly and those suffering from diabetes, immune system disorders and heart and lung diseases are particularly at risk.

PROTECTION AND TREATMENT

Vaccination offers good protection against influenza and is recommended for those at risk of developing complications. The vaccine is only designed to combat the specific strain of virus that researchers believe will be prevalent in the coming months. It does not give protection against all strains of flu. Nevertheless, it is advisable for vulnerable people, for example the elderly or those susceptible to respiratory problems, to be vaccinated. During severe outbreaks these people should also reduce contact with possible carriers.

The major antiviral treatments, which only attack influenza A strains, are the drugs amantadine—this sometimes causes side effects—and rimantidine. Antibiotics have no effect against the influenza virus, but may be given to combat any subsequent infection.

A new drug, recently licensed, is Relenza. It is a neuraminidase inhibitor that attacks the influenza virus directly. It is taken by means of a nasal spray, and if given within two days of the start of an attack it can reduce the severity and duration of symptoms by 24 hours.

Pleurisy

The pleura is a double membrane that lines the cavity of the chest and surrounds the lungs. The space in between the two skins is filled with fluid, which provides lubrication as the lungs expand and contract. In pleurisy, this membrane becomes inflamed, usually following another infection such as pneumonia. The main symptom is a sharp pain felt in the chest when breathing in. Treatment is by prescribing antibiotics for the underlying infection and taking painkillers for the pain.

? Did you know?
In a normal year, influenza accounts for around 4,000 deaths in the UK and 10,000 in the USA, but these figures can rise to extraordinary levels when there is an epidemic. In 1918, for example, "Spanish flu" caused 20 to 30 million deaths worldwide over the next three years.

CHEST X-RAYS
Women who smoke are prone to diseases of the lungs. Routine chest X-rays may identify problems at an early stage so that medical help can be given.

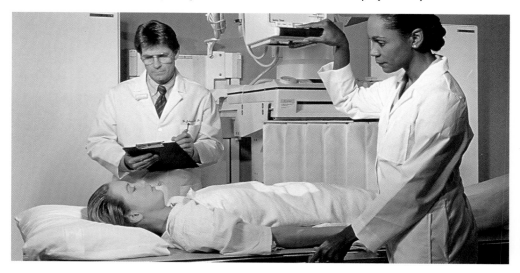

Bronchitis

There are two forms of bronchitis: acute and chronic—though repeated attacks of acute bronchitis may develop into the chronic form. Acute bronchitis usually develops suddenly, following a viral infection such as a common cold or influenza, and usually in the winter. It may also be triggered by air pollution, which causes increased sensitivity of the respiratory tubes. Bacteria invade the bronchi—which are the tubes that branch off the windpipe (the trachea) in the lungs—and the area becomes inflamed.

SYMPTOMS

Initial symptoms include a mild fever and a dry, hacking cough which, after a few days, starts to produce greenish-yellow sputum, the colour indicating that the mucus is infected. Breathing may be affected by a characteristic wheezing and shortness of breath, and coughing may be painful. There may also be a rise in temperature. This stage lasts for a few days, then the fever dies down. The coughing may persist for 10 days or so. In chronic bronchitis sputum is coughed up on most days for at least three consecutive months in at least two consecutive years (p. 216).

Anyone who is at risk from complications of respiratory disease—the young, the elderly and those suffering from diabetes, immune system disorders and heart and lung diseases—should consult their doctor if they develop the symptoms of bronchitis. So, too, should anyone who experiences breathing difficulties, particularly smokers and people living in an area with a high level of atmospheric pollution.

TREATMENT

Using a humidifier and drinking fluids both help to relieve the symptoms. Antibiotics will probably be prescribed to combat the bacteria. If there is still severe breathlessness after three days, if blood is coughed up or a high temperature persists then you should consult your doctor immediately.

Self-help treatments

- ♀ Bed-rest.
- ♀ NSAIDs (nonsteroidal anti-inflammatory drugs).
- ♀ Steam inhalations.
- ♀ Cough medicine containing expectorants to loosen the mucus and ease the cough.

ENVIRONMENTAL AND OCCUPATIONAL LUNG DISEASES

The environment and the workplace are responsible for many life-threatening respiratory problems, and more are being recognized each year. Fortunately, preventive measures are also improving. The three main types of problems are: pneumoconiosis, extrinsic allergic alveolitis and occupational asthma (p. 217).

Disease	Causes and symptoms
Pneumoconiosis	Caused by the inhalation of minute particles of mineral dust, the three main types are: asbestosis (from inhaled asbestos fibres); silicosis (from silicon dioxide, or "quartz" particles); and coalworker's pneumoconiosis ("black lung disease" from coal dust). In silicosis and asbestosis the lung tissue becomes progressively more fibrous over a period of two to 20 years; asbestosis can develop at any time from 10 to 40 years after exposure and commonly people with this develop lung cancer. Breathlessness and oxygen starvation increase until the lungs can no longer operate. The conditions are usually fatal and the only treatment is oxygen therapy.
Extrinsic allergic alveolitis	Hypersensitivity to an allergen causes the alveoli at the base of the lungs to become inflamed, with fibrous tissue forming in the area. The allergens are found in inhaled organic dust, and include bacteria, fungal spores and proteins from other organisms. The reaction may be acute, or progress slowly over many years. If acute, there may be fever, tiredness, tightness in the chest and coughing and wheezing; in other cases there may be weight loss, increasing coughing and clubbing (rounding) of the tips of the fingers and toes. Treatment involves stabilizing the condition with bronchodilators and anti-inflammatory drugs.

COPD

Cigarette smoking is the main cause of the most common chronic condition affecting the lungs. Chronic obstructive pulmonary disease (COPD, which encompasses previous labels such as chronic bronchitis and emphysema) affects more women than ever before, as a result of the increase in women smoking or living with a smoker. COPD causes 30,000 deaths a year in the UK (4 percent of all female deaths). Other less important risk factors include environmental pollution, occupation, diet and genetic inheritance.

COPD is diagnosed from a history of chronic progressive cough, with or without mucus production, breathlessness and wheezing. In advanced cases when severe obstruction is present in the airways, the blood vessels in the lungs can become constricted. This puts pressure on the right side of the heart and can lead to heart failure, which can require treatment with diuretics and heart-stabilizing drugs. A number of things are going wrong in the lungs in this condition: some predominate in one sufferer, some in another.

ASSOCIATED CONDITIONS

These include chronic mucus overproduction (chronic bronchitis), which in cigarette smokers largely results from mucous gland enlargement in the bronchi (central conducting airways). Progressive obstruction of the airways can also occur, caused by a combination of inflammation and scarring in the smaller airways and loss of elasticity of the lungs because of emphysema. This is measured by tests of airway function such as the forced expiratory volume (FEV). Bronchiolitis, inflammation of the walls of the bronchioles (terminal smaller airways) can progress to fibrosis—permanent narrowing—of these tubes. This adds to the permanence and irreversibility of COPD.

Emphysema is the name given to permanent destruction of the air spaces within the bronchioles. It can be caused by cigarette smoking. In less than 1 percent of emphysema cases the condition affects younger people and is caused by the lack of Alpha-1-antitrypsin, a protein in the walls of the air sacs. Symptoms of emphysema vary but generally include difficulty in breathing with a long expiration phase; severe breathlessness, especially after even light exercise; wheezing; weight loss, but retaining a barrel chest shape; and tiredness.

PREVENTION AND TREATMENT

North American and earlier UK studies confirm that stopping smoking can help lung function. However, the risk of mortality is not back to the same as a non-smoker until 10 years or more after stopping. This emphasizes the need to stop smoking as early as possible.

Inhaled drugs can be useful in helping with symptoms of wheezing, and infections can be treated with antibiotics. Influenza and pneumococcal vaccines should be recommended. In severe cases, oxygen therapy at home is extremely useful. This involves inhaling oxygen from a cylinder by means of a mask, for up to 12 hours a day.

A programme of pulmonary rehabilitation exercises may be suggested, to maximize lung function and build up exercise tolerance. Some studies have shown that a high intake of antioxidants and fish may reduce the risk in smokers. With good management, COPD sufferers can be stabilized. Avoiding cigarettes, regular exercise and the correct medication are essential components of a management plan, as is regular review by a doctor.

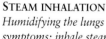

What to watch for

♀ Breathlessness, especially when walking or lying down, which causes sleeping problems.
♀ Constant wheezing with production of as much as a cupful of mucus each day.
♀ Increased weight through lack of exercise.
♀ A blue colouring of the face and fingers (cyanosis), as a result of the lack of oxygen in the blood.
♀ Swelling in the ankles, which indicates problems with circulation.

STEAM INHALATION
Humidifying the lungs relieves symptoms: inhale steam from a bowl of boiling water.

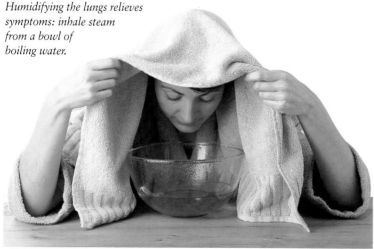

Asthma

See also:

1/BEING A WELL WOMAN
Healthy body systems p. 35

3/GENERAL HEALTH ISSUES
Anxiety-related disorders p. 108

6/TREATMENTS & THERAPIES
Conventional treatments
pp. 282–283
Complementary therapies p. 292

Asthma is a respiratory condition in which the small muscles controlling the diameter of the airways have a tendency to go into spasm, together with inflammation of the lining of the airways. The airways narrow and excessive mucus is produced. Asthma is particularly common in developed countries, where 10 percent of children and young adults may be affected. The primary cause of asthma is unknown as yet, although attacks can be precipitated by many environmental and other stimuli, such as unaccustomed physical exercise.

SYMPTOMS

Sufferers experience tightness in the chest, coughing, wheezing and shortness of breath which, without treatment, may last for several hours. When asthma is very severe—status asthmaticus, or severe acute asthma—it can be considered life-threatening and hospitalization is usually required.

Because asthma is caused by inflammation of the airways, some sufferers will wheeze most of the time. There is a vicious circle: the lining of the tubes swells and secretes mucus which constricts the airways, reducing the amount of air that can pass through them. At the same time the lining becomes more sensitive to various trigger factors that increase the constriction.

EXTRINSIC ASTHMA

This type of asthma is triggered by allergens, most often pollen, dust mite droppings and salivary protein on cat hairs. This asthma is also called atopic, meaning that the allergens affect a different part of the body from the point of contact.

Other causes of extrinsic asthma may be irritants such as tobacco smoke, exhaust fumes, household cleaners and burning fuels; respiratory infections such as acute or chronic bronchitis or a cold; exercise, especially in cold weather; some drugs, typically aspirin and NSAIDs; sulphate preservatives; emotional stress; and chemicals and organic substances found in the workplace (occupational asthma).

Immune cells called eosinophils are activated by the allergen and respond more fiercely the next time it is encountered. They are also more likely to be activated by other allergens as well. This type of asthma usually starts in childhood, and often persists into later life, but rarely develops after the age of 35.

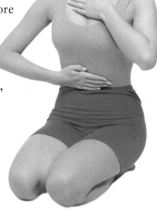

MAXIMIZING LUNG EFFICIENCY
To practise deep breathing, rest one hand on the chest and one on the stomach. The hand on the stomach should rise first, while the hand on the chest should hardly move.

WHAT HAPPENS
Breathing difficulties experienced in asthma are as a result of a constriction of the respiratory tubes. This constriction is caused by the spasmodic contractions of the muscle in the walls of the bronchioles (tubes), or by their inflammation. The tubes may become blocked by the excessive production of mucus.

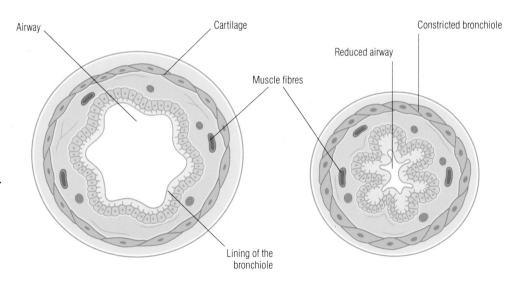

Airway

Cartilage

Muscle fibres

Lining of the bronchiole

Constricted bronchiole

Reduced airway

Normal bronchiole

Asthmatic bronchiole

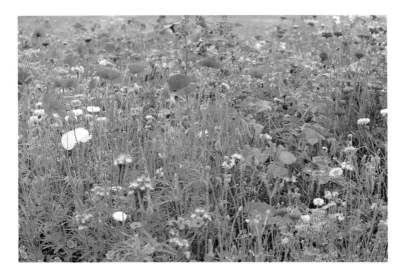

bronchodilator causes improvement in the results. Skin-patch tests may then be carried out to see if an allergen is responsible.

TREATMENT AND SELF-HELP

Generally, the aim of asthma treatment is to manage the condition rather than to cure it. The exception is desensitization therapy, in which the patient's tolerance to an allergen is raised by increasing exposure to it in a series of injections. However, this procedure carries the risk that there may be a potentially fatal reaction to the allergen.

One of the most important ways of managing asthma is to avoid triggers by taking steps to keep yourself away from the substances responsible. For example, stay indoors on days when the level of a pollen to which you are allergic is high, or wear a mask outside; avoid cats and dogs if you are allergic to proteins on animal hair; wash curtains and bed covers frequently in very hot water if the house-dust mite is responsible for your asthma, and dust with a damp cloth so that dust is collected rather than spread around. Choose wood floors and blinds rather than carpets and curtains where possible. Investing in a high-efficiency particulate-arresting (HEPA) or double-filtered vacuum cleaner may also be worthwhile.

If skin tests do not reveal any allergies, you will have to identify your trigger factors yourself. The best way to do this is to keep a diary in which you describe asthma symptoms, grading them on a scale of one to ten, and correlate them with outside factors. For example, note if wheeziness increases when walking alongside a busy road, or when using a particular domestic cleaning product. However, bear in mind that individuals often have more than one trigger factor, and that a hypersensitivity to new trigger factors can develop.

SUMMER ALLERGIES
Many species of plant can trigger asthma attacks, but you can learn to avoid the worst. Wind-pollinated flowers produce more and smaller pollen grains than insect-pollinated flowers. Your reaction to pollen granules will also be worse if they are damp, since the water carries them to the lungs.

INTRINSIC ASTHMA

If no specific allergen is found, the disease is called intrinsic asthma. This type usually develops later in life, possibly after the age of 35, and is more common in women than men. Attacks of intrinsic asthma will be triggered by stress, emotional crises or physical exercise. Although the disease is treatable and controllable in most cases, it is still responsible for an alarming number of hospital admissions and around 6,000 deaths each year.

HOW ASTHMA IS DIAGNOSED

The doctor will take a history of symptoms and will arrange respiratory function tests that measure the amount of air that the lungs can expel. If allergy is suspected, blood and mucus tests may also be carried out.

The main tests use a peak flow meter and a spirometer. The patient blows into the peak flow meter, which records the maximum rate at which air can be expelled—this is the peak expiratory flow rate (PEFR). The spirometer measures how much air can be expelled in one second—the forced expiratory volume in one second (FEV1)—and also the time it takes to empty the lungs of air after a breath—this is the forced vital capacity (FVC).

These tests are performed before and after a bronchodilator inhalation is given to widen the bronchioles, and asthma is diagnosed if the

DRUG TREATMENT

Once diagnosed, asthma should be monitored by a doctor. It can be controlled successfully by drugs, which can both prevent and treat an attack. Sufferers will be encouraged to use a peak flow meter at home, as a way of monitoring their health, and should take appropriate action when thei condition worsens. When asthma affects you more frequently, it may be

MITES AND ASTHMA
Allergy to faeces of invisible house-dust mites can trigger asthma attacks. Efficient vacuum cleaning and regular washing of bedding can help reduce adverse reactions.

The world threat from TB

Tuberculosis (TB) is caused by the bacterium Mycobacterium tuberculosis, which is spread in the droplets sneezed or coughed out by those in whom the disease is active. More rarely, it can be present in milk (bovine tuberculosis). In most people the bacteria will multiply to form a pocket of infection, but this will be healed by the immune system and surrounded by scar tissue. It is estimated that about 50 percent of the population in poorer countries and around 5 to 10 percent in the industrialized world harbour the bacteria.

When the immune system starts to falter, as a result of age, infection, immune system disorders such as AIDS, malnutrition, some drug therapies, infections and other disease, the bacteria may begin to spread through the bloodstream, causing fatigue, weight loss, loss of appetite, fever and night sweats. Then tubercles—nodes of affected tissue— form in the lungs and in other organs, and blood-flecked sputum is coughed up. Without treatment, tuberculosis is fatal in about 50 percent of those affected.

There are several reasons why TB has become a problem once more:
♀ International air travel has increased the risk of exposure.
♀ Both the increase in drug use and AIDS have increased susceptibility to the bacteria (AIDS sufferers have a 10 percent chance each year of contracting active TB, while others have only a 10 percent lifetime risk).
♀ A new strain of the bacterium has emerged, called multiple-drug-resistant TB (MDR-TB) as drugs so far have little effect on it.

The risk of TB is highest among people such as volunteer workers and young travellers in underdeveloped countries, who spend long periods in overcrowded, badly ventilated conditions and have not been vaccinated.

If you suspect you may have been exposed to TB, you should consult your doctor. A multiple puncture tuberculin test or a Mantoux test will be carried out to check whether there has been any previous exposure to the tuberculosis bacterium. You may be a candidate for treatment with a drug such as isonaziad to prevent the bacteria from becoming active.

necessary to inhale corticosteroid drugs on a daily basis, to reduce inflammation; oral corticosteroids may be used as well but tend to produce more side effects than when inhaled. Metered-dose bronchodilators are also inhaled, either to prevent an attack—before exercise, for example, in exercise-induced asthma—or to provide relief during an attack. Salmeterol, a long-acting bronchodilator, can be used to prevent overnight attacks. A new group of drugs known as leukotriene modifiers has proved effective in relieving the symptoms of an attack. In practice, a combination of drugs is likely to be given, tailored to individual needs.

SELF-HELP TECHNIQUES

There are various self-help techniques to lessen the severity of an asthma attack and reduce sufferers' anxiety during one. These approaches all focus on breathing and on helping the sufferer to be in control. The exercises, also suitable for children, may be learned from a physical therapist and should be practised daily.

As well as inducing a feeling of calm and control, the exercises maximize the efficiency of the lungs. They concentrate on breathing out using the diaphragmatic muscle to force the maximum amount of air from the lungs. The body's natural craving for air then assists the in-breath.

Alternatively, other exercises include those of the Buteyko method, which aim to increase the lungs' tolerance of carbon dioxide by a programme of shallow breathing exercises. Yogic breathing exercises (p. 293) may also be used by asthma sufferers. Many yoga classes begin with 10 to 20 minutes of breathing exercises, but you need to be taught how to do them. In all these

approaches it is vital that you should not become anxious about your breathing, since this will be counterproductive.

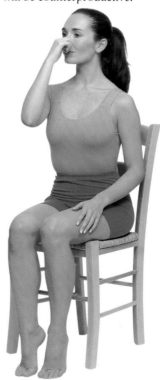

YOGIC BREATHING
Controlled breathing techniques, for example breathing through each nostril alternately, can have a powerful calming effect.

Lung cancer

See also:

1/BEING A WELL WOMAN
Healthy body systems
    p. 35

3/GENERAL HEALTH ISSUES
Problems of the mind pp. 98–99

6/TREATMENTS & THERAPIES
Treatment plans pp. 262–267
Conventional treatments p. 276;
    pp. 278–281

If smoking had never been invented, lung cancer would be relatively rare. As it is, it is now the third highest cause of cancer-related death in women, after breast and colorectal cancer—a situation that is regarded as serious by medical practitioners. As the number of women who smoke continues to increase so does the number with lung cancer. There has been a noticeable rise, too, in nonsmoker's cancer among women, which may be related to environmental factors.

There is some evidence that women may be more vulnerable to lung cancer: in other words, a woman who smokes could be more likely to do damage to lung cells than a man with the same smoking habits and history. Hormones have also been linked to the cancer. Research has shown that cells in lung cancers in women are twice as likely as those in cancers in men to have receptors for oestrogen and progesterone—two hormones that can stimulate tumour growth.

The symptoms of lung cancer are primarily a cough, especially with the production of sputum, which may be blood-stained; difficulty in breathing; pain in the chest or centre of the back; difficulty in swallowing; and loss of weight for no obvious reason.

There is good news for a woman who stops smoking, even if she has been a heavy smoker for years. After 15 years she will reduce her risk

Should you see a doctor?

You should consult a doctor if you have one or more of the following symptoms, which may relate to different types of cancer:

♀ A persistent sore in the mouth.
♀ A constant sore throat.
♀ A lump, white spot or scaly area on the lip or in the mouth.
♀ A swollen lymph node in the neck, armpit or groin that remains for longer than three weeks.
♀ Moles, freckles or warts that change colour or shape, or bleed.
♀ Unusual bleeding or discharge between periods, especially during or after menopause.
♀ Thickening or lumps in the breast.
♀ Difficulty in swallowing or a lump on or near the thyroid gland.
♀ Rectal bleeding or changes in bowel habits (which are unconnected to diet or lifestyle changes).
♀ Urinary difficulties such as pain when passing urine, frequency, weak flow or blood in the urine.

of developing lung cancer to nearly the same level as that of a lifelong non-smoker. However, a non-smoker who has a partner who smokes runs twice the risk of getting lung cancer.

SMOKERS' LUNGS
Tobacco smoke and nicotine build-up in the lungs stimulate the production of cancerous cells in the lining of the bronchi and bronchioles (the airways branching off from the bronchi). The smoke also destroys the walls of the alveoli (the tiny air sacs in the lungs), causing them to coalesce so that the available surface area for gas exchange is reduced.

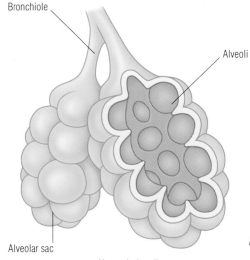

Bronchiole

Alveoli

Alveolar sac

Normal alveoli

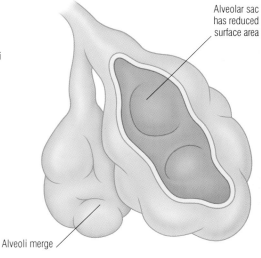

Alveolar sac has reduced surface area

Alveoli merge

Alveoli in smokers

LIVING WITH CANCER

Although at present only a minority of people with lung cancer can be completely cured, various research and clinical trials are under way to find different ways of applying the various current treatment methods.

Surgery is usually only possible if an early diagnosis is made and the tumour is fairly small. Some treatments are aimed at easing pain and discomfort rather than curing the disease. For example, laser surgery may be used to shrink a tumour that cannot be removed completely but which is blocking an airway. In some people a small metal tube, called a stent, may be inserted to keep the airway open. There are various ways of minimizing the side effects of radiotherapy and chemotherapy (see box below), such as nausea and vomiting and constipation.

Palliative care for lung cancer, which is designed to improve the quality of life rather than cure the disease, can also be very effective in controlling pain and other symptoms.

Emotional difficulties linked to lung and other types of cancer are not easy to talk about and are often hardest to share with those close to you. You may find the help you need is available from a trained counsellor specializing in cancer. Your doctor should be able to put you in touch with a counsellor or a self-help group, which can also provide support and advice.

TYPES OF LUNG CANCER AND TREATMENTS

Adenocarcinoma—which affects mucus-producing cells in the airway linings—is the most common type of lung cancer in women. Squamous cell carcinoma is the most common in men and accounts for about half of all cases of lung cancer. It develops in the cells that line the bronchi (airways), which lead from the trachea (windpipe) to the lungs. Large cell carcinoma is the least common. The three types are often referred to collectively as non-small cell cancers, to distinguish them from small cell lung cancer, which accounts for around a quarter of all lung cancer. Small cell lung cancer spreads rapidly through the lungs and to other parts of the body. It is usually inoperable by the time it has been diagnosed and is therefore treated in a different way.

Steps to diagnosis A chest X-ray will usually show whether cancer is present, but other tests will confirm the diagnosis and give more detailed information that is required before any decision can be made about treatment. A sample of sputum will be analysed in the cytology lab. A test called a bronchoscopy may be performed under local anaesthetic to allow the doctor to look inside the lung and do a biopsy (take a tissue sample). Alternatively, the doctor may perform a mediastinoscopy, which involves inserting a small telescope via an incision in the neck to look at the chest and lymph nodes and take samples. Lung biopsies may be done with the aid of X-rays or a CT scan.

Surgery The treatment plan will be based on the results of all these tests. An operation to remove the tumour may be the best option for non-small cell cancer. This may involve removing all or part of an affected lung. In some treatment trials, radiotherapy and/or chemotherapy may be used together with surgery in various combined treatments. Surgery is rarely the right treatment for small cell cancer, since it is unlikely that the cancer will be confined to the lung and so it would be impossible to remove it with an operation.

Radiotherapy This can be very useful for relieving pain and in situations where a tumour is causing other problems, such as blocking an important blood vessel or causing a

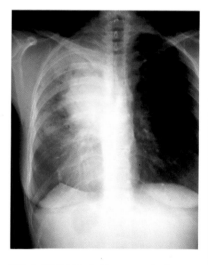

X-ray revealing an area of lung cancer (red).

lung to collapse. It is also being used in new ways in clinical trials, such as giving it in several daily doses for people with non-small cell cancer or combined with chemotherapy for some people with small cell cancer.

Chemotherapy Anticancer drugs that destroy the tumour cells or inhibit them from multiplying are the best option for treating small cell cancer. The choice of drugs, dosage and frequency of treatments will depend on circumstances and local policy.

SKIN PROBLEMS

Genetics, hormones, drugs, allergies and a wide variety of environmental factors can contribute to the range of afflictions that influence the look, feel and condition of your skin. These can all cause problems for women at any age.

See also:

1/BEING A WELL WOMAN
Essentials of good health p. 26
Healthy body systems p. 42

5/ILLNESSES & EMERGENCIES
Skin problems pp. 230–233

6/TREATMENTS & THERAPIES
Conventional treatments
pp. 272–277
Alternative medicine pp. 298–311

> **! Caution**
>
> Resist the temptation to try to hide pimples with heavy layers of make-up. This may irritate already sensitive skin. Skin can also become even more sensitive as a result of cover-up medication. It should not be used for more than three months; if there is no improvement in that time, discuss the problem with your doctor.

Acne

The skin condition known medically as acne vulgaris, which produces blackheads, whiteheads, pimples and red pustules, can distress those people who have it. Most sufferers are teenagers, with more boys than girls affected at this age. This undesirable change in their appearance can seriously undermine teenagers' self-confidence. They can become very self-conscious or even clinically depressed as a result. Some teenagers of both sexes will continue to have the condition into adulthood, particularly as the disease is becoming more common among people in their 20s and 30s.

Acne is most common at times of hormonal upheaval, and the body's sex hormones play a role in triggering the symptoms (except in pregnancy when acne tends to improve). A rise in hormone levels, in particular the male hormone testosterone, leads to an increase in the production of sebum, an oily substance

Self-help plan

♀ Be gentle with your skin.
♀ Establish a daily skincare routine that cleanses, moisturizes and nourishes your skin.
♀ Choose unscented, mild cleansers, and apply them gently.
♀ Avoid cosmetics, lotions or creams (including sun protection) that block pores or cause an allergic reaction.
♀ Wear sunscreen all year round. Avoid waterproof sunscreens, since these may block pores.
♀ If pimples appear, don't pick at them.
♀ Don't use abrasive skin-peeling methods (for example masks or face scrubs), which can damage sensitive skin.
♀ Don't go to sleep without thoroughly removing make-up—or your pores will remain clogged for eight hours or more.

SEBACEOUS GLANDS
The sebaceous glands are found alongside hair follicles in the layer of skin called the dermis, which lies under the epidermis. When they over-produce sebum, they become clogged and a whitehead or a blackhead forms on or just under the surface.

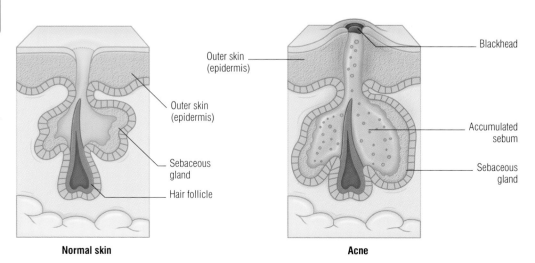

Outer skin (epidermis)

Outer skin (epidermis)

Sebaceous gland

Hair follicle

Blackhead

Accumulated sebum

Sebaceous gland

Normal skin

Acne

secreted by the sebaceous glands in the skin, to help keep it moist and supple. Acne results when these glands go into overdrive, producing excessive amounts of sebum which then block a hair follicle. The trapped sebum can form a whitehead under the surface of the skin, or if it reaches the surface it becomes discoloured on contact with air, causing a blackhead. Infection may set in, making the pimples inflamed with pus and very sore.

Some women develop skin eruptions like this for a few days each month just before their menstrual period. The progestogen-only contraceptive pill can also cause acne.

Unfortunately, the eruptions tend to be in the most visible areas—on the face and sometimes the neck, the top of the chest and back. These areas have more sebaceous glands than other parts of the body.

WHAT A DERMATOLOGIST MAY DO

Your doctor can prescribe antibiotics, either as skin creams or pills, which may need to be taken for several months for the maximum benefit.

Vitamin A derivatives taken as capsules are one of the most effective treatments for acne, but because they are very powerful and can have serious side effects, they are reserved for severe acne that does not respond to any other treatment. Known as Roaccutane, they are only available from hospital dermatology clinics. Usually creams and gels containing vitamin A derivatives will be tried first to reduce the formation of sebum plugs in the follicles and encourage the sebum to drain away. These treatments should not be used if you are pregnant, since in some cases excess vitamin A can cause birth defects.

Because of the hormone content of certain birth control pills, they can improve acne in some women. However, with other pills the acne can get worse.

OVER-THE-COUNTER REMEDIES

There are many creams, lotions and gels available to treat acne. They contain substances called keratolytics—usually benzoyl peroxide—that loosen the top layer of skin so that it can be rubbed off and unblock the pores. The remedies are also antibacterial and so help to suppress the inflammation caused by infection.

Most topical agents should be used once or twice a day after cleaning and drying the skin. They may make your skin sting a little and will leave it dry, so always use a light moisturizer after application.

? Did you know?

♀ Acne is not caused by eating chocolate, fried food or too much junk food (although for your general health, it's best to keep these to a minimum and increase your intake of fresh fruit and vegetables).

♀ Dirty skin does not cause blackheads and pimples (but it can contribute to them if you do not have a good daily cleansing routine).

♀ Your sex life has nothing to do with whether or not you develop acne.

♀ Most people grow out of acne (it usually disappears after adolescence).

♀ You don't have to put up with acne (there are ways to help you control it—seek advice from your doctor).

ROSACEA

This skin disorder was once thought to be a form of acne but since neither whiteheads nor blackheads develop it is now considered to be a different condition. It mostly affects fair-skinned women and some men in middle age and later.

The skin across the nose and cheeks, and sometimes the forehead, eyelids and chin, becomes inflamed, with enlarged blood vessels. If the inflammation is severe the area may swell up and eventually the swelling on the nose may become permanent. There may be tiny spider veins on the cheeks or the face may become taut, red and shiny. The cause is unknown (it may be genetic) and the effects can be distressing psychologically. The usual treatment is long-term antibiotics in pill or capsule form, or topical creams may be prescribed to keep the condition under control. You will be advised to cover up in the sun and to wear a suitable sunscreen all year round.

HELPING YOURSELF

You may be able to discover which factors are likely to make your skin more sensitive or the symptoms worse by keeping a diary of the food and drink you have and when you have them. Triggers can be alcohol consumption, exposing your face to the sun, too-hot drinks or spicy foods. For some people cheese and caffeine may also make the condition worse. You may be able to improve your skin by being very careful with daily moisturizing and cleansing routines and by using only mild products. You can try applying light nonallergenic make-up (for sensitive skin) to lessen the appearance of the condition.

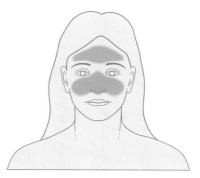

Areas affected

Eczema

The symptoms of atopic eczema vary, but generally the skin becomes dry and scaly and unbearably itchy. Blisters may develop and eventually burst, leaving you with red oozing patches that dry into crusts. Scratching the skin makes the condition worse.

If you have suffered from eczema since you were very young, or if you or anyone else in your immediate family also has asthma, hay fever, perennial rhinitis (year-round hay fever symptoms) or a food allergy, then your skin condition may result from an atopic allergy—an inherited tendency to develop allergies to a wide range of substances in the environment that are normally harmless. Symptoms develop because the immune system reacts to these substances or allergens by triggering a series of defensive measures when the presence of the allergen is detected.

Many people grow out of atopic eczema by the time they reach the age of 30, although it may return. The usual places where it reappears are in natural skin creases (such as at the inner elbow or back of the knee), on the lips and around the nipples of young women, often at times of stress.

One of the main difficulties with atopic eczema is identifying the allergens to which you are reacting, especially since they may well be substances that do not come into direct contact with your skin. One of the more common allergens is the droppings of house-dust mites. These mites live in carpets, other soft furnishings and bedding, and feed on your body's dead skin flakes. Other allergens include animal hair and fur; other animal traces such as saliva; feathers or down in pillows; and pollen from grass or trees.

The situation may be made more complicated if you also develop allergies to new substances as a result of long-term exposure to them. This kind of reaction, called contact dermatitis, can occur in people with a prior condition of atopic eczema, but it can also affect people who have not had the condition before.

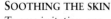

SOOTHING THE SKIN
To ease irritation, use bath and shower products instead of soap, and apply a cream or gel after washing. Always use products without perfumes.

DIAGNOSIS

The fact that most people who have atopic eczema as children eventually grow out of it means that diagnostic tests (including skin and blood tests) are not usually necessary. However, they may be done if your doctor suspects your problem is the result of contact eczema.

Pompholyx eczema affects the hands and feet, particularly the areas where sweating is prevalent—the palms, sides of the fingers, toes and soles. Small itchy blisters form under the skin. They usually break and ooze, which may lead to a secondary infection. Outbreaks are common in hot weather and during stress.

Discoid eczema is an adult illness in which round scaly patches form on the skin. They are usually atopic. The patches itch and look like highly contagious ringworm, a fungal infection that may come from infected animals or people. Ringworm requires antifungal treatment. Discoid eczema is treated with moisturizers and steroid creams.

Varicose eczema may occur if you have severe varicose veins or had a deep vein thrombosis. The area above the ankles swells, the skin is tense and shiny, then becomes scaly and changes colour. It needs medical attention to prevent an ulcer from forming.

POSSIBLE TREATMENTS

If you have only a few patches of eczema or they only appear now and again, fairly simple treatment will usually keep them under control. One of the easiest steps you can take is to avoid cosmetics and keep your skin well moisturized. There are various products available over the counter as well as by prescription in the form of bath and shower additives, cream and gels, which clean the skin and ease dryness and irritation. You may have to experiment to find the one that works best for you. Mild steroid creams, also available with or without prescription, can be applied when the skin is irritated, or your doctor may prescribe stronger ones to be used for a limited period if the eczema flares up badly.

Some people with atopic eczema have lower than normal levels of an essential fatty acid called gamolenic acid, and your doctor may prescribe a course of evening primrose oil to

CONTACT DERMATITIS

Dermatitis includes a range of inflammatory skin disorders with symptoms similar to eczema. However, in adults, it is more often the result of a reaction to some substance the skin has come into direct contact with. The skin becomes hot and red, dry, scaly and itchy and may blister then ooze and form crusts. In contact or irritant dermatitis this can be seen on the areas of the skin exposed to the allergen, most often the hands, face, ears, neck and earlobes.

Sometimes you may begin to react to a product or substance that you have encountered previously without any problems because your skin has become sensitive to it over time. This can happen with cosmetics and skincare products, shampoos, bath and shower additives, perfumes, sunscreens, detergents and fabric conditioners and also with a wide range of other

SENSITIVITY
Many household products can cause skin rashes, scaling or blistering. You need to identify which product is causing the problem and buy an alternative.

potential allergens such as nickel—in jewellery or fastenings in jeans and other clothes—or rubber.

Occupational dermatitis can affect people who work with substances such as chemicals or dyes over long periods of time and eventually become sensitive to them. Sometimes these people may develop other allergic conditions such as asthma if they continue in regular contact with the allergen.

If the trigger is not obvious it may be identified through skin-patch testing in a hospital dermatology or allergy clinic. Solutions containing possible allergens are placed on your skin and covered for a few days: itchiness and redness at any site indicates that you are allergic to the substance concerned.

The only real cure is to avoid the allergen, but emollients and weak steroid creams can be used to relieve the dryness and itching.

correct the problem, but this does not work for everyone. You may find it helps to wear natural fibres such as cotton or silk next to your skin (although wool may aggravate the condition). Try to resist scratching the itchy areas. You can scratch yourself unconsciously at night, so protect yourself by wearing thin cotton gloves when you sleep.

HERBAL MEDICINE
Herbal treatment is specific to the individual, adjusted to your food intolerances, stress levels and environmental factors. You may be given topical ointments such as calendula to soothe and moisturize the skin, or camomile to ease pain and itching. Herbal teas made from marigold, camomile, red clover and burdock may have anti-inflammatory properties. *Echinacea*, nettle and

yarrow may help the immune system, and cooling compresses of burdock, chickweed, marigold, witch hazel or yellow dock may reduce inflammation or heal blisters. Chinese herbal remedies can be effective in treating childhood eczema. Consult your doctor or dermatologist if considering herbal treatment.

TRACKING DOWN THE ALLERGEN
Keeping a diary may help you relate your symptoms to specific allergens or stress points. On each day, describe the state of your eczema then note what you ate and drank, the smells you came into contact with, the soap you washed your hands with and other possible triggers. Over time you may see a pattern emerging. If your skin gets suddenly worse or shows no improvement by your late 20s, you may have developed contact eczema: discuss this with your doctor.

HERBAL INFUSIONS
Some herbal teas can reduce your reaction to allergens. Up to three cups a day of dandelion or burdock (Arctium) tea may reduce inflammation.

225

See also:

3/GENERAL HEALTH ISSUES
Anxiety-related disorders
p. 108

4/HORMONAL HEALTH
Endocrine system problems
pp. 142–143

5/ILLNESSES & EMERGENCIES
Skin problems pp. 230–231

6/TREATMENTS & THERAPIES
Conventional treatments
pp. 272–277
Alternative medicine pp. 298–299

Psoriasis

Although psoriasis can develop in infancy, it more commonly appears between the ages of 15 and 25, but it can also appear for the first time later in life. While psoriasis cannot be cured, it often subsides for long periods of time and various treatments can help the sufferer to keep it under control.

When you have psoriasis you develop pinkish-red, raised and scaly patches, which have a silvery sheen, on the skin. These patches, which may be large or small, are called plaques and are the result of an abnormality in the way skin cells replace themselves. Normally, skin cells are replaced by new ones every 28 days or so but in people with psoriasis the turnover happens up to seven times faster than it should, so that cells reaching the skin surface are not properly formed. The result is itching and flaking, and inflammation of the underlying blood vessels, which makes the skin look red.

TYPES OF PSORIASIS

Plaque psoriasis commonly affects the knees, elbows, trunk, scalp and hairline. The nails may become pitted and thickened and may separate from the nailbed. Fortunately, psoriasis does not often affect the face. For many sufferers the worst part of the condition is the way it looks.

Flexural psoriasis appears on the moist areas of the body: under the breasts, in the groin area or on the genitalia. In another type, pustular psoriasis, small pustules develop on the palms or soles of the feet. People with psoriasis usually find that both sides of the body are affected in a symmetrical way. Psoriasis may start after a throat infection. This form is called guttate psoriasis and should resolve itself in two or three months.

The causes of psoriasis are not fully understood, although certain triggers have been identified. It may be set off by a streptococcal infection or by hormonal changes brought about by birth-control pills or the menopause. Alcohol consumption and some drugs such as ibuprofen and beta-blockers also seem to act as triggers in some people. Stress may aggravate the condition although it is not thought to cause it directly.

PSORIATIC ARTHRITIS

This is a complication that affects only a small minority of people with psoriasis, perhaps 5 percent, most of whom are women between the ages of 40 and 60. Pain and swelling in the hands and feet and other joints, as well as in the spine, are experienced before or after the appearance of the skin plaques.

The activity of the arthritis is usually independent of the skin disease. The inflammation and pain can be treated with NSAIDs (non-steroidal anti-inflammatory drugs) and in more severe cases with anti-inflammatory agents such as sulphasalazine and methotrexate.

WHAT YOUR DOCTOR CAN DO

If you only get small patches of psoriasis now and then, you may treat it yourself with over-the-counter remedies from the pharmacy. If you do consult your doctor you will find that many of these treatments are also available by prescription, including moisturizers, creams, shampoos, scalp lotions and bath lotions containing tar and mild corticosteroid creams. More intensive treatments, such as skin preparations containing vitamin D analogues or a cream called dithranol, can effectively

AFFECTED AREAS
The areas of the body most susceptible to plaque psoriasis are the scalp, elbows and knees, but the condition can spread over the torso.

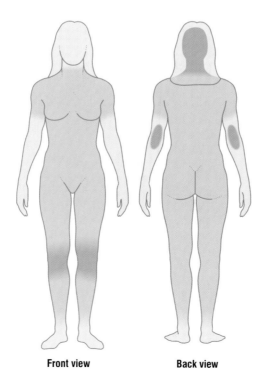

Front view   **Back view**

SKIN CHANGES
The epidermis (outer layer of skin) sheds its upper layer of cells continually, but in a psoriasis sufferer new cells reach the surface much more quickly than in normal skin. Dead and living cells begin to accumulate at the surface.

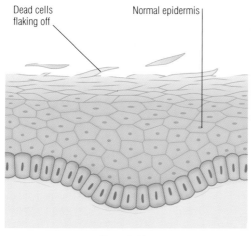

Normal skin

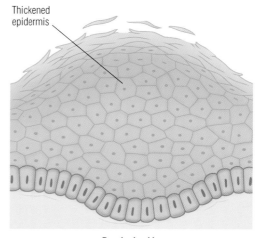

Psoriasis skin

suppress symptoms. It is often necessary to weigh the benefits against possible side effects —skin irritation and increased sensitivity—and how easy you find the treatment to use.

Severe psoriasis that does not respond to medical treatment may improve with a course of therapy involving a combination of drugs called psoralens and ultraviolet (UV) light, or UV treatment on its own. Methotrexate is used orally to control severe psoriasis, nail psoriasis and psoriatic arthritis. Some treatments can be given on an outpatient basis or you may have to stay in hospital for a few days.

Drugs that have an effect on the immune system, such as cyclosporin, can help to control the abnormal skin cell turnover, but you will need to be monitored for side effects—anything from stomach or intestinal disorders to skin rashes. This will involve blood tests and blood pressure checks as the effects of these drugs are not confined to the skin.

SELF-HELP TREATMENTS
Women with psoriasis may benefit from finding a self-help group where other sufferers share their experience and knowledge. Self-help treatments include spending time in the sun, which enables the body to manufacture vitamin D, sometimes combined with mineral baths or phototherapy under ultraviolet light.

Herbal remedies can also be used to soothe the itching associated with the condition— burdock (*Arctium*) can be made into a herbal drink; evening primrose capsules can be taken orally or rosemary and sage shampoos can be

used to clear the scalp condition. Diet may also help to control outbreaks. Oily fish, such as mackerel, herrings or sardines, or cod-liver oil may help to reduce the itching, and vitamins A and B complex can sometimes help the skin to heal. Concentrated vitamin E can be massaged into the scalp once or twice a week. However, it is probably more helpful to record your body's reactions to foods and other situations to see if you can find what triggers psoriasis in your case.

Sunlight and skin reactions

Many psoriasis sufferers find that exposing their skin to sunshine or to an ultraviolet lamp helps to clear plaques, but for some people it can also make psoriasis worse. You must be cautious and take care to protect yourself against sunburn, especially if you have had any treatment that increases your sensitivity to UV light.

Photodermatitis is caused by sensitivity to sunlight. Tiny blisters or bumps appear on the parts of the skin exposed to the sun. The skin sensitivity may occur from chemicals in a sunscreen, perfume or an antibiotic, or from exposure to resins from plants such as wild parsley or giant hogweed.

Urticaria, which is also called hives or nettle rash, causes the skin to become acutely sensitive. Cold, heat or sunlight can cause it, or a bite or a sting, or a food allergy. Stress or anxiety or even hormonal changes can make it worse.

See also:

1/BEING A WELL WOMAN
Healthy body systems p. 42

Skin markings

There are various minor skin disorders that affect the appearance of the skin but are not serious medical conditions. Some, like liver spots, are associated with ageing. If they make you feel self-conscious, there are treatments available for those conditions that cannot be disguised with cosmetics.

You and your melanocytes

Two forms of melanin colour the skin, hair and eyes: eumelanin produces shades of brown or black; pheomelanin is the pigment of red hair. No matter what your skin colour, we all have the same number of melanocytes (cells that absorb ultraviolet rays and convert them to harmless infrared ones). The more melanin you have, the further the melanocytes spread out to protect the skin when it is exposed to sunlight, which is why fair-skinned people (with less melanin) are more susceptible to sunburn than darker-skinned people. The number of melanocytes reduces with age, making the skin more susceptible to ultraviolet rays that damage the genetic make-up of skin cells, and this can cause skin cancer (pp. 232–233).

RASHES AND MARKS
Rashes and other skin disorders may be symptoms of various infectious diseases, such as measles and chicken pox, or a serious allergy, such as to strawberries or shellfish. Differences occur in where the rash is on the body (for example, mostly on the hands or on the moist areas of skin) and in the appearance and colour of the blisters or other spots. The rashes may also vary in the degree of itchiness or pain they cause.

SPIDER VEINS

Spider veins are tiny blemishes that appear on skin exposed to harsh weather, including cold and wind.

LIVER SPOTS

Liver spots are like freckles and develop mostly on the hands, becoming more obvious in middle age.

URTICARIA

Known also as nettle rash or hives, urticaria results in white or yellowish swelling with an inflamed outer area.

GERMAN MEASLES

In rubella (German measles) a rash develops on the face and trunk, but may sometimes be unnoticeable.

SHINGLES

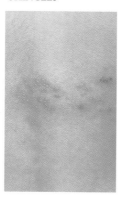

The rash caused by the herpes virus usually affects one side of the body only, causing painful blisters.

SPIDER VEINS

These tiny, hairlike blood vessels become visible on the upper or lower legs and sometimes on the face. The cause is not known, although they often run in families. Since more women have them than men, the hormones oestrogen and progesterone may play a role in their development. They tend to appear at times of hormonal change such as puberty, menopause, pregnancy and after childbirth, or when a woman is taking birth control pills.

The cheeks of fair-skinned people are a common site for spider veins, caused by exposure to weather extremes. Wearing skin protection in the sun or wind can prevent them. They are harmless and easily covered with cosmetics. If they are unsightly, you may want to talk to your doctor about having them removed by laser therapy or sclerotherapy.

LIVER SPOTS

Caused when the skin's pigment (melanin) collects in patches, liver spots (medically called lentigo) look like oversized freckles and develop mostly on the backs of the hands and the face. Since they are most noticeable in middle and later life, they are also known as age spots.

Liver spots are normally light brown in colour and flat and are completely harmless. It is thought that they result from long-term exposure to the sun, and will certainly get darker over time without sunscreen protection. They can usually be covered quite effectively with cosmetics or they can be removed by cryosurgery—a method in which the tissue is frozen with liquid nitrogen.

VITILIGO

Vitiligo is a condition in which some of the melanocytes—the pigment-producing cells in the skin—stop working, and round milky-coloured patches appear. The contrast is particularly noticeable on the face, neck, backs of the hands and arms, although patches can affect the genital area too. It is not known why the melanocytes malfunction in this way, although an autoimmune disorder may be involved.

The pale areas of skin gradually increase making you more vulnerable to sunburn, so you need to use a high protection factor sunscreen and stay out of the sun as much as possible. If you have light skin and can avoid getting a tan, this will make the contrast between the affected and normal skin less obvious. A few people find the condition improves with treatment with UV light, but this does not work for everyone.

NAIL ABNORMALITIES

Nails are made of keratin, the same protein that makes up skin and hair. It is normally tough and can resist most things. Nails can soften if immersed in water for any length of time so it is best to protect them with rubber gloves when you are washing up dishes or doing similar chores.

There are many possible reasons why nails become misshapen or discoloured. In skin conditions such as eczema or psoriasis nails tend to become loose or pitted, and occasionally more serious conditions such as heart or respiratory disorders can affect the way they grow. The colour of the flesh beneath the nail, called the nailbed, can be a sign of a circulatory problem such as anaemia. A greenish discoloration of the nail may be a sign of bacterial infection.

If there is a noticeable change in your nails you should consult your doctor. It may indicate something needs medical attention in another part of your body.

Diets or treatments Although there is no truth to the old wives' tale that calcium in the diet strengthens nails, hollows, ridges or white flecks may be indications of dietary deficiencies in iron, calcium, zinc or vitamin A.

Inflammation of a nailfold, called a whitlow, is probably caused by a bacterial infection, in which case antibiotics may be needed, or the herpes simplex virus, which may require antiviral treatment. In severe cases, minor surgery may be needed to drain the inflammation.

Nail clipping While the nails themselves are made of dead cells, they elongate as a result of the living tissue in the matrix under the half-moon. Regular trimming of fingernails and toenails will keep them healthy. Take care not to cut the cuticle as this can allow infection in. It is better to follow the shape of the flesh on the finger or toe rather than to cut straight across. This will prevent the nail from growing into the flesh and causing an ingrown toenail. This occurs because the edges grow faster than the centre, or alternatively the abnormal growth may be triggered by an accident.

Toenails, like feet in general, benefit from wearing shoes that follow the shape of the foot rather than squashing them.

Older people may need help with nail clipping, as may diabetics and those who are very overweight. They should seek the advice and help of a chiropodist.

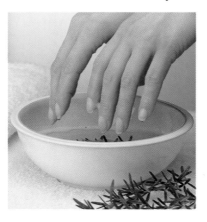

HERBAL CARE
Dry or brittle nails may benefit from a soak in water to which dried horsetail and comfrey have been added.

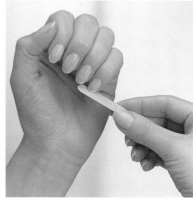

SHAPING YOUR NAILS
It is best to file your nails following the shape of the fingertip. File regularly to avoid unsightly breakages.

See also:

1/BEING A WELL WOMAN
Healthy body systems p. 42

Being safe in the sun

Although most people enjoy being out in the sunshine, the fact is that ultraviolet radiation from the sun is not good for your skin. According to dermatologists, even a light tan is a sign that skin damage has occurred.

Ultraviolet radiation occurs in various different wavelengths. Virtually none of the shortest wavelength (UVC) reaches the Earth's surface and so is no danger to the skin. Although UVA (with the longest wavelength) makes up approximately 95 percent of the solar radiation that reaches your skin, it is less harmful than UVB radiation, which is what burns the skin. Nevertheless, prolonged exposure to UVA light can cause skin damage such as photoageing and may play a role in triggering some types of skin cancer.

Sun, and how much is good for you, is controversial. The psychological benefits of sunshine and its role in encouraging vitamin D synthesis, essential for strong bones and good health, have to be balanced against the risk of skin cancer. Dermatologists generally recommend staying out of the sun. Sunburn can develop within hours of your skin being exposed to the sun. The redness and tenderness are part of the body's attempt to repair damage caused by UVB radiation to the DNA in cells

Tanning beds

Modern tanning beds deliver only UVA (not UVB) radiation and many people believe that they don't damage the skin. In fact, regular sessions can cause photoageing and may increase the risk of skin cancer in susceptible people. People with fair skin and a lot of moles are at the greatest risk of developing skin cancer and should avoid tanning altogether. Everyone should be aware that tanning beds damage the skin when deciding whether to use them. Safety guidelines should be on display or explained to you by tanning bed operators.

in the epidermis. If the repair is incomplete, it can cause cells to mutate, and if these abnormal cells continue to multiply, the long-term consequence may be a melanoma (p. 233).

CHECK THE EFFECTS

Even if you do not sunbathe, skin that is frequently exposed to the sun—on your face and arms, for example—will show signs of photoageing such as thickening, wrinkles and freckles. You can see this for yourself if you compare the way your skin looks on your face with the

COVER UP

A successful campaign in Australia raised awareness of the sun's dangers and is helping to reduce the high skin cancer rate there. The clear message said: slip on a shirt, slap on a hat and slop on the sunscreen. The wearing of sunglasses and skin-protective swimwear has been accepted enthusiastically by children whose parents grew up in the "tan is beautiful" era and are now suffering the effects.

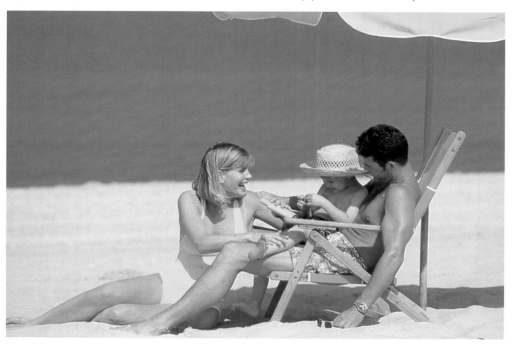

skin that is normally covered—your bottom, for example. It will have smoother, younger-looking skin (unless, of course, you sunbathe in the nude). Photosensitization is the name given to an allergic reaction that occurs when a cosmetic or perfume you are wearing causes a rash in the sun.

WHY A TAN IS BAD NEWS

When your skin is damaged by UV radiation, defensive measures are set in motion by your body to try to prevent further injury. The outer layer of skin becomes thicker and melanocytes (p. 228) release melanin which is responsible for your tan. People with dark skin have more of this pigment than pale-skinned people and are therefore better protected against the ill effects of UV light. However, a tan only gives protection roughly equivalent to a low SPF (sun protection factor) sunscreen (about SPF 2 or 3). The tan is not enough to prevent further damage and you can certainly still burn even after you have already developed a tan.

After the age of about 30 you have fewer melanocytes, so you will not tan as easily and you may find you are not able to stay in the sun as long as you once did.

SKIN PROTECTION FACTORS

Ideally you should never go out, even on a cloudy day, without wearing a sunscreen that protects against both UVA and UVB, and you should avoid sunbathing altogether. Sunscreens are graded by factors—the higher the SPF, the greater the protection. If you could normally stay in the sun for half an hour without burning, a sunscreen of factor 15 could conceivably extend that time to seven and a half hours (15 x 0.5), but sunscreens are not a substitute for avoiding excessive exposure.

Sunscreens either absorb or reflect the UV rays and the chemicals in them differ. Some waterproof types can clog the pores of the skin and can cause adverse reactions, especially for people with oily skin.

All sunscreens need to be reapplied constantly while you are in the sun, especially after swimming or exercise that makes you sweat.

You should be aware that SPFs are not standard in all parts of the world. If you are travelling to other countries, take the products that you use at home and don't rely on being able to buy them on arrival at your destination.

SUN SENSE

There are many sensible precautions you can take to minimize damage caused by the sun and reduce your risk of developing skin cancer. You should, for example, never sunbathe in the summer months when the sun is at its most intense—between 11.00 am and 3.00 pm. It is also advisable to put on a sunscreen—at least SPF 15, every day, before applying cosmetics. This will help protect your skin against UVA radiation. Sunscreen should be worn even in the shade, since some UV light will still be reaching your skin. Even on cloudy summer days, UV radiation can penetrate all but the thickest cloud cover and get through the ozone layer. This layer in the stratosphere limits the amount of UVB radiation reaching the Earth's surface, but there are areas within it that are being rendered less effective by pollution.

You must be particularly careful at high altitudes where the UV radiation is more intense, and on beaches or by water where the sunlight is reflected on to your skin even when you are in the shade. Wear a long-sleeved T-shirt or shirt and a hat with a wide enough brim to provide shade for your face and the back of your neck. This is particularly important if the hair on the top of your scalp is thinning or if you have had certain types of therapy to treat a disease (p. 233).

Drink plenty of water to keep your body hydrated in the sun. Don't let sea or poolwater dry on your skin after bathing.

Dry yourself well and then reapply sunscreen.

If you do get burned, apply calamine lotion immediately, to cool and soothe the skin . You may also need painkillers if the burning is very painful.

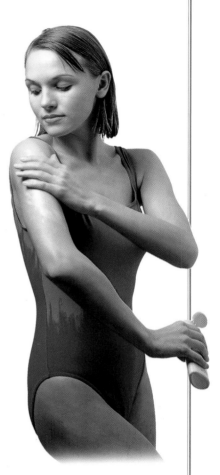

PROTECT YOURSELF
Don't rely on a sunscreen to protect you unless you apply it frequently while you are in the sun. Fair-haired, red-haired and fair-skinned people are especially vulnerable. Be aware that skin creams and cosmetics for the face may say "protects against UV rays" but if there is no SPF given you need a sunscreen too.

See also:

6/TREATMENTS & THERAPIES
Treatment plans pp. 266–269
Conventional treatments
pp. 272–283

Skin cancer

By far the most serious disorder caused by the sun is skin cancer. It is one of the most prevalent cancers in many parts of the world and its incidence is increasing. There are three types of skin cancer—basal cell, squamous cell and melanoma—named according to which cells of the epidermis are affected, and all are related to overexposure to the sun.

Although it is the least common, melanoma, which is the proliferation of the melanin-producing cells, is the only skin cancer likely to be fatal if not caught and treated in time. The other two types mostly affect older people, especially those who have spent a lot of time out of doors over the years, perhaps because of their jobs or a hobby such as golf or gardening.

All skin changes should be seen by a doctor. Treatment in all cases is likely to involve cutting away the affected area of skin under local anaesthetic, and sending a sample to the lab for analysis to confirm the diagnosis. With basal or squamous cell cancer, this may be all that is necessary, but additional treatment may be needed for melanoma.

BASAL CELL CANCER

This is the most common skin cancer and you are unlikely to get it before the age of 60. It generally appears on the face, especially in the inner corner of the eye, around the nose and on the neck. The first sign is a slow-growing pearly lump or nodule the colour of normal skin. If it is not treated, over time the affected area grows larger, the tissue breaks down and an ulcer that does not heal forms in the centre. It may eventually reach 6 mm ($^{1}/_{4}$ in) in diameter. It is relatively easily to treat, either with surgery or, if it is small, with a skin-freezing technique that uses liquid nitrogen to kill the affected cells. In the rare instances when it spreads, it can also be treated with radiotherapy.

SQUAMOUS CELL CANCER

Squamous cells are flat, scale-like cells and the first sign of this type of cancer is the appearance of scaly patches. Fair-skinned older people are most prone to this skin cancer, which is about four times less common than basal cell cancer and usually occurs in those who have been exposed to the sun over many years. It may also be caused by certain substances used in manufacturing and industry, such as tar, arsenic and petroleum derivatives.

At the start it can look like a scaly, raised, solid nodule that grows quickly—it can double in size in six months—located usually on the face, top of the ears, the scalp (on someone who is bald and rarely in women), the back of the hands, the upper chest and the back of the shoulders. The cancer has a high rate of cure

WHO IS AT RISK?
Almost anyone can develop skin cancer, but you are most at risk if you have more than 100 moles on your body (if you are a young person) or more than 50 moles if you are older; have several moles of unusual size, shape and colour; have fair, freckled skin that burns easily and rarely tans; have a family history of melanoma; and have lived in hot, sunny climates, especially during early childhood.

BASAL CELL SIGNS

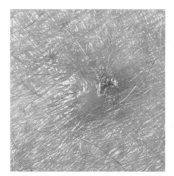

A slow-growing, small lump or nodule near the top of the nose area and the area between the eyes. Over time, if not treated, it gets larger and an ulcer may form in the centre.

SQUAMOUS CELL SIGNS

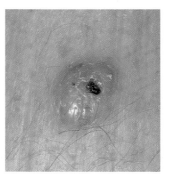

Although uncommon, this type of skin cancer appears as a scaly, raised nodule on those parts of the body that have been exposed to the sun. It can double in size in six months.

MALIGNANT MELANOMA SIGNS

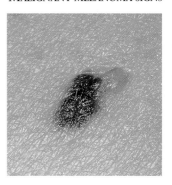

An odd-looking mole or freckle is the usual site of a melanoma—in women it may be on the calves. The edges of the mole are ragged and the colour can be various shades of tan, black or red.

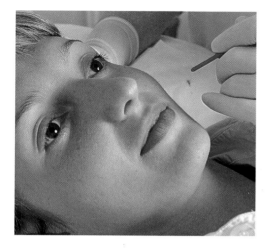

when treated at an early stage. The usual treatments are surgical removal, cryotherapy with liquid nitrogen, or laser surgery to remove the affected tissue. Radiotherapy may be used if the cancer is in an area difficult to treat surgically.

SOLAR KERATOSES

These are warty, rough, red scaly patches which occur mainly on the face, neck, hands or forearms, and sometimes the scalp, of people who have spent many years working out of doors. The patches are not in themselves cancerous but those people who develop them may have a higher risk of developing squamous cell cancer at or near the site of the keratoses, especially if they continue to be exposed to the sun. They are easily removed with cryotherapy or can be treated with chemotherapy drugs.

MALIGNANT MELANOMA

This form of skin cancer is different from the others in that it is more serious and if not treated can spread to other organs—notably the liver, lungs, bones and brain—and is then fatal.

Malignant melanoma can affect young people, although it is extremely rare before puberty. It is essential that you see a doctor immediately if you notice any changes in a mole or freckle. The chances of a cure are much higher if melanoma is treated in the early stages.

In women, the most common site of a malignant melanoma is on the calf; in men, it is on the trunk, especially the back. In older people it can also appear on the face. You should be especially careful if you are fair-skinned, have lots of moles or had several experiences of sunburn as a child or later. All these factors increase the risk, although melanoma is not necessarily

associated with sunburn. Smoking is believed to be an additional risk factor. Although melanoma can appear anywhere, it is most likely to develop around an existing mole.

EARLY SIGNS

Skin cancer doctors have devised an alphabetic guideline to help people recognize possible early signs:

A—Asymmetry or alteration in the appearance of a mole.

B—Border of the mole changes, or there is bleeding from a mole.

C—Colour change, especially if the mole darkens or develops several different pigmentations.

D—Diameter increases to more than that of a pencil end (about 6 mm/ 1/4 in).

E—Enlargement, the mole appears to be getting bigger or seems thicker.

TREATING MELANOMA

A doctor may remove a suspicious mole so that it can be examined microscopically in a lab. Treatment will depend on whether or not the cancer has spread to other tissues. If it is melanoma and it has not spread, it will be surgically removed under a local anaesthetic, although a larger area of skin may have to be removed than with other types of skin cancer. Advanced melanoma that has spread may be treated with chemotherapy as well. This type of tumour does not respond to radiation therapy.

You will be carefully monitored over the following months and years, as about one in three people has a recurrence of melanoma. You will be advised to make sure that you protect your skin very carefully with clothing or sunblock whenever you are out in the sun.

When cancer spreads

Treatment for many cancers is intended to cure the condition and succeeds in doing so more often than many people realize. Whether it consists of surgery, chemotherapy, hormone therapy, radiation therapy or a combination of these different approaches, the aim of potentially curative (as opposed to symptom-relieving) treatment is to get rid of all the cancerous cells in the body. However, it takes time to tell if this aim has been achieved.

There is as yet no way of identifying and targeting microscopic cancer cells that may have migrated from the original site. This is why anyone who has been treated for cancer must have regular check-ups. If there is any sign of the cancer recurring or the appearance of a secondary cancer in a new place, further treatment will be necessary.

Different cancers tend to spread in different ways—malignant melanoma can spread everywhere via the bloodstream and lymphatic system and squamous cell cancer can spread locally to lumph nodes. New tumours that result from an original one somewhere else in the body are known as secondaries or metastases. In those instances when curative treatment is not a realistic prospect, treatment that will alleviate symptoms and prolong life is often possible.

See also:

1/BEING A WELL WOMAN
Essentials of good health p. 16
Healthy body systems pp. 40–42
A healthy mind pp. 44–49

Hair disorders

The importance of hair to a woman may vary but it can play a big part in the way she feels about herself. Everyone has roughly the same number of hairs on their head throughout their life. The look, texture and volume of hair is influenced by a number of factors, including heredity, your age, your diet, and your general state of physical and mental health.

In its natural state, hair is either dry or oily, thick or fine, curly or straight, or any variation of these. It may be affected by how you treat it. Colouring your hair or using a very hot hairdryer may dry and weaken it, for example, and it is likely to split at the ends if you don't have it trimmed regularly.

Each hair, made up of dead keratin-containing cells (the same protein in nails), grows from a follicle just under the skin and is supplied with oil from nearby sebaceous glands and fed by tiny blood vessels (p. 222). Hair comes and goes constantly—the average growth rate is about 1.25 cm (^{1}/$_2$ in) per month and a hundred or more strands fall out each day. Normally this makes no difference to the 100,000 or so on the average head. As you grow older you are likely to find that your hair becomes dryer and coarser. After the menopause, you may have less of it.

Hair growth stimulator

Application of minoxidil (first used for high blood pressure) may stimulate hair growth in a small number of women with androgenic (male-pattern) hair loss. Applied for at least four months, it is effective for as long as it is used. Patients with high blood pressure must be monitored, and it may cause dermatitis. The hair produced is fine. It is not commonly available through the NHS and can be expensive.

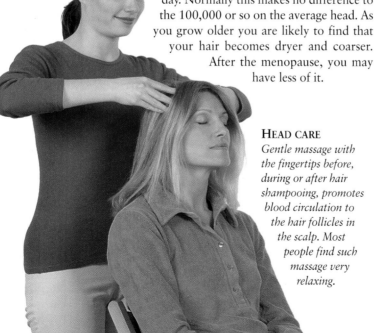

HEAD CARE
Gentle massage with the fingertips before, during or after hair shampooing, promotes blood circulation to the hair follicles in the scalp. Most people find such massage very relaxing.

PREGNANCY AND AFTER

In women most hair changes are related to hormones. The dramatic hormonal changes that are a normal part of pregnancy have a noticeable effect on your hair—and not just the hair on your head. As well as becoming drier or oilier, your crowning glory will almost certainly become thicker; this is because pregnancy temporarily interrupts the normal cycle of hair loss and replacement, and you shed much less than you normally would each day.

Once your baby is born, you compensate by losing hair at a sometimes alarming rate, a process which can continue for up to two years. This is normal and does not mean you will end up bald or have thinner hair than before.

When you are pregnant you may notice that your body hair is becoming more profuse or growing where it never did before, and if you are naturally fair it may turn darker. All these changes will reverse themselves.

CAUSES OF HAIR LOSS

Abnormal hair loss is associated with a lack of protein or certain vitamins and minerals in the diet, or with a specific health problem such as thyroid disease or anaemia. If this is the case, hair loss is unlikely to be your only symptom and you should see your doctor for a proper diagnosis.

Alopecia areata is the medical name for the most common type of patchy baldness. Several patches may occur together. The condition may be precipitated by stress, or by severe shock or trauma. It is generally temporary, although a small number of people lose all the hair from their head and body and it doesn't grow back. Alopecia areata is thought to be an autoimmune disorder. It can be treated by steroids, immune suppressors, minoxidil (see box, left) and ultraviolet light therapy. However, these do not all work in every case.

Hair loss or hair thinning can also be caused by illnesses that alter the balance of certain hormones, such as hypothyroidism. The underlying cause will need to be investigated and treated. A mild excess of male hormones can cause hair thinning on the front and top of the scalp, while a severe excess can cause loss of hair from the temples. Either type of hair loss should be evaluated by your doctor. Some drug treatments may cause hair loss, especially chemotherapy for cancer. Additional drugs may be given at the same time that can sometimes prevent this side effect.

A fungal infection such as ringworm can cause hair loss, but it can be treated with anti-fungal medication. Vitamin deficiency and severe undernourishment/malnutrition related to eating disorders, and obsessive hairpulling, most usually from the scalp but also from eyebrows or eyelashes, will need psychological help.

DANDRUFF

The cause of this irritating condition is thought to be a hypersensitivity to a yeast we all have on our skin. It is not a hygiene or dry skin problem and it can affect anyone. It comes and goes, may be accompanied by itching and may be related to a time of stress or ill health. Anti-dandruff or dry-scalp shampoos can help but in severe cases your doctor may prescribe anti-yeast shampoos and a topical steroid solution or foam.

AN EXCESS OF HAIR

The medical term "hirsutism" means having or developing an excessive amount of body hair and not always on those parts where it is customary. On a woman it can affect the chin, upper lip, chest, stomach, back and thighs.

The extra growth may be caused by over-production of male sex hormones (androgens) which are also present in a woman's body. Just as men have some oestrogen, women have some testosterone. Usually hirsutism is the result not of increased levels of this hormone but an increased sensitivity to even normal levels of it. However, some people naturally have more hair than others—Japanese and Chinese women have very little body hair while Mediterranean women tend to have more.

If the amount of body hair starts to increase or changes in texture see your doctor, especially if you are also having irregular periods. It could indicate a condition such as polycystic ovary syndrome, needing investigation.

Other rarer conditions might be responsible for similar changes. Increased body hair and no menstruation are two symptoms of Cushing's syndrome caused by a disorder of the adrenal gland or by long-term steroid use (for asthma or rheumatoid arthritis, for example). Women with eating disorders such as anorexia nervosa

---

HAIR REMOVAL TREATMENTS

Small amounts of unwanted hair, especially on the face, can be removed using a technique called electrolysis, which destroys the blood supply to a hair follicle by passing a weak electric current into it with a needle. It is a slow process and may be uncomfortable. Ask about the likely effectiveness, cost and duration of treatment before committing yourself. Laser hair removal is less painful but very expensive and may result in up to 80 percent permanent hair loss after multiple treatment sessions. Technology is improving rapidly in this area, but be sure to review the anticipated results, cost and length of treatment. In all cases choose a fully trained specialist experienced in the technique.

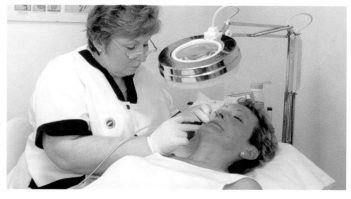

Electrolysis may be slightly painful, but done correctly it is harmless.

---

or bulimia often start to grow additional hair as they lose weight. This is the body's defensive response to compensate for the absence of an insulating layer of fat.

Sometimes, women may notice a slight increase in the amount or texture of their body hair after the menopause because of hormonal changes. Treatment with HRT can help to reverse this effect. In older age maverick hairs sprout from areas on the face, also the result of hormones. Pulling out individual hairs with tweezers may result in irritation, so you may prefer electrolysis treatment (see box above).

If you are dark-haired, excess body hair will be more obvious than if you are fair or red-headed. You might consider cosmetic bleaching or wax removal and there are various self-application kits you can buy.

AREAS AFFECTED
The face, chest, stomach, back and thighs may all have excess body hair.

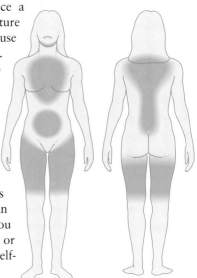

PROBLEMS OF THE SENSES

The senses are vital to your quality of life. Illnesses or infections that affect the ears, nose, throat and eyes may isolate you from the world around you if they are not treated quickly. Most people will suffer some sensory loss with age, but this can be minimized with care.

See also:

1/BEING A WELL WOMAN
Healthy body systems pp. 42–43

6/TREATMENTS & THERAPIES
Treatment plans pp. 262–269

Ear problems

Most people have no problems in their ears until they notice that their hearing becomes less sharp late in life. However, certain illnesses and infections can arise which may affect your hearing and balance.

OTOSCLEROSIS

A fairly common condition, more often occurring in women than men, otosclerosis affects the three tiny bones in the middle ear, called the auditory ossicles, which connect the eardrum to the hearing part of the inner ear, the cochlea. The innermost of the three bones, the stapes or stirrup, becomes progressively thicker, so that it cannot vibrate as much and therefore transmits less sound so you become increasingly deaf.

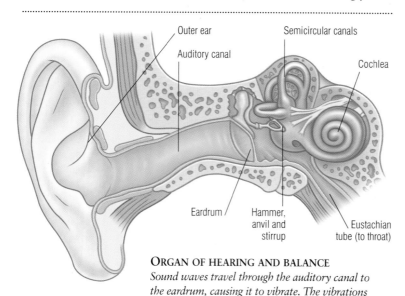

ORGAN OF HEARING AND BALANCE
Sound waves travel through the auditory canal to the eardrum, causing it to vibrate. The vibrations are amplified by the tiny ossicles in the middle ear, causing vibrations in the fluid of the inner ear.

Labels: Outer ear · Auditory canal · Semicircular canals · Cochlea · Eardrum · Hammer, anvil and stirrup · Eustachian tube (to throat)

Other symptoms include tinnitus—ringing in the ears (see opposite). The thickening occurs more quickly during pregnancy and may be oestrogen-related. In most people, both ears will eventually be affected. The only available treatment is surgery, in which the stapes bone is replaced by a synthetic graft, but there is a risk of deafness and a hearing aid may still be required. Women who have this condition are usually advised not to use hormone replacement therapy (HRT).

MASTOIDITIS

The mastoid process is a part of the temporal bone, which is just below and behind the ear. It is honeycombed with air cells that connect with the middle ear. If an infection here spreads inside the bone then it causes the inflammation called mastoiditis. The symptoms are earache, fever, ringing in the ears and hearing difficulties. Antibiotics should clear up pus or bacteria. In some rare cases a mastoidectomy operation will be necessary, draining the pus and removing the infected bone.

LABYRINTHITIS

The inner ear (labyrinth) includes three fluid-filled, semicircular canals that contain the sensors for balance. Labyrinthitis is an infection of the canals that may be either viral or bacterial. A virus causing a throat infection may travel up the eustachian tube to the middle and inner ears, causing symptoms such as a loss of balance, vertigo or dizziness, nausea, vomiting and hearing loss. The infection generally clears up by itself in a few weeks. You should have bed rest and take drugs to treat the nausea. Bacterial labyrinthitis is characterized by the same symptoms as the viral type but should be treated with antibiotics immediately as it can lead to deafness and, if it should spread to the brain, to the development of meningitis (p. 250).

TINNITUS

An extremely distressing condition that may be either temporary or permanent, tinnitus occurs when the auditory nerve is subjected to interference so that sounds ranging from a deep roar or buzz to a high-pitched whine are heard intermittently or continuously in one or both ears. The usual cause is damage to the cells in the inner ear, through an infection, a head injury, an underlying health problem such as high blood pressure or even the use of certain drugs (such as aspirin and some antibiotics).

Temporary tinnitus from an infection generally clears up quickly. Tinnitus that will not go away may interfere with all aspects of life, and coping strategies may be learned to "turn off" the unwanted sound, particularly if it affects your sleeping. Yoga and self-hypnosis techniques may ease the irritation of tinnitus, and masking devices and hearing therapists can be a great help.

DEAFNESS

There are two types of deafness. Conductive deafness is caused by a disruption of the mechanism by which sound waves are transmitted through the outer and middle ear. In sensorineural deafness there is a failure in the transmission of nerve impulses from the inner ear to the brain. This includes hearing loss with age, Ménière's disease (see right) and exposure to loud noise (see below). A build-up of ear wax in the outer ear is the most common cause of conductive deafness; the wax should be syringed out at your doctor's surgery. The other main cause is an infection of the middle ear, called the otitis media, which in adults normally clears up with antibiotics. Children, however, can develop a chronic build-up of fluid in the middle ear, causing temporary hearing loss. A doctor may decide to drain the ear.

A gradual loss of hearing occurs with age as the inner ear slowly becomes less efficient at translating sound waves into nerve impulses. The rate at which this happens can be increased by circulatory disorders that reduce the blood supply to the ear, such as high blood pressure, heart disease and atherosclerosis; by hereditary factors; and by exposure to loud noise. The condition is irreversible, but a hearing aid can be worn to amplify the sound waves entering the ear.

MÉNIÈRE'S DISEASE

Accumulated fluid in the semicircular canals, and sometimes the cochlea, damages the inner ear cells, causing Ménière's disease. It tends to become more apparent in middle age and is slightly less usual in women than men. Symptoms are deafness in one ear, vertigo or dizziness, nausea and high-pitched tinnitus. Drugs may control the symptoms and the condition may be slowed by restricting fluid intake and taking diuretics.

Motion sickness

This problem is caused by disorientation of the organ of balance in the inner ear. The following tips can help:
♀ Drive the car yourself or sit in the front passenger seat. Sit upright with both feet flat on the floor. Make sure the seat belt isn't too tight.
♀ Don't try to read maps; instead focus on a point on the horizon. A neck cushion will keep your head upright.
♀ Avoid rich food, alcohol and sweet drinks when travelling.
♀ Make frequent stops on the journey if possible.
♀ Keep a window open, or stay on deck on a boat.
♀ Breathe in deeply through your nose and out through your mouth.
♀ Try wearing acupressure wristbands.
♀ Remember that over-the-counter antinausea pills may make you drowsy.

SOUND SENSE AND STEREOS

Excessive noise permanently damages the nervous tissue and pathways in the inner ear, leading to deafness. The signs of damage are ringing in the ears that fades in a few hours, a reduced ability to hear higher frequencies and ear pain.

If you use stereo headphones at high volume, have powerful in-car or home stereo systems or spend time in noisy clubs you will be exposed to noise levels well in excess of 85 decibels. You risk injury at a decibel level over 80. A typical rock concert is about 100, a pneumatic drill at 1 m (3 ft) records 120—which can be felt as actual pain. Operators of all high-noise equipment should wear ear protection.

The nose and mouth

See also:

1/BEING A WELL WOMAN
Essentials of good health
pp. 16–19
Healthy body systems pp. 42–43

6/TREATMENTS & THERAPIES
Treatment plans pp. 262–269

Although the nose and mouth areas are usually subject only to minor problems, these can make life uncomfortable and affect your general health and well-being.

SEPTUM PROBLEMS

Occasionally, people are born with the nasal septum—the plate of bone and cartilage that separates the two nostrils—off centre. This may also arise from damage to the nose later in life. The condition may affect breathing, but it can be corrected surgically.

Long-standing cocaine use or, in rare cases, using steroid nasal sprays over a long period, can cause perforation—a hole in the septum—which surgery can correct.

NASAL CONGESTION

The accumulation of excessive mucus can make breathing difficult and affect your sense of taste and smell. Congestion can occur during pregnancy but for most other people a cold is the usual cause. Persistent congestion, called catarrh, may be allergic rhinitis, triggered by pollen, dust and pollutants. Smokers are more susceptible to

nasal congestion, since the smoke destroys the tiny hairs that line and protect the nasal passages. You can ease congestion by inhaling steam over a bowl of hot water with a towel over your head. This loosens the mucus which you can then blow out through the nose. Avoid dairy products, which increase mucus formation. Decongestant drops or sprays can give relief but should not be used for more than a week, since the mucous lining of the nose may be damaged.

Congestion can spread to your sinuses, causing pain that may be severe. Sinusitis can also be triggered by an abscess in a tooth. It can lead to laryngitis or an ear infection and may become a chronic problem. The usual treatment is decongestants and antibiotics but in some cases surgery may be performed to improve the drainage of the sinuses.

NOSEBLEEDS

Bleeding from the nose is generally caused by damage to the blood vessels in the delicate lining of the nasal passages. The damage may be caused by trauma—a blow to the nose, for example—or by repeated nose picking, sneezing or excessive nose blowing.

Sometimes a nosebleed can be a sign of hormonal changes in the body—in pregnancy and adolescence—or it may be a reaction to prescribed drugs such as warfarin, which reduces blood clotting to help prevent strokes, allergies and polyps. Atherosclerosis (a disease of the arterial wall) can sometimes cause spontaneous nosebleeds, especially in the aged. Blood vessels can become enlarged during illnesses that cause a fever, making a nosebleed more likely; nosebleeds can happen, too, with high blood pressure, though this is less common.

To deal with a nosebleed, pinch the nose just beneath the point where the bone turns into pliable cartilage. Hold for at least 10 minutes with your held tilted forward and breath through your mouth. Don't rub or blow your nose for several hours or you will dislodge the clot that has formed.

You should consult your doctor if nosebleeds are persistent so that any underlying disorder can be ruled out. The doctor may seal the damaged blood vessel by means of an electrical current (a procedure known as cauterization).

Caution

If a nosebleed starts after a blow to the head, this may indicate a fractured skull. The blood may also cause a breathing problem for you. You should go to hospital immediately, preferably accompanied by a friend or member of your family.

CLOSE COOPERATION
Lips and cheeks, teeth and gums, the tongue, palate and salivary glands all work together as the first stage of the digestive system. Local infection and structural disorders affect the senses of smell and taste, which in turn may detract from the enjoyment of eating.

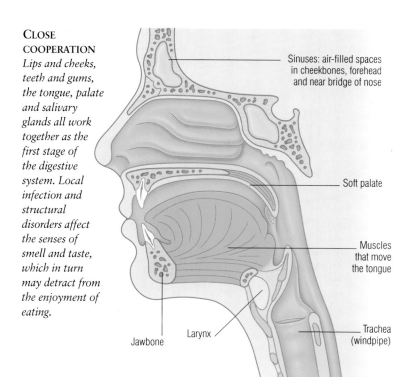

Sinuses: air-filled spaces in cheekbones, forehead and near bridge of nose

Soft palate

Muscles that move the tongue

Trachea (windpipe)

Larynx

Jawbone

SNORING

Vibration of the soft palate at the back of the mouth is not uncommon but, if someone who doesn't usually snore suddenly starts, it may signify a breathing problem. A congested nose, advancing age, excess weight, smoking, alcohol abuse, use of sleeping pills and general ill health all tend to lead to snoring.

Apnea—temporary cessation of breathing while snoring—can be more serious, especially in someone with an existing heart condition. Apnea itself may cause cardiac arrhythmia and elevated blood pressure, resulting in a feeling of tiredness and reduced attention span during the day. A study of women who snore regularly concluded that they are 33 percent more likely than nonsnorers to develop heart disease and 46 percent more likely to develop hypertension.

Light snoring can often be prevented by sleeping on the side rather than on the back, or by sleeping without a pillow, to straighten out the airway. Heavy snorers tend to snore in whatever position they sleep.

NASAL POLYPS

Polyps are soft, jellylike, benign tumours that are attached to a mucous membrane by a thin stalk. In the nose, polyps are normally caused by chronic inflammation from an allergy, such as hay fever, although by no means all hay fever sufferers develop polyps. Polyps may be associated with chronic sinusitis and asthma—symptoms include a blocked, full feeling in the nose, a reduced sense of smell, headaches, pain and nasal discharge. Treatment is by steroids, taken by nasal spray.

DRY MOUTH

Probable causes are thirst, breathing through the mouth and fear or anxiety. Anaesthetics and some prescription drugs—antidepressants for example—may reduce saliva. This in turn can lead to dental problems. Persistent thirst (plus other symptoms) may indicate diabetes.

MOUTH ULCERS

Small, white, painful lesions with a red margin form in the mouth because of stress, bacteria, infections or occasionally a deficiency of folic acid and vitamin B_{12}. Ulcers often affect women premenstrually and can be treated by a number of over-the-counter preparations.

Temporomandibular joint syndrome (TMJ)

The jaw and skull meet at a joint in front of the ear where a disc of cartilage, plus muscles and ligaments, allow movement of the jaw. In some women the disc slips out of place, producing pain at the joint, a clicking sound as the jaw moves, headaches and earache. This condition (TMJ) has a range of causes—accidents producing whiplash, stress that leads to unconscious grinding of the teeth, especially at night, a bad bite (where the bottom teeth don't meet the top teeth correctly), or rheumatoid arthritis—so treatment varies.

Immediate relief can be provided with a warm, damp compress to the area. Drugs such as NSAIDS should alleviate pain. If emotional stress is part of the problem, counselling or relaxation may be appropriate.

CARING FOR YOUR TEETH AND GUMS

The aim of tooth care is to remove plaque—the primary cause of tooth decay and gum inflammation. Plaque comes from the foods you eat. If you have false teeth pay scrupulous attention to cleansing, since plaque build-up can affect your sense of taste and smell.

Brushing your teeth at least twice a day, or preferably after every meal, helps prevent plaque build-up. It is more effective to use short, up-and-down movements. Don't forget your tongue. Soft-bristled brushes are kind on tooth enamel but need to be changed every three to four months.

Using a fluoride toothpaste and mouthwash will keep plaque at bay and freshen your breath. Using dental floss will also be beneficial. Floss between your teeth and down to the gum, then form a "C" around the side of the tooth and floss gently up to its top. Repeat on the other side and front and back. Do not over-floss as this can abrade the teeth or cut the gum, allowing bacteria to enter.

It is advisable to visit your dentist regularly for check-ups.

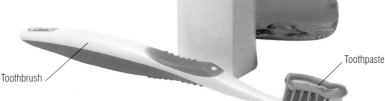

Mouthwash

Dental floss

Toothbrush

Toothpaste

Vision problems

Many people are born with eyesight that is less than perfect and most people's eyesight will degenerate with age. Both long- and short-sightedness are errors of refraction—the process by which the surface of the cornea in the eye and the lens bend light rays so that they focus at a point on the retina. If the degree of refraction does not match the length of the eye, the image will not be sharp.

LONG- AND SHORT-SIGHTEDNESS

In long-sightedness, or hypermetropia, the light rays are naturally focused behind the retina because the length of the eye is too short. When you are young, if the hypermetropia is not too extreme, the ciliary muscles round the lens can easily change the shape of the lens to adjust this—a process known as accommodation—but as the eye becomes less elastic this ability to accommodate deteriorates. Distance vision may remain good but close vision becomes increasingly difficult. If it is not corrected hypermetropia can cause headaches and general blurred vision when the eyes are strained, which is why all those who use computers at work are recommended to have regular eye tests.

In short-sightedness (called myopia) the light rays are focused in front of the retina because the length of the eye is too long. As a result close-up vision is good, but distance vision is deficient. Myopia tends to run in families, becomes evident during adolescence and stabilizes by adulthood.

Both myopia and hypermetropia are corrected by glasses or contact lenses that have opposite qualities from those of the lenses in the eyes that are causing the problem: people with myopia have glasses with concave lenses, and those with hypermetropia have glasses with convex lenses. Myopia can also be improved with laser treatment, which reshapes the cornea, although it cannot restore elasticity to the eye.

CATARACTS

The lens of the eye is made of protein fibres and is normally translucent. With age, or in some other circumstances, the protein fibres undergo changes in structure that make the lens more or less opaque. Around half of people over the age of 60 have some degree of cataract but the

See your doctor

♀ If your eyesight is frequently blurred.
♀ If you get constant headaches.
♀ If you see haloes of colour round lights at night.
♀ If your eyelids begin to droop suddenly.
♀ If there are blind spots in your field of vision.

Little black floaters

Dark specks, lines or cobwebs sometimes appear to be moving about in the front of the eyes. They are seen more often when you look at a light, plain background, such as the sky.

Floaters are not usually serious and often appear after you have rubbed your eyes. However, the sudden appearance of floaters should always be investigated by an optometrist, especially if you also see flashes of light. This is because the floaters may be a symptom of detachment of the retina—the retina becomes separated from the tissue surrounding it after a tear and vitreous fluid leaks out. The floaters are specks of blood that have escaped into the vitreous fluid.

The problem is not uncommon in the elderly, since the vitreous fluid tends to degenerate with age. It is also a risk for people who are very short-sighted or have had an eye injury.

effect on their vision may be minor, since the process of opacification may be confined to the edge of the lens. The changes can also be caused by too much ultraviolet radiation, for example from sunlight, cigarette smoking, eye injuries, long-term use of steroids and diabetes. Heredity may also be a contributory factor. More rarely, children may be born with cataracts.

Cataracts develop very slowly and the effects on the eyesight differ in different people—there may be blurring of the vision, short-sightedness, and some distortion in colour perception.

Cataracts are diagnosed by an eye test, in which eye drops are used to enlarge the pupils and the lenses examined with an ophthalmoscope. They are then treated by surgery. This surgery is very safe—complications, such as infection or retinal damage, occur in only about one in 2,000 cases. A local anaesthetic is given and a small incision is made in the eye. The lens and focal length are measured with ultrasound, then either the whole lens is replaced by a plastic one or the implant is fitted inside the lens after the old protein fibres have been removed. Antiinflammatories and steroids are given as eye drops, and recovery is usually complete within six weeks.

GLAUCOMA

The damage caused by glaucoma is the result of increasing pressure within the eye. This is created by a build-up of aqueous humour, which is unable to flow away as normal because there is a blockage in the drainage channel. The excessive amount of fluid compresses blood vessels that supply the optic nerve, causing the nerve fibres to degenerate. If the use of medicines fails to lower pressure then surgery may be necessary to unblock the drainage channel or to create an artificial channel for the aqueous humour.

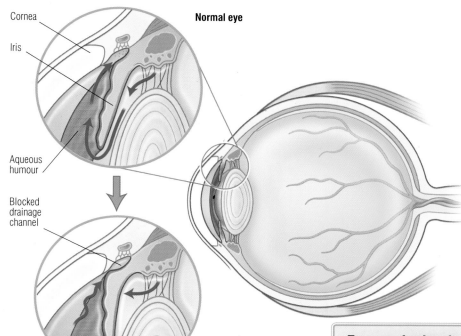

Cornea

Iris

Aqueous humour

Blocked drainage channel

Normal eye

Eye with glaucoma

GLAUCOMA

The main part of the eye behind the lens is filled with a fluid called the vitreous humour. The space between the iris and the cornea is filled with the aqueous humour. This fluid is constantly renewed and drains away through spongy tissue (the trabecular meshwork) between the iris and the cornea. When this drainage system becomes blocked, the pressure of the fluid (the intraocular pressure) builds up and the blood vessels that supply the optic nerve become compressed. The nerve can then degenerate and vision is gradually impaired.

There are various reasons why the drainage system can break down—trauma to the eye, long-term steroid use, diabetes and, rarely, a defect present at birth. However, in most cases the condition falls into one of two main groups: primary open angle glaucoma (POAG) or primary angle closure glaucoma (PACG). POAG is the most common form of glaucoma. It is a slow, progressive condition occurring mainly in the over 50s and rarely seen in the under 40s. It is often not detected until "blind spots" start to appear in vision, usually in peripheral vision.

In PACG, an increase in intraocular pressure slowly closes the angle between the cornea and

the iris, forcing the iris against the drainage system. When the system is finally blocked, the intraocular pressure rises suddenly, over a few hours, causing an acute attack of glaucoma.

SYMPTOMS

Symptoms may be minor (blurred vision and haloes seen around lights) or severe (intense pain, nausea and vomiting). An acute attack of glaucoma is a medical emergency, since there is a risk of permanent damage to the eyesight. PACG tends to run in families and affects long-sighted people and those of Asian descent more than others; it rarely affects people under the age of 50.

Because glaucoma of both types can progress undetected until a late stage, optometrists routinely check intraocular pressure during eye tests, and it is recommended that all those over age 50 have regular eye tests for this purpose. If glaucoma is suspected, the diagnosis is confirmed by an ophthalmologist. ▸

Eyes and migraine

Many but not all migraine sufferers experience visual symptoms. Usually these are part of the "aura"—visual and sensory disturbances experienced by about a fifth of migraine sufferers that precede the onset of the characteristic headache. There are flashes of light, bright zig-zag lines in either central or peripheral vision, blind spots, and blurred vision. These symptoms normally last for up to an hour until the headache starts.

In some people, however, the symptoms die down and the headache does not follow. This condition is known as ophthalmic migraine, and is caused by a spasm in the blood vessels supplying the eye.

You should consult your doctor if you suffer from visual disturbances—whether or not a migraine headache follows them—to rule out the possibility that another condition may be responsible, and to obtain medication to control the problem.

Colour blindness

Defects in colour vision are usually inherited, though on rare occasions trauma or conditions such as optic neuritis or macular disease may be responsible (acquired defective colour vision). For this reason, medical advice should be sought if colour vision starts to deteriorate.

Colour blindness affects about 12 percent of men but only around one in every 200 women. This is because the gene responsible is linked to the X chromosome. However, a woman carrying the gene will pass the faulty gene on to her descendants. (In the case of women who suffer from colour blindness, both X chromosomes carry the fault.)

There are various types of colour blindness, of which the most common is an inability to distinguish red and green. The nature of the vision defect depends on which category of colour receptors, or cones, in the retina is affected: one group of cones detects red, another green, and a third detects blue.

Colour blindness is rarely a problem, since most sufferers learn to adapt to their situation. Exceptions include driving and some occupations, such as navigation.

LOSS OF VISION
In macular degeneration the central part of the retina at the back of the eye becomes overlaid with scar tissue. This creates a circular area of blindness in the centre of the visual field. It does not lead to complete blindness since vision is still retained around the edges of the visual field.

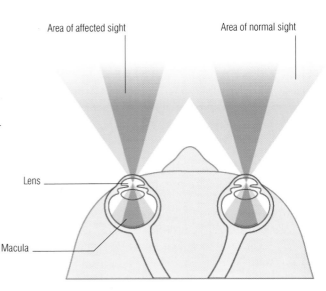

Area of affected sight   Area of normal sight

Lens

Macula

TREATMENT

The treatment of glaucoma depends on the stage that the condition has reached. In its early stages, eyedrops are used to control intraocular pressure: these may be beta-blockers, epinephrine or prostaglandins. Laser surgery is now often used to reduce intraocular pressure by increasing the size of the drainage system, but the effect of this is sometimes only temporary. An artificial drainage duct can be inserted in an operation called a trabeculectomy, but it is usually necessary to continue to use eye drops.

MACULAR DEGENERATION

The macula is the central part of the retina at the back of the eye. Its light receptors distinguish detail at the centre of the visual field—for example, when reading or driving. It is common for the tissues of the macula to degenerate with age and allow fluid leakage, in age-related macular degeneration (ARMD). However, in some people ARMD progresses more quickly, leading to a loss of central vision. You will notice a central blind spot, so that reading becomes more difficult and you have difficulty recognizing people's faces.

The risk of ARMD is highest in those over 60, though some younger people who are very short-sighted may be affected. Other risk factors include gender—women are affected more

often than men—a family history of ARMD, smoking, and race—white people are affected more often than those of African descent.

ARMD can be detected by an optometrist—so it is important that all those at risk have regular eye tests. The diagnosis will be confirmed by an ophthalmologist. In some cases it may be possible for ARMD to be treated by laser surgery, in which the fluid leakage is sealed off. Other cases may not be treatable but since peripheral vision is unaffected the eyesight is not lost completely.

DIABETIC RETINOPATHY

The high levels of glucose in the blood of people with diabetes can cause a complication called diabetic retinopathy. In the early stages, or background retinopathy, the glucose causes small blood vessels in the retina to become blocked or leak. The result may be some loss of vision but often there are no symptoms for a long time. However, as the condition worsens, new blood vessels start to grow in the retina—this stage is known as proliferative retinopathy. The new vessels are fragile and tend to leak fluid, and scars may also form on the retina, causing it to detach. Without treatment, these problems can cause blindness. (In people with type 2 diabetes only the macula may be affected, causing a loss of central vision that affects reading.)

Once detected, diabetic retinopathy can be controlled by keeping glucose levels to within narrow limits. If the condition has progressed to proliferative retinopathy, it may be treated by laser surgery to seal the retinal blood vessels and prevent new ones from growing. However, it is vital that all diabetics monitor glucose levels carefully and have their eyes tested regularly by an ophthalmologist to prevent the condition from developing.

DRY EYES

A condition called dry eye syndrome is now recognized, in which the quantity and quality of the tear fluid that naturally bathes the eye declines. As a result the eye becomes irritated and feels gritty, it becomes difficult to cry and to wear contact lenses, and over time the sufferer may become very sensitive to light. Eventually the cornea may become scarred, affecting vision. The symptoms are made worse by smoking, dust and exposure to substances to which an individual is allergic.

Dry eye syndrome is extremely common, and it is estimated that about two-thirds of people over the age of 65 are affected to some degree. The condition is most common in women who are either pregnant or who have passed the menopause. In most cases the cause is a reduction in the efficiency of the glands that produce tears—a result of ageing. Other causes include a reaction to drugs, such as antihistamines, that reduce secretions, and also infections of the glands of the eyelids.

However, in a large number of cases, 90 percent of them women, the cause is an autoimmune disorder called Sjögren's syndrome, when the antibodies attack the body's own glands. Some people with the condition only have symptoms of dry eyes and mouth, while others also have symptoms of connective tissue disorders, such as rheumatoid arthritis and SLE. Although most Sjögren's sufferers are postmenopausal some are younger, and their children have an increased risk of suffering from heart defects. For this reason, symptoms of dry eye syndrome should be reported to a doctor without delay.

The treatment of dry eyes depends on its cause. Antibiotics are given in the case of infection, and artificial tears are used to relieve the irritation. In some cases small plugs can be inserted into the tear ducts in order to retain tears in the eyes. Sjögren's syndrome is treated by NSAIDs (nonsteroidal anti-inflammatory drugs) and steroids.

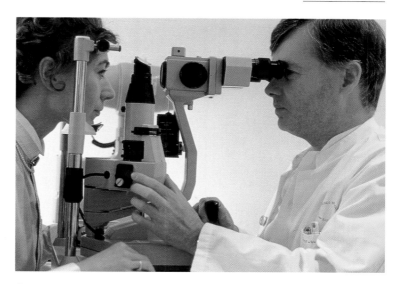

ALLERGIC CONJUNCTIVITIS

The symptoms of conjunctivitis are a reddening and swelling of the membranes of the eyes and eyelids, which often comes on suddenly, together with itching, a burning sensation and a discharge, which may be watery or sticky. However, similar symptoms, in particular the itchiness and discharge, can also be caused by bacterial and viral infections (p. 247), so you should consult your doctor to rule these out before starting to use any over-the-counter anti-allergy preparations.

The allergens responsible for the condition are generally the same as those that cause hay fever—pollen, mould spores, and animal or insect proteins, as from animal hair and the droppings of the house-dust mite—but may also include cosmetics, shampoos, perfumes, contact lenses and contact lens solutions. Eye drops containing antihistamine will be prescribed or, in severe cases, corticosteroids.

DROOPING EYELIDS

It is not uncommon for the eyelids to start to droop—called ptosis—in old age, as a result of the weakening of the muscles that hold them in place. However, ptosis may also be sign of a number of serious conditions. It may be the result of a muscle weakness caused by a condition affecting the muscles, such as the autoimmune disorder myasthenia gravis, or by a condition that affects the nerves. A brain tumour or cerebral aneurysm (damage to an artery in the brain) may cause drooping eyelids and you should consult your doctor if the condition develops suddenly.

EYE TESTS
You should make sure you have regular eye tests, particularly if there is a history of eye problems in your family. Some conditions, such as glaucoma, may show no symptoms in early stages, so can be detected only by an eye examination.

243

ACUTE INFECTIONS

Women are particularly susceptible to infections that strike suddenly. You should see your doctor as soon as possible since these infections need prompt treatment to prevent them spreading. Without medical attention the infections may quickly worsen and can become chronic.

Pelvic problems

Because your reproductive and urinary systems are so close to each other, infections can affect both. Such infections are most common in your 20s and 30s but may also occur at and after the menopause.

CYSTITIS

Women are more susceptible than men to cystitis—inflammation of the bladder—which can lead to kidney damage if not treated promptly. Cystitis is usually caused by E. coli bacteria that live in the bowel without causing harm until they are transferred to the bladder or urethra.

Triggers of cystitis include poor hygiene, pregnancy, sexual intercourse, putting off urination and some forms of contraception. Some women experience recurrent attacks around the time of their period. The usual symptoms are an urgent need to urinate, with only a little amount of urine to pass, a burning sensation during urination, and cloudy or sometimes bloody urine. If the inflammation has spread up the ureters to the kidneys, there may be fever, backache, nausea and vomiting.

At the first sign of cystitis, take a painkiller and flush out the bacteria by drinking 275 ml ($^1/_2$ pint) of water immediately and then every 20 minutes for two hours. Over-the-counter cystitis remedies, taken at certain times over 48 hours, can be used to reduce the urine's acidity. If the symptoms persist or if you have signs of a kidney infection, see your doctor. If a check of a urine sample shows bacteria, a short course of antibiotics may be prescribed.

SELF-HELP MEASURES

There are a number of measures you can take to prevent cystisis. Drink plenty of plain water and cut down on tea, coffee and alcohol (which stimulate urine production but may irritate the bladder). You could also try drinking cranberry juice which stops E. coli bacteria sticking to the bladder wall.

Empty your bladder regularly, particularly before and after sex, and always wipe from front to back after a bowel movement. Do not use perfumed soaps and avoid bubble baths, vaginal deodorant or douches. Wear cotton underwear, stockings rather than tights, and avoid tight jeans or trousers.

URETHRAL SYNDROME

This is the name for chronic inflammation of the urethra. It is much more common in women than in men and has cystitis-like symptoms. The cause of the inflammation is often unknown, since usually there are no bacteria present in urine, and kidney function and urinary tract

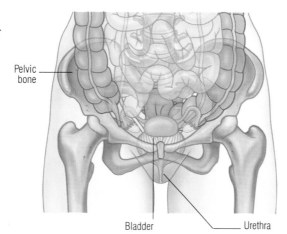

PELVIC AREA
The bladder is lower down the pelvis in a woman than in a man, and the urethra—through which urine is passed—is only one-fifth as long. As a result, women have more urinary tract infections.

Pelvic bone

Bladder   Urethra

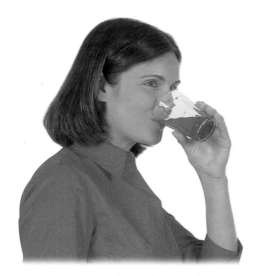

CRANBERRY JUICE
As well as having a number of substances that stop the growth of bacteria, cranberry juice can raise the acidity of the urine, helping to kill bacteria in the kidneys and urinary tract.

Kidney failure

Swelling of tissues, listlessness, nausea, rapid breathing, diarrhoea and difficulty in urinating are all symptoms of kidney failure. It can be caused by diabetes, scleroderma, lupus, high blood pressure, by traumatic injury or congestive heart failure. It is a rare complication of pregnancy. Whatever the cause, it needs prompt attention to prevent damage to the organ.

anatomy are normal. Urethral syndrome may occur in women at or around the time of the menopause, and may be due to lack of oestrogen. The vulval tissues become thinner and there is less vaginal moisture. The vulva and urethra (which lies close by) become vulnerable to trauma and irritation. The vulva may also be sore, making intercourse painful.

There is no specific treatment, although urethral syndrome may be eased with the same self-help measures as cystitis. You should also use a vaginal lubricant during sex and avoid any foods causing irritation, such as chocolate, spicy or acidic foods, mature cheese, tomatoes, alcohol, caffeine, nicotine and carbonated drinks. A doctor may prescribe oestrogen or steroid creams to soothe the inflammation.

CHANGES IN THE URINE

In a healthy body urine is normally pale in colour and has little odour. It can be discoloured by foods such as rhubarb, beetroot or blackberries, but returns to normal within 24 hours. However, you should see your doctor if you experience dark-coloured or red urine (which may be a side effect of a drug or viral infection) or dark yellow urine (which indicates overconcentration, and a lack of fluids).

You should also consult your doctor if you have cloudy, smelly urine (which is usually caused by a urinary tract infection) or blood in the urine (which may be caused by a kidney infection). Low levels of urine may indicate kidney problems, a kidney stone or severe dehydration, whilst high levels of urine could be a symptom of diabetes mellitus. In either case you should see a doctor.

KIDNEY STONES

Medically termed renal calculi, kidney stones are crystals formed by chemicals in the urine. They can vary in size from a grain of salt to a marble. Some people seem to be more prone to making stones than others, although it is not known why. Stones are much more common in men. The formation of kidney stones is associated with hot climates, drinking too little fluid, and frequent urinary tract infections.

Small stones may be passed out of the body in the urine and in fact most stones pass naturally if large quantities of water are drunk. Larger stones can cause serious problems. A severe, sudden pain starts in the small of the back and spreads down and round the front of the abdomen to the groin. The pain may come and go for minutes or hours (most stones pass in the urine within a few hours). There may also be nausea, blood in the urine, and frequent, painful urination. If stones become lodged in the bladder, there may also be incontinence.

Diagnosis is by ultrasound or X-ray. If the stones are large, or if there is an infection present, surgical treatment may be necessary to prevent damage to the kidney. A non-invasive technique called extracorporeal shock wave lithotripsy (ESWL) may be used to shatter the stones into small fragments that can be passed in the urine.

KIDNEY STONES
To prevent stones from recurring, as they do in 50 percent of cases, you should drink at least eight large glasses of water a day, avoid large doses of vitamin D and dairy products and cut down on protein foods.

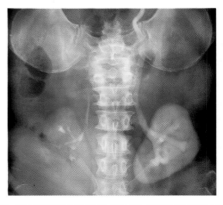

Yeast infection

This condition—also known as candidiasis, thrush or monilia—is caused by a yeastlike fungus called Candida, which is normally present in the vagina and in the mouth in small quantities. Usually it is kept in check by the naturally occurring bacteria, but this delicate balance is easily upset, and the fungus then grows out of control. Candida most commonly infects the vagina but may also affect the mouth or the skin. It is a very common and irritating infection with severe itching as the primary symptom.

Broadspectrum antibiotics are a common cause, since they may destroy the friendly bacteria, allowing the yeast to grow. Steroids or immunosuppressive drugs may also allow the yeast to proliferate. Candida feeds on sugar, so untreated diabetes (which causes high blood-sugar levels) and hormonal changes during a menstrual period, pregnancy or menopause (which affect the sugar levels in vaginal tissues) increase the risk of infection.

SYMPTOMS AND TREATMENT

In the mouth Candida infection produces sore, yellowish patches; on the skin it may infect damp folds and form an itchy rash. Vaginal yeast infection causes a thick, white discharge resembling cottage cheese, and with an unpleasantly sweet and "bready" smell. The vagina and vulva are sore and itchy and urination is painful.

Applying natural live yogurt to the vaginal area may relieve the symptoms, perhaps by increasing the acidity of the vaginal area. Over-the-counter remedies, such as pills, antifungal creams or pessaries, kill off the yeast. Even so the infection can take up to a week to clear up. You should not use local anaesthetic creams formulated for itching as these can cause sensitivity and make the condition worse.

If an over-the-counter treatment does not work, see your doctor. A yeast infection should be properly diagnosed as it can be similar to other vaginal infections. The doctor will do an internal examination and take swabs of the discharge for laboratory analysis. Once the diagnosis is confirmed, the doctor can prescribe an antifungal treatment. Candidiasis is not strictly a sexually transmitted disease but it can be passed on from sexual partners. Men rarely experience symptoms but if you have recurrent attacks your partner may need to be treated too.

SELF-HELP MEASURES
To prevent the recurrence of Candida infection, take cool baths or showers in hot weather. Avoid using perfumed soaps, bubble baths, vaginal deodorants or bath oils. Wear cotton underwear and loose clothes (especially on warm days) that allow air to circulate. You may find it helpful to reduce your intake of foods that contain sugar and yeast (bread, for example).

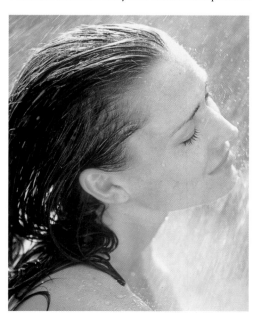

Sexually transmitted diseases

Sexually transmitted diseases (STDs) can be difficult to detect in women, since many have nonspecific symptoms, such as vaginal discharge, pelvic pain, genital itching and pain on intercourse. However, they can cause long-term damage. For example, chlamydia can lead to infertility, while hepatitis and genital warts (fleshy lumps around the genitals) can increase the risk of cervical cancer.

There are over 25 different types of STDs. Women most at risk are young adults, people from ethnic minorities and the socially and economically disadvantaged. If you suspect that you may have an infection, you should act promptly and visit a genitourinary (GU) or STD clinic, where you will be able to consult an expert. You will have a physical examination, and blood and urine tests. Many STDs can be treated with antibiotics or antiviral drugs if they are caught early enough. You should notify your sexual partner(s) so that they can be tested—and possibly treated—too. (The clinic may offer to do this for you.) You should avoid sexual contact until the infection has cleared up.

Eye problems

See also:

1/BEING A WELL WOMAN
Healthy body systems p. 42

5/ILLNESSES & EMERGENCIES
Problems of the senses
pp. 240–243

6/TREATMENTS & THERAPIES
Treatment plans pp. 262–269

There are various eye infections that can cause anything from mild discomfort to a more serious threat to your eyesight. Eye infections are easily passed on to others through touch—at schools or colleges, for example.

CONJUNCTIVITIS

The conjunctiva is the transparent membrane covering the white of the eye and inside of the eyelids. Inflammation of the conjunctiva is called conjunctivitis or pink eye. It can be caused by a bacterial or viral infection or an allergy (to cosmetics or pollen, for example). The eyes are red, sore and itchy, with a gritty tight feeling. With an allergy or viral infection there is a watery discharge; with a bacterial infection there may be a sticky yellowish discharge that dries at night, making the eyelids difficult to open. This crust can be removed with water (which has been boiled and then cooled) applied with a cotton wool ball.

Viral conjunctivitis may last several weeks but usually gets better on its own. Sometimes, as with the herpes virus, it is serious and can cause permanent damage. Antibiotic eye drops or ointment can clear up a bacterial infection, while antihistamine or anti-inflammatory eye drops relieve symptoms caused by an allergy.

STYES

If an eyelash hair follicle becomes infected, a painful, inflamed abscess, or stye, appears at the base. It develops a white head of pus that bursts within a few days, relieving the pain. The eyelash then falls out. A warm compress three times daily can help the pus discharge and the infection can be treated with an antibiotic ointment. Never squeeze a stye: this can spread the infection to other hair follicles. Styes usually subside within a week, but tend to recur in diabetics or, sometimes, in teenagers or women under stress.

BLEPHARITIS

Blepharitis, also known as seborrhoeic dermatitis, or inflammation of the eyelid, is often associated with dandruff. The eyes may be sore, itchy, and have flaky eyelids. The flakes of skin can cause conjunctivitis. If the eyelids become infected they develop small blisters which cause the lashes to fall out. The eyelids should be cleaned carefully with a cotton bud dipped in cooled, boiled water. Medicated shampoos will treat any dandruff. Your doctor may prescribe an antibiotic eye ointment. If the eyelid becomes ulcerated, the infection may spread to the cornea, which must be treated immediately.

CORNEAL ULCER

The cornea (outer part of the eyeball) may be infected and develop ulcers. Some of these infections are quite easy to clear up but if the infection is by the herpes virus and leads to an ulcer, the virus may enter the eyeball. You should contact your doctor immediately.

ACUTE IRITIS OR UVEITIS

In rare cases, the iris (the coloured part of the eye) may be infected, often due to other conditions, such as tuberculosis or syphilis. This condition can also be associated with autoimmune joint diseases. Symptoms include one pupil becoming smaller than the other, red eyes, blurred vision and pain. Early treatment is vital, as it may cause long-term visual problems, such as corneal ulcers, glaucoma and cataracts.

A doctor can prescribe steroid and dilating drops to reduce the inflammation. Persistent cases need steroid injections into the soft tissues around the eyes.

KEEPING EYES HEALTHY

You can keep your eyes healthy by following a few simple precautions. In smoky or otherwise polluted atmospheres your eyes may become irritated and red. Do not rub them as this can spread infection. Bathe them afterward with cooled boiled water.

Cleanliness is vital: never share towels or face flannels; and do not wear eye make-up if you have an infection. Use eye drops to flush out minute particles. Plenty of sleep can also help.

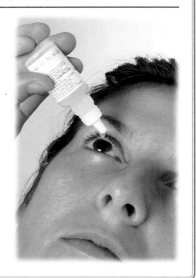

UPPER RESPIRATORY TRACT INFECTIONS

Infections that commonly affect the upper respiratory tract are known collectively as URTIs. Your ears, nose and throat are generally involved. Most URTIs make you feel miserable, but fortunately they are shortlived and harmless. However, they can easily become a more serious condition if you are run down or your immunity is impaired for any reason. Some are contagious, so you should take care not to spread any infection.

Cause	Symptoms	Treatment	Duration
Common cold			
Over 200 different viruses.	Feeling under the weather with a sore throat, a congested or runny nose, a cough and headache.	Ease symptoms with pharmacy remedies: painkillers for fever, lozenges for sore throat, decongestant for stuffy nose, and cough syrup. Take 2 g ($^1/_2$ tsp) of vitamin C daily.	Most colds last a week at the most.
Cold sores			
Caused by the herpes simplex virus, which lies dormant between attacks. They can be triggered by a cold, sun or stress; some women experience outbreaks around their period. Highly contagious.	Sores that appear around your mouth or nose. The first sign is a tautness and a tingling feeling on the skin, which develops into a small painful blister. The blister turns into a weeping sore, which dries to form a scab.	Antiviral treatments at the tingling stage can prevent the sore from developing. One self-help measure is to dab on natural live yogurt or witch hazel at the first tingle. Avoid eating nuts, chocolate and seeds.	Five to 10 days. Don't touch a cold sore, as you can spread the virus to your eyes or genitals.
Sinusitis			
Excessive build-up of mucus following a cold, which settles in the air-filled spaces in your cheekbones, forehead and near the bridge of your nose. Persistent sinusitis may be allergic rhinitis, which can be triggered by pollen, dust, and pollutants.	Pain in the face, nose and forehead, and in severe cases laryngitis or an ear infection.	Should be treated with decongestants and antibiotics, otherwise it can become a chronic problem and may require surgery to improve the drainage of the sinuses. You can ease congestion by inhaling steam over a bowl of hot water with a towel over your head. Avoid dairy products, since these increase the formation of mucus.	Up to 10 days. Don't use decongestants— either pills or sprays—for longer than one week, since they may make the congestion worse.

> **! Caution**
> If you have a congested nose, don't blow too hard or too often. This can make the congestion worse, force infected mucus back into your sinuses, or weaken the small blood vessels in your nose, causing nosebleeds. Applying too much pressure when blowing can rupture an eardrum.

Cause	Symptoms	Treatment	Duration
Ear infections			
After a cold or allergic reaction, catarrh or inflamed mucus may block the eustachian tube, which connects the middle ear to the nasal cavity.	Loss of balance, dull throbbing pain and nausea indicate an infection of the middle ear (otitis media). If untreated, the eardrum can rupture and cause hearing loss.	Decongestants and paracetamol can help to ease discomfort, but severe pain needs medical advice. A middle ear infection can be treated with antibiotic or steroid ear drops.	A week.
Pharyngitis			
Throat infection triggered by a virus or streptococcus bacteria (known as a "strep throat"). If it is a recurring problem it may be caused by smoking or an allergy, such as hay fever.	Back of the throat hurts when swallowing, voice becomes hoarse, and glands under the jaw become enlarged. Headache.	Drink plenty of fluids, gargle with dissolved aspirin, suck throat lozenges, use local anaesthetic products (from pharmacies) for pain. Antibiotics may be needed for the bacterial infection.	A week to 10 days.
Laryngitis			
Usually follows a cold but can be caused by straining the voice box (from too much talking or shouting) or smoking. The swollen larynx restricts the airflow through your vocal cords, causing a temporary loss of voice.	Hoarse voice and an irritating cough.	Should be treated like a mild attack of flu: stay in bed, take paracetamol and eat lightly. Rest your larynx completely by not talking for a couple of days.	If hoarseness or loss of voice last for more than a week, consult your doctor, since laryngitis can be a sign of cancer in rare cases.
Infectious mononucleosis			
Very common viral infection of the white blood cells (lymphocytes or mononuclear cells), also known as glandular fever. It is passed on through close contact, mainly kissing, and is especially common in teenagers and young adults.	Fever, a sore throat, enlarged tonsils and swollen lymph glands in the neck, armpits and groin may develop over four to six weeks. General malaise and lethargy, and a measles-like rash may appear on the body, arms and legs.	No specific treatment. If a "mono" sufferer takes the antibiotics ampicillin or amoxicillin, a red, blotchy rash may appear. The infection can enlarge the spleen and spread to the liver, causing jaundice or hepatitis.	It can take six months to recover. Relapses are common and it is vital to have plenty of rest, since chronic fatigue syndrome (p. 206) can occur.
Tonsillitis			
Highly contagious infection. Tissue at the back of the throat is covered in tiny white pus-filled spots.	Severe sore throat, swollen neck glands, a cough, fever and fatigue. Can be caused by bacteria or a virus.	Stay in bed, drink plenty of fluids, gargle with aspirin, eat soft foods. A bacterial infection needs antibiotics.	10 days. If a quinsy (tonsil abscess) forms take antibiotics.

See also:

6/TREATMENTS & THERAPIES
Treatment plans pp. 262–265
Conventional treatments
pp. 272–277

Meningitis

Meningitis is an inflammation of the meninges, the delicate membranes surrounding the brain and spinal cord. The most usual cause is a virus, which is rarely severe. However, a bacterial infection can be dangerous and needs urgent diagnosis and treatment.

TYPES OF MENINGITIS

Viral (aseptic) meningitis The most common form of meningitis is rarely life-threatening. It is caused by many viruses, such as mumps, polio, varicella-zoster (related to chickenpox and shingles) and herpes simplex (which causes cold sores). The viruses are spread by coughing or sneezing or can be picked up in areas of poor hygiene from contaminated food or water. The symptoms vary from a mild flu-like illness with a bad headache to a more severe condition that resembles the bacterial form.

Bacterial meningitis This is a serious infection spread through close contact, such as kissing, sneezing and coughing. The most common symptom is a severe headache, usually associated with an intolerance of bright lights. The

sufferer may also feel feverish, have a stiff neck, feel nauseous and vomit. Local outbreaks can occur among groups gathering in restricted space. One type of infection, meningococcal meningitis, tends to affect children and young adults, while another, pneumococcal meningitis, is found more often in people over 45 years of age. Hemophilus influenzae meningitis is less common today, since babies are now routinely immunized with the Hib vaccine.

One in 10 people have the meningococcal bacteria in their throat and nasal passages without realizing it. The infection, which mostly occurs in winter, develops if the bacteria overcome the body's immune defences. There are three types of meningococcus bacteria—A, B, and C—with B being the most common and most dangerous. Although the bacteria are highly contagious, they can survive for just a few minutes outside the body and therefore can only be spread by very close contact. Because the symptoms of meningococcal meningitis develop very rapidly, you need to be aware of the danger signs (see opposite).

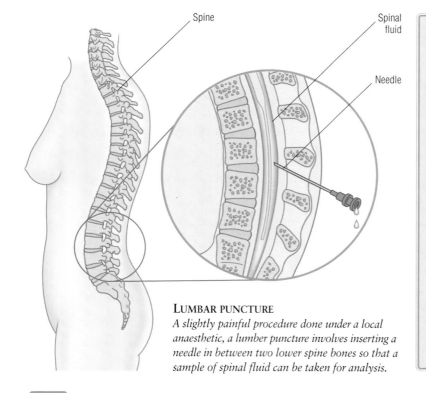

Spine

Spinal fluid

Needle

LUMBAR PUNCTURE

A slightly painful procedure done under a local anaesthetic, a lumber puncture involves inserting a needle in between two lower spine bones so that a sample of spinal fluid can be taken for analysis.

When do antibiotics work?

When you get an infection you need to know the cause so that treatment will be effective. Viral infections are common, are usually mild and clear up on their own over several days—you rarely need a doctor's help unless your immune system is challenged by chronic illness or age. Antibiotics do not work against viruses. However, they are highly effective in treating bacterial infections, which have more severe symptoms. Antibiotics can cause side effects such as diarrhoea and skin rashes.

Because of the widespread use of antibiotics, bacterial resistance is occurring. It is probably also the result of people not finishing a prescribed course of treatment. In these cases the antibiotic kills off the weakest bacteria, but the toughest ones are left to breed, mutate and become stronger, creating a resistant "superbug". This means that some diseases may no longer respond to common antibiotics.

DANGER SIGNS

Meningococcal meningitis develops quickly from minor flu-like symptoms to the severe disease. There are a number of symptoms but all of them are quite easy to detect. A severe headache, neck pain and dislike of bright light can indicate the disease. Vomiting and dizziness, accompanied by a very high temperature can also be a sign, as can a purple rash that looks like pin pricks (which can indicate septicaemia—blood poisoning). Drowsiness, convulsions and, occasionally, a loss of consciousness are also warning signs. In such cases, call your doctor immediately.

TESTING FOR MENINGOCOCCAL SEPTICAEMIA
Press the side of a glass tumbler firmly against the rash on the skin. If the rash does not fade or lose colour under the pressure of the glass, seek medical help straight away.

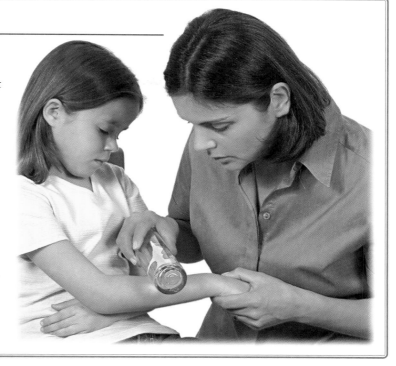

HOW IT IS DIAGNOSED

All cases of meningitis are regarded as potentially dangerous. The symptoms are so similar that it may not be immediately obvious whether the cause is viral or bacterial. For this reason meningitis patients may be given antibiotics before the infection is properly diagnosed, to give the doctors time to complete various tests. The usual method of diagnosis is a lumbar puncture (see left). Normal spinal fluid is clear, so meningitis is suspected if the fluid is cloudy and contains pus cells. Samples of blood, urine, and nose or ear secretions may also be tested.

TREATMENT AND AFTER EFFECTS

With viral meningitis there is no need for antibiotics, although they may help prevent secondary infection (see left). The usual treatment is bed rest in a darkened room, plenty of fluids to drink, and painkillers for headaches. Viral meningitis usually has no lasting effects. Infrequently it causes recurring headaches, short-term memory loss, tiredness and depression, which may need a doctor's help.

With bacterial meningitis, the patient will need antibiotics (intravenously initially, then by mouth), anticonvulsants to reduce the risk of epileptic seizures, and antinausea drugs for sickness. If bacterial meningitis is diagnosed early enough, the patient may make a complete recovery. However, it can be fatal or lead to permanent damage, particularly in the very young or old. Babies are most susceptible and the bacteria may cause deafness, mental deficiency, cerebral palsy or epilepsy, and can cause the cerebrospinal fluid to accumulate in the brain (called hydrocephalus).

PREVENTIVE MEASURES

Meningococcal meningitis is a medical emergency requiring rapid hospitalization and treatment—immediate injection of penicillin and drugs to reduce the swelling of the brain and the risk of an epileptic seizure. Because of the problem of contagion, the patient may be treated in isolation and will stay there until the infection is eradicated. Preventive antibiotics may be given to people who had intimate or direct contact with the patient within seven days of the infection.

At present, there is no vaccine for type B. All children under the age of 18 have now been vaccinated for meningitis C. From now on babies are being vaccinated and university students—at risk because large groups of young people are in close proximity—will be offered the vaccination in case they have slipped through the net.

EMERGENCY FIRST AID

Knowing what to do and being able to help promptly when a child or adult is injured can save lives. Remember that staying calm will allow you to act sensibly and give you confidence to assist in a wide range of first-aid situations described in these pages.

In an emergency

♀ Make sure the help you give does not endanger your own life.

♀ Sum up the situation quickly and act fast.

♀ Call 999 if immediate medical assistance is needed.

♀ If you suspect a head, neck or back injury do not move the person.

♀ Check the ABC first (see right) so the brain is not starved of oxygen.

♀ Place an unconscious person in the recovery position (see opposite) unless you suspect a spine or neck injury.

♀ Put pressure on an injury to stop any severe bleeding, but do not use a tourniquet.

♀ Treat the person for shock.

If someone is unconscious

This is a procedure to follow in any situation with an injured person:

SPEAK, asking "Can you hear me? Are you all right?"

SHAKE his or her shoulders gently without jerking the neck.

LISTEN for breathing by placing your ear close to the mouth.

LOOK along the chest to see if it is moving up and down.

CHECK that there are no signs of fracture, neck or spinal injury. If none,

PLACE person in the recovery position.

CHECK THE ABC
(AIRWAY, BREATHING, CIRCULATION)

If there is both breathing and a pulse, put the person in the recovery position (see opposite). Cover with a coat or blanket and talk reassuringly until help arrives. If there is a pulse but no breathing begin mouth-to-mouth ventilation (p. 254). If there is no pulse and no breathing, begin CPR immediately (p. 254).

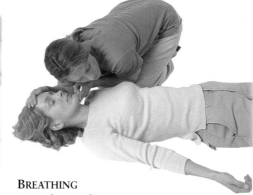

AIRWAY
The passage between the mouth, nose and throat must be clear. If the person is lying face up, press down on the forehead with one hand while lifting the back of the neck with the other. Move this hand to tilt chin up. Turn head to one side and use your first two fingers to sweep around inside mouth to remove any obstruction. Do not attempt this if a neck fracture is suspected.

BREATHING
Listen for sounds around the mouth and nose, watch for movements of the chest and place your face close enough to feel the breath on your skin.

CIRCULATION
Place the tips of your first two fingers in the depression at the side of the adam's apple and feel for a pulse.

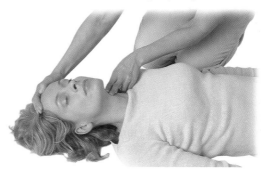

THE RECOVERY POSITION

The aim is to turn the injured person so he or she can breathe without the danger of the airway being blocked by vomit or by the tongue falling back and cutting off the air. Stay with the person until help arrives, monitoring breathing and pulse every 10 minutes.

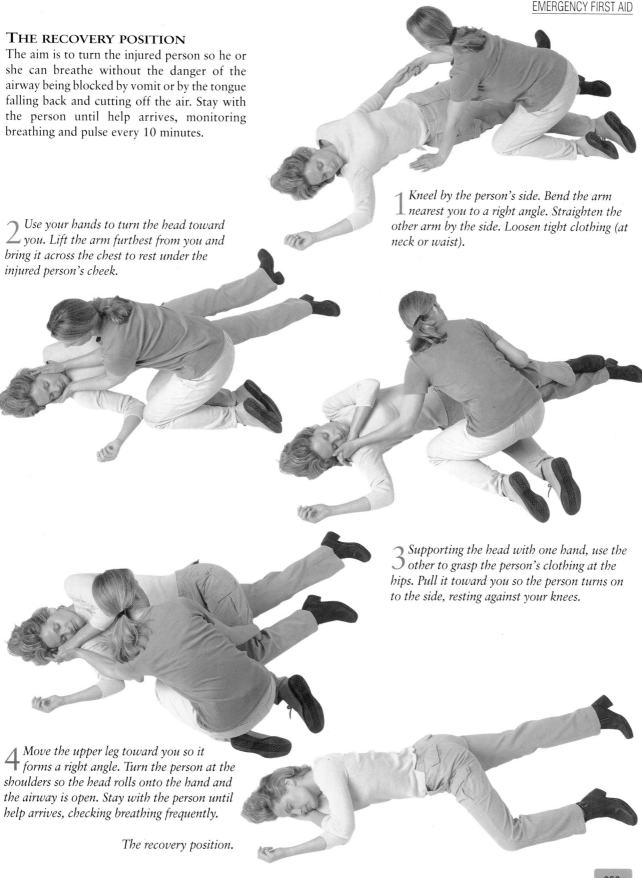

1 Kneel by the person's side. Bend the arm nearest you to a right angle. Straighten the other arm by the side. Loosen tight clothing (at neck or waist).

2 Use your hands to turn the head toward you. Lift the arm furthest from you and bring it across the chest to rest under the injured person's cheek.

3 Supporting the head with one hand, use the other to grasp the person's clothing at the hips. Pull it toward you so the person turns on to the side, resting against your knees.

4 Move the upper leg toward you so it forms a right angle. Turn the person at the shoulders so the head rolls onto the hand and the airway is open. Stay with the person until help arrives, checking breathing frequently.

The recovery position.

MOUTH-TO-MOUTH VENTILATION (when there is a pulse but no breathing)

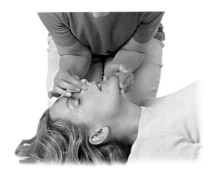
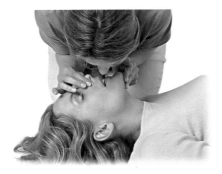
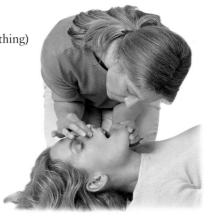

1 *Tilt the head back using two fingers under the chin. Pinch the nose between index finger and thumb. Take a deep breath and place your lips around the person's mouth, making a seal.*

2 *Blow firmly and slowly for two seconds into the mouth until you see the person's chest rise. Remove your lips and release the nose. Count to four, take a deep breath and repeat.*

3 *If the chest does not rise and fall check the airway for an obstruction. Sweep the mouth with a finger to remove anything there. Repeat ventilation procedure.*

CPR

Cardiopulmonary resuscitation is used to help someone whose breathing or heart has stopped. It combines mouth-to-mouth ventilation, in which you blow your breath into the person's lungs, with compression to help the heart con-tract and keep the blood circulation going. Compression is hard work and it is usually recommended that it be done only by a person who has been trained. Mouth-to-mouth ventilation may help the person until medical aid arrives.

CPR is required for these symptoms: skin tone pale or bluish, no sign of breathing in chest or from mouth, no heartbeat or pulse.

1 *Place your middle finger where breastbone meets ribs and your index finger above it. Slide heel of your other hand down to fingers.*

2 *Lift first hand over second, interlock fingers. Count: on 1 lean forward and press on breastbone; on 2 depress it up to 5 cm (2 in), on 3 release pressure. Repeat 15 times. Give mouth-to-mouth ventilation twice, repeat compression.*

> ! **Be alert**
> Always check if a person is wearing a pendant or bracelet marked SOS Talisman or Medic-Alert which will give instructions about what to do in an emergency. People vulnerable to shock or coma (for example, through diabetes, epilepsy, heart problems and dangerous allergies, such as reactions to nuts or bee or wasp stings) wear them; some also carry a syringe filled with adrenaline for immediate use for allergic reactions. It should be injected into the muscle of the upper arm.

Anaphylactic shock

Sudden collapse with swelling of the tongue, throat and mouth. Call 999. Check if person is wearing pendant or bracelet or carrying adrenaline injection. Follow given instructions. Loosen clothing at neck, waist and wrists, take pulse and breathing rate. Cover with coat or blanket and be prepared to give mouth-to-mouth ventilation.

Treatment for shock

When giving any form of first aid keep an eye on the injured person's face.
Signs of shock are: skin becomes pale, grey-looking, is cold and moist with sweat. If pulse is weak and rapid and breathing is fast and shallow, don't give the person anything to eat or drink.
Raise the feet and put a coat or cover across the trunk for warmth. Call for medical aid.

HEART ATTACK

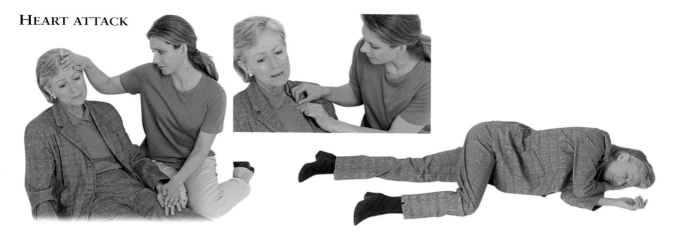

1 *If the person is conscious make her comfortable in a half-sitting position with good support to the head and shoulders. If there's no wall to lean against, the back of another person, sitting with knees bent, will substitute.*

2 *Loosen clothing around neck and waist. Call 999. Give reassurance and make a note of breathing and pulse rates. Ask if they carry any medication for heart problems; if so give this. If the person is fully awake give an aspirin tablet to chew.*

3 *If the person becomes unconscious, put him or her in the recovery position.*
If breathing stops, turn her on to her back and begin CPR (see opposite).

STROKE

Call 999. If the person is conscious lay him or her down, with head and shoulders raised and supported by rolled clothing. Turn head to one side, loosen clothing. If the person is unconscious, place in the recovery position.

FAINT

Brief loss of consciousness. Place the person flat and lift the legs to help blood flow back to the heart and head.

If the person is sitting bring the head forward between the knees.

Call 999 if person doesn't recover quickly.

> **! Be alert**
>
> If someone is unconscious:
>   SPEAK, asking "Can you hear me? Are you all right?"
>   SHAKE his or her shoulders gently without jerking the neck.
>   LISTEN for breathing by placing your ear close to the mouth.
>   LOOK along the chest to see if it is moving up and down.
>   CHECK that there are no signs of fracture, neck or spinal injury. If none,
>   PLACE person in the recovery position.

WHEN A CHOKING ADULT COLLAPSES

1 *Turn the person on to the side and give five sharp blows with the flat of your hand between the shoulder blades. Turn the person on to the side and sweep inside mouth with fingers. If obstruction is not removed, slap the back again.*

2 *If that doesn't work, turn the person face upward with head tilted back. Sit astride the person, placing the heel of one hand below the ribcage and the other hand on top. With straight arms press sharply inward and upward five times.*

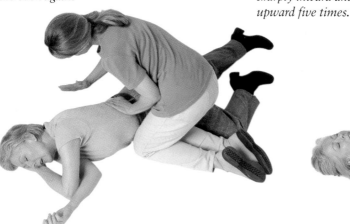

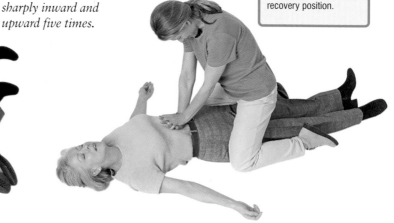

WHEN A PERSON IS CHOKING

If something is stuck in the airway breathing
will be difficult. Act quickly.

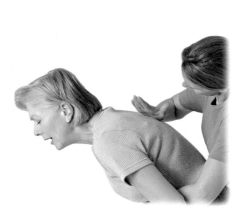
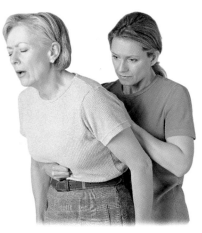
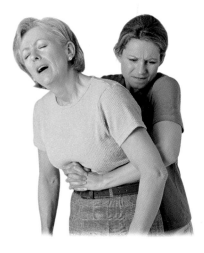

1 First get the person to breathe in
deeply then to cough forcefully.
If that doesn't work, get the person
to bend over from the waist and slap
the back sharply between the
shoulder blades.

2 If this doesn't work, do the
Heimlich manoeuvre. Stand behind
the person, make a fist with one hand
and place it thumb inward in the
middle of the abdomen.

3 Grab the fist with your other hand
and pull both sharply against the
person's body, inward and upward.
Repeat four times if necessary, but it
should force the obstruction out of the
throat like a cork out of a fizzy bottle.

IF A CHILD IS CHOKING

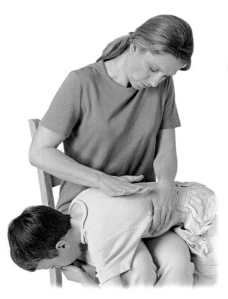
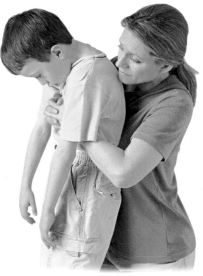
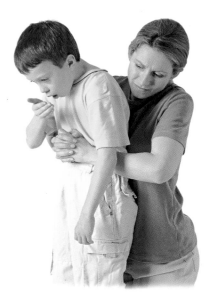

1 Sit on a chair and pull the child
across your upper legs, head and
face down. Give four quick but not too
forceful slaps between the shoulders
with the heel of your hand.

2 If the object is not dislodged, kneel
behind the child, make a fist and
grasp it with your other hand. Make
five sharp inward thrusts against the
lower breastbone.

3 If this doesn't work, move your
arms down and make five thrusts
between the ribcage and the navel.

IF A BABY IS CHOKING

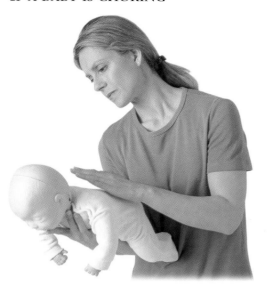
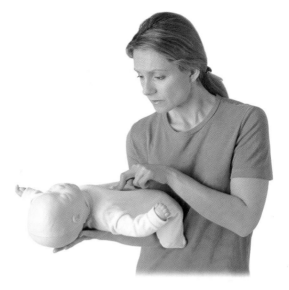

1 *Place the baby, tummy down, along your arm so the head is below the chest and your hand supports the head and shoulders. With your other hand give five firm, but not hard, slaps between the shoulder blades.*

2 *Turn the baby over and check the airway. If the object was not dislodged and you can't hook it out with your finger, repeat the first step.*

IF A CHILD BECOMES UNCONSCIOUS CALL 999

Put into recovery position and watch ABC carefully until help arrives.

EPILEPTIC FIT OR SEIZURE

Do not move the person or put anything in the mouth or between the teeth. If possible loosen tight clothing (around neck or waist), but do not restrict his or her movements. Protect the person from harm (for example, against the edges of nearby furniture or railings), staying until he or she recovers fully, usually after several minutes. Place him or her in the recovery position.

FEBRILE CONVULSION

Sponge or bathe the baby with lukewarm water to try to lower the temperature. Call the doctor.

DROWNING/RESUSCITATION

1 *Once out of the water lay the person flat and check Airway, Breathing and Circulation. Get someone to call 999. Turn the person's head to the side, sweep around inside the mouth with two fingers to clear it—it may also cause him or her to vomit water. Begin mouth-to-mouth ventilation.*

2 *If the chest does not rise and fall, check the airway again for an obstruction. If the person is choking push him or her on to the side and slap the back five times with the heel of your hand. Repeat ventilation procedure. When breathing is restored put the person in the recovery position.*

Treatment for hypothermia

When someone has been immersed in water or been exposed to extreme cold raising the body temperature is essential. Remove wet clothes and replace with dry ones. Put person in recovery position and wrap well from head to toe with anything available. Shield from the wind. Stay with person until help arrives, carefully watching breathing.

ELECTRIC SHOCK

The first objective is to break the connection between the person and the electricity without endangering yourself. Make sure your hands are dry. Switch off the current at the mains or electric point. If that's not possible, take a wooden broom handle or wooden stool, stand on paper of any sort and push the electric gadget well away from the person. Check ABC and begin mouth-to-mouth ventilation if necessary. If unconscious but breathing, place in the recovery position. Call 999.

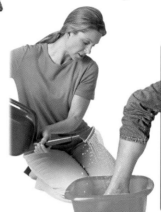

BURNS

If the burn is extensive cool the area as quickly as you can with clean water from a fine sprinkler of a hose or watering can.

> **! Caution**
> There is a high risk of infection when skin is damaged. Do not touch the injured area, do not try and burst any blisters and do not use lotions or ointments of any kind. Water is the best treatment for most injuries as it cools and cleans the area.

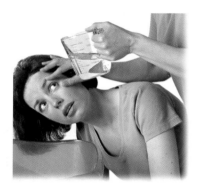

CHEMICAL BURNS OF THE EYE

If possible, place the person's face sideways to a sink under a tap so cold water runs gently into the eye for at least 10 minutes. Otherwise place the person down on his or her side, lift and turn the head and gently pour cold water into the eye for 10 minutes, making sure water doesn't run down the face or into the other eye. Seek immediate medical help.

Tips for successful first aid

♀ After cleaning a wound exposure to the air will allow the blood to clot naturally. Holding a bleeding cut under running water will prevent this happening and the blood will continue to flow.

♀ If a cut or wound is large, press the edges together with your (clean) fingers until a clot forms, then cover the cut with a dressing to allow healing to take place.

♀ If a wound is deep or has ragged edges, stitches may be needed to bring the skin together.

♀ Keep a magnifying glass in your first-aid box so you can see inside the wound clearly.

♀ Never put undiluted antiseptic on a wound.

♀ Don't use fluffy materials such as cotton wool as a dressing on small grazes and cuts. Fibres get caught in the scab that forms and bleeding will start again if you try to remove them.

BURNS TO MOUTH

Call 999. Loosen clothing round the neck. Give small sips of cold water or an ice cube to suck. Do not try to make the person be sick; if a corrosive has been swallowed, vomiting will make matters worse. Watch for signs of shock or restricted breathing and take action until help arrives. Do not give mouth-to-mouth ventilation as this may endanger you.

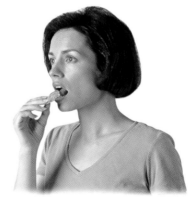

POISON

Common poisons include medicinal tablets, household and other corrosive liquids, solvents, fumes, berries, fungi and alcohol. Call 999. Check the ABC.

If the person is breathing but unconscious, place in recovery position.

If there is indication of burning in and around the mouth and the person is conscious, help him or her to drink a glass of water or milk, then put in the recovery position. Monitor pulse and breathing until help arrives.

FRACTURE

If you suspect a bone is fractured do not move the person until you have immobilized the injured area. Seek medical help.

BITES

If a bite is of animal or insect origin and skin is broken, it should be taken seriously. Wash well, allowing blood to flow, then cover with a sterile pad or sticking plaster. Contact the doctor as tetanus injection or antibiotics may be needed.

Insect bites may be swollen and red, an allergic reaction to what the insect has left in the skin. Wash area well then cover with sticking plaster.

Snakebites are indicated by pain, swelling and puncture wounds. Lay the person down keeping injured leg or arm flat. Clean area, wiping away from the wound, then bandage firmly. Seek immediate medical help.

Skull, neck and back injuries

Injuries to the skull, neck and back are serious and need expert help. Call 999. If you are alone, do not attempt to move the person. If someone can help, hold the head steady while he or she puts rolled-up clothing either side to immobilize the neck and shoulders. If the person is turned on the side and resuscitation is needed, you will need help to ease him or her on to the back. At all times you should keep the head supported and aligned with the neck and back. Check ABC every 10 minutes.

? Did you know?

A first-aid kit should be kept in a safe place in your home, accessible to you but well out of the reach of children. It need not be large, but it should contain all you need if someone is injured. If you are in doubt about what to do, call 999.

Keep in it: aspirin, paracetamol, magnifying glass, thermometer, a range of different types of bandage (roller, tubular), safety pins, sticking plasters or dressings, disposable gloves, antiseptic wipes for wound and skin cleansing, and tweezers.

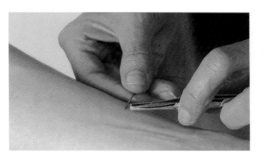

REMOVING SPLINTERS

Clean the area around the splinter with an antiseptic wipe. Press tweezers on to skin and catch protruding splinter. Gently ease it back out, in the direction it went in. If you can't see splinter end, sterilize a sewing needle in a flame. Try to get it under splinter so you can grab it with the tweezers. Clean area with antiseptic wipe.

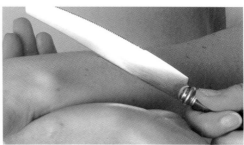

STINGS

Remove the insect's venom sac by scraping it from the skin, in one direction only, with the blunt edge of a knife or your fingernail. Don't use tweezers as these push the venom into the skin. Clean area with an antiseptic wipe and place an ice cube or pack of frozen peas on the site. Also see anaphylactic shock, p. 254.

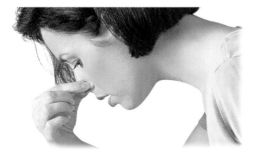

NOSEBLEED

Use your thumb and index finger to pinch the soft part of the nose (the nostrils), lean forward and breathe through the mouth. Hold position for 10 minutes so that a clot forms. Don't touch or blow the nose for several hours to prevent further bleeding.

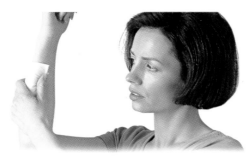

CUT THAT WON'T STOP BLEEDING

Place under cold running water for a few seconds, then raise the arm above chest height, cover the injury with a clean lint-free dressing or sticking plaster and apply direct pressure with your other hand or fingers until the bleeding has stopped.

! Caution

Stopping the blood flow in an artery at pressure points in the upper arm or groin by pressing artery against the bone needs strength and is only done as a final resort when indirect pressure on the wound itself fails. Do not use a tourniquet, and do not compress artery for more than 15 minutes. Both can stop blood flow entirely.

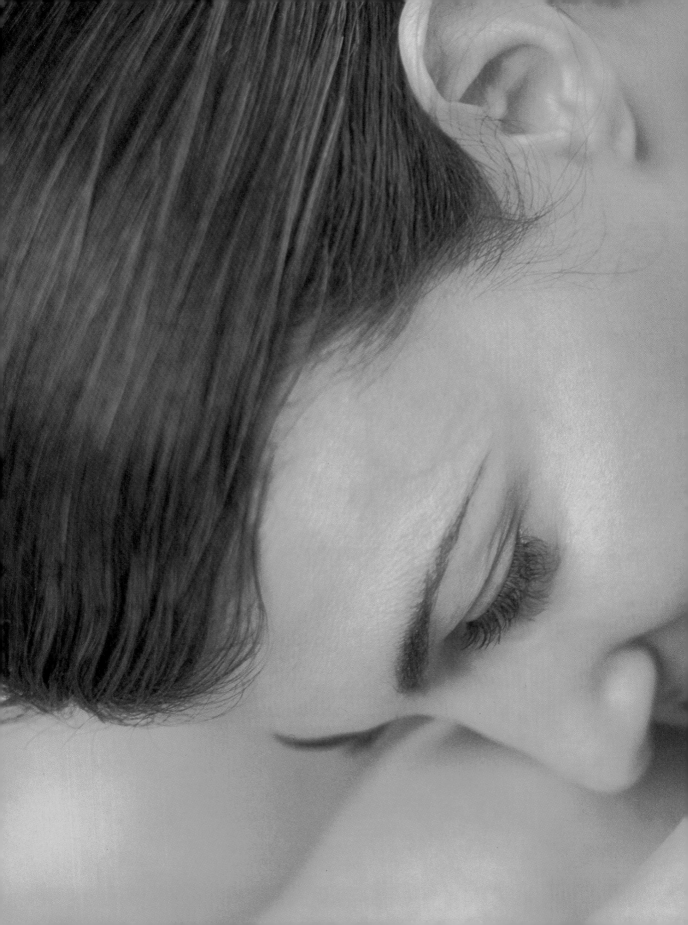

TREATMENTS AND THERAPIES

Treatments for illness may involve you seeing many different professionals and it helps to understand what each does and what the drugs they may prescribe are for. Orthodox medical treatment is often backed up by talking therapies such as psychotherapy or physical therapies like osteopathy. Complementary therapies and alternative treatments such as acupuncture can work alongside conventional treatment or be used for preventive health care—and pure pleasure. Yoga, Pilates and t'ai chi, for example, are excellent for relaxation, posture and muscle-toning, inducing a sense of calm and well-being that makes you look as good as you feel.

TREATMENT PLANS

When you seek help from the world of medicine because you are ill or simply undergoing a life stage like pregnancy you benefit from having as much information relating to your condition as possible. Then you can make decisions about your care and know what to expect.

Finding out the facts

See also

1/BEING A WELL WOMAN
Healthy body systems pp. 30–43
A healthy mind pp. 44–49

Once you've made your appointment with the doctor about a problem needing investigation, you enter an environment in which professional skills will be used to find the best way to treat your condition and answer your questions. Whether you are pregnant or uncertain about one or a collection of symptoms you have, you have every reason to expect that you will receive optimum care. In a busy surgery or hospital, however, there may not be the time to find out all you need to know immediately and you should prepare ahead.

UNDERSTANDING YOUR RECORDS

In normal circumstances the relationship you have with your doctor is confidential and what is said between you should not be disclosed to a third party unless it is as part of ongoing treatment. You have the right to access the records that your doctor keeps on you, and to check their accuracy. In many instances the data on the records may be written in medical language that is hard to understand. Ask for an explanation if need be. You can have a third person present to fill in any details you may have missed, especially if what the doctor has to say is complicated and involves a range of investigations and specialists.

You will want to know possible risks of the proposed treatment as well as the benefits. It is important that you understand the suggested plans and the scale of time of the treatment. Unless the situation is described as an emergency, you should not feel hurried into making decisions. You should find out whether a second opinion is an option and whether you have a choice of treatment.

YOUR MEDICAL TEAM

Your doctor will explain the diagnosis and discuss with you the treatment and who will be responsible for you. In many conditions the expertise of a wide range of professionals will be called on to play a part in your return to good health. Find out who should be your point of contact during treatment if you need advice or more information.

Get a clear explanation of anything you sign. Consent forms should indicate exactly the medical or surgical treatment you agree to and consider acceptable if you are under anaesthetic. Make sure your family, partner or caregiver has your written instructions should you be unable to make decisions.

SUPPORT SERVICES

If you have difficulty coming to terms with the diagnosis and treatment, or have other concerns, find out the services that may be available to help you. You may need psychological and social back-up to deal with your own anxieties and fear, family matters or to support your partner during this time.

MAKING A PREGNANCY PLAN

Family-centred obstetrics brings together the mother-to-be, her partner and family, health-care provider (the hospital) and support staff (midwives) so screening and diagnostic tests are explained and understood. Care should encompass your health concerns, such as gestational diabetes and blood pressure, your wishes, such as the type of birth you want and who may be present, through to problems such as domestic violence or giving a baby up for adoption.

INVESTIGATIVE TESTS

Doctors may carry out or arrange a wide variety of tests which either diagnose or confirm diagnosis. Some treat women's conditions at the same time. Certain tests may be performed as part of regular check-ups. Making sure you know exactly what the test involves prepares you and makes it less stressful.

Type	Purpose	Where done /anaesthetic
Amniocentesis	Antenatal screening.	hospital/mild tranquillizer
Arthroscopy	Joint problems.	hospital/general or local
Balloon angioplasty	Unblocking artery.	hospital/general
Barium enema	To check colon and intestines for abnormalities.	hospital/none
Biopsy	To obtain tissue sample for laboratory examination: breast (needle); cervical (curette); endometrial; skin (scalpel); vulval.	hospital/ local hospital/ local hospital/local surgery, hospital/ local hospital/ local
Blood	Range of tests to diagnose or rule out disorders: complete blood count; coagulation; glucose; enzymes and electrolytes (for heart, liver or kidney damage); uric acid; cholesterol; triglycerides; albumin and globulin (abnormal protein levels); thyroid; antenatally (anaemia, rubella, rhesus factor, hepatitis, STDs); syphilis; bilirubin (red cell level).	hospital/none
Blood pressure	To check that it is not above 140/90 (adults, pregnant women), and for those with a family history of high blood pressure.	surgery/none
Cervical smear	Simple method of obtaining cervical cells for lab analysis.	surgery/none
Colonoscopy	To get an inside view of large intestine using an endoscope (flexible fibre-optic tube). Enema or laxatives given first to clean out colon.	hospital/light sedation
Colposcopy	Routine optical examination of vagina and cervix after cervical smear shows some abnormality. May be combined with biopsy.	hospital/none
Computerized axial tomography (CAT) scan	Evaluates soft tissue (after stroke or haemorrhage, for cysts, abscesses, tumours) using X-ray to produce 3D image. Contrast dye may be given intravenously to enhance detection of abnormalities.	hospital/none
Coronary angiography	Detects blockages in heart arteries. Dye is injected and its flow through the arteries pictured. Women are less often offered this test as part of heart investigation, and so should request this.	hospital/general

Continued overleaf

Type	Purpose	Where done/anaesthetic
Cystometric tests	Estimate bladder function.	hospital/none
Cystoscopy	Examination of bladder using a fibre-optic passed along urethra. May be combined with biopsy or cautery treatment.	urodynamic unit of hospital/local or general
DEXA	Dual energy absorptiometry X-ray used to assess bone density (eating disorders, osteoporosis).	special hospital unit/none
ECG and stress ECG	Electrocardiogram traces activity pattern of heart at rest. A stress ECG is done while walking or jogging on a treadmill. Either may be done in conjunction with thallium scanning.	hospital cardiac unit, surgery/none
Echocardiography	Ultrasound to detect blockage in single blood vessel, using reflected heart waves to generate an image. Also used to look at chambers and valves of heart.	hospital cardiac unit/none
EEG	Records electrical activity in brain.	surgery, hospital/none
Endoscopy	Method of visually examining inside of body using flexible fibre-optic instrument called an endoscope. May be combined with biopsy, injected radio-opaque dye X-ray and surgery.	hospital/general
Exercise stress test	Also called a stress ECG or exercise tolerance test, this assesses blood available to heart during exercise.	hospital cardiac unit/none
Fluorescent angiography	Test for macular degeneration by evaluating blood vessel pattern in eye. Special dye is injected into arm vein.	ophthalmologist's office/none
Hystero-salpingogram	Method of assessing whether Fallopian tubes are open and shape of uterus, in infertility investigation.	radiology unit of hospital/light
Hysteroscopy	Endoscope is inserted via vagina and cervix. Problems found by test may be treated by infertility specialist at same time.	gynaecology unit of hospital/general
Immunoassay	Test for antibody concentration in immune system disorders.	hospital/none
Intravenous pyelogram	X-ray of kidney and bladder; dye is injected into arm vein. May be done instead of cystoscopy.	urodynamic unit of hospital/light sedation
Laparoscopy	Minimally invasive surgery for diagnosing and treating reproductive system problems.	gynaecology unit of hospital/general
Laparotomy	Abdominal surgery to detect, diagnose or treat conditions. Incision is 10–13 cm (4–5 in) long, above pubic region.	hospital/general
Lumbar puncture	Spinal tap to obtain sample of spinal fluid for analysis.	hospital/light sedation
Lung function test	Check capacity of lungs, airflow and oxygen/ gas exchange.	surgery, hospital/none

Type	Purpose	Where done/anaesthetic
Magnetic resonance imaging (MRI)	Noninvasive method of viewing and photographing inside of body, using no radiation or contrast dyes. Best MRI for breast is 1.5 tesla system.	radiology unit of hospital/light sedation if necessary
Mammograph or mammogram	X-ray of breast to detect cancer or other abnormalities.	radiology unit of hospital/none
Moiré shadow photography	Non X-ray technique to detect spinal contours.	hospital/none
Pelvic examinations	Often routine check-ups of reproductive organs. May combine an external, internal (speculum), bimanual (gloved finger inside vagina, hand pressing outside), and rectovaginal (gloved fingers in vagina and rectum).	surgery/none
Physical examination	This is not done routinely except in private medicine. Good time to raise health concerns.	surgery/none
Postcoital test	Much like cervical smear, to obtain cervical mucus after intercourse as part of infertility investigation.	surgery or hospital infertility unit/none
Proctoscopy	Examination of anus and rectum to assess bowel conditions.	hospital/none
Radionuclide scan	Technique to assess density of gallstones.	radiology unit of hospital/none
Sigmoidoscopy	As proctoidoscopy, but uses flexible lighted tube to view lower part of large intestine.	hospital/light sedation
SPECT	A radiologic test to look at blood flow in brain.	radiology unit in hospital/none
Stool tests	Sample is examined for blood, mucus, bacteria, fat or bile.	pathology/none
Thallium scanning	Radioactive material is injected into a vein in conjunction with exercise ECG. Not common in women.	hospital/none
Tonometry	Measure of pressure of fluid in eye to diagnose glaucoma.	ophthalmologist/eye drops
Ultrasound	Internal view of body using high-frequency sound waves recorded on screen to form a picture. Wide range of uses.	surgery, hospital/none
Urine tests	Regular part of antenatal care or physical examination. Also to analyse for blood, infection, glucose, acidity or alkalinity.	surgery/none
VER	Visual evoked response is used to detect retina reactions in different conditions (bright lights, flashes etc).	ophthalmologist's surgery/none
X-rays	Electromagnetic radiation image for medical or surgical diagnosis. As X-rays can damage tissue a woman who suspects she is pregnant should not be X-rayed.	hospital unit/none

SEEING A SPECIALIST

Medical care involves the skills of a range of qualified practitioners who work as a team in planning and carrying out tests and treatment. Consultation and other services may be available at a hospital or large group practice. A range of professional staff, based at hospitals or health centres, may also treat or be involved with the treatment of patients following a doctor's recommendation.

Medical specialists

Audiologist	Specializes in the study and treatment of hearing defects.
Cardiologist	Diagnoses and treats disorders and diseases of the heart.
Dermatologist	Diagnoses and treats skin disorders and diseases.
Embryologist	Specializes in the development of the foetus from implantation to maturity.
Endocrinologist	Diagnoses and treats disorders and diseases of the glands and hormones.
Gastroenterologist	Diagnoses and treats diseases and disorders of the stomach and the digestive tract.
General practitioner	The doctor you visit first. Assesses and treats symptoms. May refer you to a specialist.
Geneticist	Specialist in links between genes and disease. Advises on congenital diseases.
Geriatrician	Specialist in ageing and its problems.
Gynaecologist	Diagnoses and treats diseases and disorders of the female reproductive organs; also advises on family planning and treats infertility. See also Urogynaecologist.
Immunologist	Specializes in the immune system, its ability to fight disease, foreign antibodies, its overreaction to allergens and its tendency to reject implants and organ transplants.
Nephrologist	Diagnoses and treats disorders and diseases of the kidneys (renal medicine).
Neurologist	Diagnoses and treats diseases and disorders of the brain and the nervous system.
Obstetrician	Specializes in the care and treatment of pregnant women and their babies during pregnancy and birth. Many obstetricians are also gynaecologists.
Oncologist	Specializes in the treatment of cancer; may be clinical, medical or paediatric.
Ophthalmologist	Specializes in the structure, functions and diseases of the eye.
Otolaryngologist (ENT)	Specializes in disorders of ears, nose and throat, and of linking channels and sinuses.
Paediatrician	Diagnoses the diseases, disorders and development of children from birth to post-puberty; may specialize—paediatric endocrinology, immunology, neo-natal medicine.
Physician	General doctor who may also specialize: for example an occupational physician is concerned with working practices and the health of the people employed.

Psychiatrist	Diagnoses and treats mental and emotional illness. A neuropsychiatrist deals with psychological symptoms and neurological disorder.
Psychologist	Specializes in diagnosis and treatment of abnormal human behaviour. Health psychology is a related speciality.
Pulmonologist	Diagnoses and treats disorders and diseases of the lungs and chest.
Radiologist	Orders and interprets X-rays, ultrasound, MRI and CAT scans, and diagnostic tests.
Rheumatologist	Diagnoses and treats disorders and diseases of the joints.
Urogynaecologist (women) **Urologist (men)**	Diagnose and treat disorders and diseases of the bladder and urinary tract, and also operate on the related structures of the urinary/reproductive system.

Surgical specialists

Anaesthetist	Specializes in giving anaesthetics before an operation and monitoring the patient's condition during it, adjusting the dosage if necessary; treats effects of surgical shock; provides pain relief post-operatively. Anaesthetists often run clinics for pain control.
Cardiothoracic surgeon	Operates on the heart and the great vessels around it. May also be called a cardiovascular surgeon.
Cosmetic surgeon	See plastic surgeon.
ENT (ear, nose and throat)	See otolaryngologist.
General surgeon	Diagnoses and treats a range of illnesses using surgical techniques. Most surgeons specialize in one area of the body, but a general surgeon may operate on any part— most often areas within the torso not covered by a hospital specialist, such as an inflamed appendix, a hernia or intestinal problems.
Neurosurgeon	Operates to treat disease or trauma to the brain, spinal cord and nervous system.
Oral and maxillofacial surgeon	Specializes in the surgical treatment of diseases and problems of the mouth, teeth and jaw; oral surgeons are trained both in medicine and dentistry.
Orthopaedic surgeon	Uses surgery to treat bone defects and disorders, whether caused by disease, injury (trauma) or age.
Otolaryngology surgeon	Surgically treats ear, nose, throat and sinuses.
Paediatric surgeon	Specializes in operating on children, from birth to post-puberty.
Plastic surgeon	Reconstructs damaged skin tissues after trauma, disease or an operation, as well as removing facial blemishes, such as port wine stains, or correcting features (cosmetic).
Vascular surgeon	Specializes in disorders and diseases of the blood vessels, such as varicose veins. A cardiovascular surgeon specializes in heart and blood vessel problems such as aneurysms, ischaemia and atherosclerosis.

Continued overleaf

Other medical personnel

Cytologist	Specializes in cells and their study in the laboratory.
Epidemiologist	Studies the distribution of disease between different groups of people, areas and environments to pinpoint possible causes and identify those ethnic, geographical and lifestyle groups that appear to be vulnerable to any particular condition.
Geneticist	Specializes in the testing of genes for inherited diseases or tendencies.
Haematologist	Specializes in the study of blood and bone marrow, identifying the type, character, and number of blood cells and other constituents of blood, to assist in the diagnosis of many diseases. They test for compatibility between the tissues—bone marrow cells, for example—supplied by a donor, and the immune system of the recipient.
Immunologist	Specializes in the study of immunity—immune response, antibodies, vaccinations.
Midwife	Assists in pregnancy, childbirth and follow-up care.
Nurse practitioner	May do cervical smears, breast examination, give vaccinations and other injections.
Nurse specialist	Has received extra training in a specific area: oncology (cancer), breast care, infertility.
Occupational therapist	Treats people disabled by physical and mental problems to help them relearn specific physical activities, to achieve possible independence in everyday life. When a disability is permanent, the occupational therapist will suggest various aids and alterations to the home that will assist with maintaining mobility.
Pathologist	Works in the laboratory and studies the cause, nature, effects on the tissues and progress of diseases to help in their diagnosis and to determine the possible prognosis. A neuropathologist is concerned with the nervous system.
Physical therapist	Specializes in rehabilitation using massage and exercise methods to treat physical problems, such as paralysis, chest problems and musculoskeletal disorders (including pelvic floor).
Physiotherapist	Specializes in physical rehabilitation using manipulation, massage and exercise methods to treat problems such as paralysis, chest diseases and musculoskeletal disorders (including pelvic floor and bladder).
Podiatrist	Specializes in the health and the care of the feet and the treatment of problems such as calluses, corns and deformities.
Radiographer	Does X-rays, breast screening, ultrasound, other diagnostic tests, for a radiologist.
Speech therapist	Diagnoses and treats acquired or developmental communication disorders, such as difficulties with speaking, reading, writing or understanding, using a programme of exercises and also working with family and friends.

Useful medical terms

When you read the entries in this book or come in contact with different personnel at a doctor's surgery or in a hospital, it is useful to know the technical and other words that may be used to describe a condition or an element of it. If you are in doubt about something you are told, always ask for it to be repeated so you understand its meaning.

Acute Describes an illness or disorder that has a sudden onset, course and resolution. Some acute disorders can become chronic—for example, several attacks of acute bronchitis can leave a patient with chronic bronchitis; and an acute, sharp, stabbing pain can become a chronic, nagging, persistent pain.

Benign Non-malignant and usually considered harmless; generally used to describe a tumour, but may also describe a disease.

Chronic Describes a disease or disorder that develops gradually, is of long duration and may cause permanent damage or change to a part of the body. Chronic pain is a dull, persistent, throbbing pain that may or may not follow an episode of acute pain.

Cyanosis A bluish tinge of the skin, especially the lips and fingernails, seen when there is insufficient oxygen circulating in the blood.

Cyst A growth or swelling containing a liquid or semi-solid matter. Cysts can occur in any tissue, but are most common in skin, breasts and ovaries. They are not malignant, but may be unsightly and recur or need to be removed because they press on vital organs.

Diagnosis Describes the process of identifying a disease and its cause. A doctor makes a differential diagnosis—a list of possible problems—from the signs and symptoms described by the patient and through a medical examination. A diagnostic procedure may then be done—such as blood and urine tests, X-rays, a cervical smear, ultrasound or other scan—in order to confirm the diagnosis.

Febrile Describes fever and a high temperature (well above 37.0°C/98.6°F). A febrile convulsion is a convulsion or fit caused by an abnormally high body temperature.

Follicle A small sac or gland. They are found, for example, at the base of a hair, in the intestines and the reproductive organs. A hormone, called follicle stimulating hormone (FSH), from the anterior pituitary gland, stimulates an egg-producing follicle in the ovary during each menstrual cycle in women, and sperm production in the testes in men.

Lesion An area of damaged tissue anywhere in the body. Cuts, bruises, rashes, abscesses, cysts, tumours and ulcers are all examples of lesions.

Malaise A non-specific, generalized feeling of tiredness with aches and pains and a sense of being unwell that often precedes an infection and accompanies a chronic disease.

Malignant A term to describe serious, progressive and sometimes fatal diseases or disorders. For example, a cancerous tumour that grows rapidly, spreads and invades other tissues is known as a malignant tumour. Certain infections such as smallpox and disorders like hypertension are more virulent than others and are said to be malignant forms of disease as they can be fatal if left untreated.

Palpation Describes a method of examination with the hands to feel the surface structures and the internal organs. The hands are said to palpate the particular area of the body.

Psychopharmacology The use of drugs to treat mental states.

Psychosomatic Term for a physical disorder that has been caused or made worse by a psychological element.

Sepsis A term used to denote infection of the body or a part of the body. The common causes are bacteria, viruses and, in some cases, fungi, which causes inflammation.

Systemic An illness or drug that affects the whole body rather than a part of it. For example, systemic lupus erythematosis affects the connective tissue throughout the body.

Tissues The entire body is composed of various types of tissue, consisting of cells that have particular characteristics. Examples include circulatory tissue, epithelial tissue, connective tissue, muscle tissue and nerve tissue.

Toxicology The study of poisons and their effects on the body.

Tumour Any swelling of body tissue, such as a cyst, abscess or a new growth. A tumour is normally described as being benign (non-cancerous) or malignant (cancerous).

CONVENTIONAL TREATMENTS

The basis of conventional treatment is scientific—a combination of medical understanding and pharmaceutical research. Prevention or cure starts with the family doctor and may involve various specialists who work as a team to restore health in their patients.

See also:

2/SEX & SEXUALITY
Sexual infections
pp. 72–75

4/HORMONAL HEALTH
Pregnancy and motherhood
pp. 170–179

5/ILLNESSES & EMERGENCIES
Digestive system problems p. 192
Respiratory problems p. 213

Safe travelling

Health protection will be needed if you are planning to travel to Asia, Africa or South America. You should consult your doctor or a specialist travel clinic six to eight weeks in advance of departure to discuss which vaccinations or prophylactic treatment might be applicable. Many need time to become effective. While some countries may advise you to have polio, tetanus, typhoid and hepatitis A jabs, no vaccinations are compulsory other than yellow fever in certain places. Some people carry a certificate showing the vaccinations they have had, since some countries require it before you can enter. This, however, is rare nowadays. If you do not have a record of these, vaccination may be forced on you, a risky procedure in countries where HIV and AIDS are widespread.

If you are travelling to places where contagious disease is rife and sanitation is doubtful—such as parts of Africa and the Indian subcontinent—you should consider short-term protection against hepatitis A (HAV) and hepatitis B (HBV) with immune serum globulin. If necessary, the injection can be given within 14 days of exposure to prevent infection. If you are a frequent traveller it is better to be vaccinated.

VACCINATION

The purpose of introducing a tiny amount of virus or bacterium into the bloodstream is to activate your immune system to produce antibodies to it so that should you then come in contact with the disease itself your body will be able to fight it off. As the effects of communicable diseases can be devastating, vaccination—or immunization as it is also known—is effective preventive medicine.

Artificially inducing immunity starts in childhood, since babies are particularly vulnerable to a range of infections. The different vaccinations, and when they are given, are shown in the box (left). Some are given in combination, others as single injections. Some, like tetanus, need a booster every 10 years. As immunity can develop on its own, as in TB, a skin test is done first. With pertussis (whooping cough) and

AGE-RELATED PROTECTION

While getting a disease gives lifelong immunity, you also risk the consequences. By being vaccinated, you improve your chances of staying healthy and fighting infection.

Vaccination	Age	Vaccination	Age
Polio	2–4 months 3–5 years 14–19 years	Tuberculosis (TB)	10–13 years
DTP (diphtheria, tetanus, pertussis)	2–4 months 3–5 years 14–19 years	Hepatitis B	3 doses: 2nd, 1 month after, 3rd, 6 months after the 1st. High risk groups: drug users and haemophiliacs
MMR (measles, mumps, rubella)	12–15 months and 3–5 years	Tetanus	aged adult
Meningitis C	2, 3, 4 months	Pneumonia	aged adult
Hib	2, 3, 4 months	Influenza	aged adult

REDUCING JET LAG

Be prepared for jet lag if your journey takes you across three or more time zones. The speed and distance covered may temporarily disrupt your internal clock, known as the circadian rhythm, influencing sleeping and waking.

To calculate the days before your body will adjust to your new time zone, divide the number of time zones by two if going east; for west, divide them by one and a half.

Long flights can also increase your risk of thrombosis. To prevent this, as well as jet lag, drink plenty of fluids (plain water, fruit juice) on the plane. Avoid alcohol which is dehydrating.

Preventive treatments are available for previous thrombosis sufferers.

On arrival, try to fit in with the local time as quickly as possible—eat the relevant meal, and sleep when everyone else does. Jet lag can reduce your awareness levels—you should be careful if you intend driving a car.

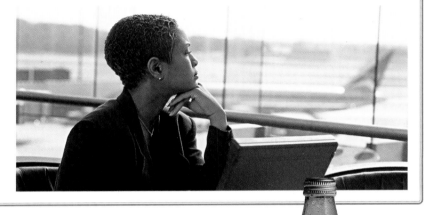

Are you medically fit to fly?

An unfit passenger is anyone with a disease that impairs the ability of the heart and lung to oxygenate the blood or its flow through the circulatory system. Infants with acute respiratory problems or premature babies have increased risks.

Problems may arise during a flight if any of these apply to you:

♀ Cardiovascular diseases (angina, myocardial infarction, high blood pressure).
♀ Respiratory diseases (emphysema, pneumonia).
♀ Surgery (chest, abdominal, ear and face) within two weeks of flying.
♀ Blood disorders (anaemia, atherosclerosis, deep vein thrombosis).
♀ Gastrointestinal diseases (peptic ulcers, acute gastroenteritis).
♀ Contagious diseases (TB, hepatitis, chickenpox, measles, German measles).
♀ Over 28 weeks pregnant (doctor's certificate needed).
♀ Ear or nose conditions (acute middle ear infection, sinusitis).
♀ Diabetes (severe diabetes mellitus).
♀ Recent stroke or heart attack.

MALARIA PROPHYLAXIS

There is no vaccination against malaria, the disease carried by the female anopheles mosquito and which is a danger in all tropical and subtropical countries. Around 1,000 people a year come back from a trip abroad with it, an increasing proportion of them with the most serious type, plasmodium falciparum, which is potentially fatal.

You should get expert advice as to which prophylactic pills are appropriate for your destination; some may not be suitable if you are pregnant or have specific health problems. You need to take the ones recommended before you go, while you're away, and for four weeks after you return. You may need to take more than one type, some of which are available over the counter. None offers total protection, so while travelling use an effective insect repellent, cover areas which attract bites (arms, scalp, neck and feet) if outdoors in the evening, and sleep under a mosquito net at night.

Don't hesitate to see your doctor if you feel ill after a trip: the illness generally appears after two to three weeks, but can show itself three months after you have been in a malarial area. Symptoms are a constant throbbing headache which can't be relieved by analgesics, fatigue, low-grade fever and nausea. Do mention the possibility of malaria when you see him or her.

WATER CURE
Keeping your body well hydrated during a flight may protect you from the debilitating effects of jet lag.

> **! Caution**
> Children and adults can develop a slight fever after vaccination. Make sure you have plenty of fluids and precautionary paracetamol (for infants, give the dose recommended by your paediatrician).

diphtheria, boosters are not generally advised. With such infections as rubella (German measles) immunity may last only five years; a blood test will reveal if antibodies are present.

DRUG TYPES AND THEIR USES

On these charts you will find drugs grouped into main categories along with their possible side effects and when they should not be taken (contraindications). The names given are generic—they refer to a drug's official name, rather than a proprietary brand name. The list is not exhaustive: it would be virtually impossible to include all drugs available for prescription or over the counter in pharmacies.

> **! Caution**
>
> Make sure you ask your doctor about any drug that you are prescribed and read any information provided by the drug company. Take precisely as directed, and report any side effects you may experience to your doctor immediately. Over-the-counter drugs are also labelled with information on their ingredients, usage and side effects. Make sure that you read and understand the labels.

Drug	Use	Action	Side effects	Contraindications
The skeletal system				
Antirheumatics: chloroquine; gold; methotrexate; non-steroidal anti-inflammatories (NSAIDs); mesalazine.	Rheumatoid arthritis; juvenile arthritis; systemic lupus erythematosus.	Modify disease process. Reduce inflammation.	Nausea; vomiting; diarrhoea; skin rashes; blood disorders; mouth ulcers; eye damage.	Kidney or liver disorders; pregnancy.
Hormone replacement therapy: oestrogens; SERMS (raloxifene).	Osteoporosis; menopausal symptoms.	Maintain the level of oestrogen.	Nausea; weight changes; oedema; depression; headaches; rashes.	Pregnancy; oestrogen-dependent cancer; thromboses (DVTs).
Immunosuppressives: prednisone; azathioprine; sulphasalazine.	Rheumatoid arthritis; psoriatic arthritis; systemic lupus erythematosus.	Suppress the immune system; reduce inflammation.	Kidney damage; changes in blood pressure; nausea; susceptibility to infections.	Kidney disease; pregnancy; high blood pressure; infectious disease.
Muscle relaxants: dantrolene; baclofen; diazepam; quinine.	Damaged spinal cord, muscle spasm; cramp.	Reduce muscle tone either systemically, centrally or locally.	Drowsiness; nausea; lethargy; dry mouth; blurred vision.	Peptic ulcer; liver damage; cerebrovascular disease; psychiatric problems.
Bisphosphonates: etidronate disodium, tiludronic acid.	Osteoporosis.	Inhibit osteoclast (breakdown of bone) activity.	Nausea; diarrhoea.	Renal disorders; pregnancy; breastfeeding.
The nervous system				
Muscle relaxants: dantrolene; baclofen; diazepam.	Multiple sclerosis.	Reduce muscle tone either systemically, centrally or locally.	Drowsiness; nausea; lethargy; dry mouth; blurred vision.	Peptic ulcer; liver damage; cerebrovascular disease; psychiatric problems.
Anticonvulsants: carbamazepine; phenytoin; sodium valproate.	Epilepsy; some mood disorders e.g. manic depression.	Decrease the excitability of the brain.	Drowsiness; liver damage.	Liver disorders; bone marrow dysfunction; porphyria.
Tricyclic antidepressants: amitriptyline; doxepin; nortriptyline; imipranine; desipramine.	Depression (some tricyclic antidepressants also have sedative properties).	Believed to increase brain levels of adrenaline, noradrenaline and mood-enhancing serotonin.	Dry mouth; constipation; blurred vision; drowsiness; drop in blood pressure when changing position.	Recent heart attack; irregular heartbeat; severe liver disease; suicidal tendencies.
Selective serotonin reuptake inhibitors: fluoxetine; paroxetine.	Depression (when sedation not required).	Increase serotonin levels by inhibiting it being taken back into nerve endings.	Nausea; vomiting; diarrhoea; weight loss; headaches.	Mania; epileptic fits; liver and kidney problems.
Monoamine oxidase inhibitors: phenelzine; isocarboxazid.	Depression, especially with hysteria and hypochondria; if other drugs not effective.	Cause increase in levels of neurotransmitters in brain.	Low blood pressure; dizziness; fatigue; dry mouth; constipation; weight gain.	Liver disease; cerebro-vascular problems; rise in blood pressure (due to food).
Lithium carbonate.	Manic depression; recurrent depression.	Stabilize mood.	Nausea; diarrhoea; weight gain; thyroid disorder.	Kidney and heart disorders.

Drug	Use	Action	Side effects	Contraindications
The nervous system cont.				
Anticholinergics: trihexphenidyl; orphenadrine.	Parkinson's disease.	Reduce tremor in Parkinson's disease.	Dry mouth; vision problems; difficulty in passing urine.	Glaucoma.
Antipsychotics: pimozide; sulpiride; flupenthixol; Atypical antipsychotics: Olanzapine; risperidone.	Schizophrenia; manic depression; delusion. Schizophrenia.	Reduce the excitability of nerve pathways in the brain. Antipsychotic.	Drowsiness; dry mouth; Parkinson's-like symptoms. Weight gain; dizziness; Parkinson's-like symptoms.	Bone marrow disorders; liver and Parkinson's disease. Cardiovascular disease; epilepsy; pregnancy.
Hypnotics: nitrazepam; diazepam.	Insomnia; stress; anxiety; senile dementia.	Affect the part of the brain controlling wakefulness.	Drowsiness; confusion; dependence.	Respiratory, liver and psychiatric problems.
Donepezil; rivastigmine.	Alzheimer's; dementia.	Reversible acetylcholinesterase inhibitor.	Diarrhoea; nausea, fatigue; cramps; peptic ulcers.	Pregnancy; breastfeeding.
The endocrine system				
Hormone replacement therapy: oestrogens; progestogens.	Menopause.	Maintain the level of oestrogen.	Nausea; weight changes; oedema; depression; headaches; rashes.	Pregnancy; oestrogen-dependent cancer; thromboses (DVTs).
Hormone: insulin.	Diabetes mellitus.	Ensures glucose enters the cells, so restoring fat and carbohydrate metabolism.	Hypoglycaemia—too much insulin; hyperglycaemia—too little insulin.	
Hormone: carbimazole.	Hyperthyroidism; thyrotoxicosis; goitre; exophthalmus.	Decreases the production of thyroxine by the thyroid gland.	Enlarged thyroid gland; headaches; nausea; hair loss; low immunity; loss of thyroxine production.	Low white blood count; infectious disease.
Hormone: thyroxine.	Hypothyroidism (myxoedema); cretinism; thyroid cancer.	Replaces missing production of thyroxine hormone by thyroid gland.	Weight loss; angina; arrhythmias; cramp; headache; restlessness; sweating.	Cardiovascular disorders; adrenal gland disorders.
Corticosteroids: prednisone; dexamethasone; hydrocortisone; fludrocortisone; betamethasone; beclomethasone.	Addison's disease; adrenalectomy; inflammatory disorders; asthma; eczema.	Inhibit the body's reaction to damage or disease, so reducing inflammation.	Long-term treatment—fluid retention, hypertension, Cushing's syndrome, osteoporosis, depression, diabetes; sudden cessation—rapid fall in blood pressure; topical use (on skin)—thinning of skin; worsening of infection.	Use of systemic steroids requires careful monitoring; exposure to chickenpox; topical and inhaled steroids—rosacea, acne, skin infections, psoriasis, tuberculosis.
The blood and circulatory system				
ACE (angiotensin-converting enzyme) inhibitors: captopril; enalapril.	Heart failure; high blood pressure.	Dilate arteries and veins and reduce the amount of fluid in the circulation.	Dizziness; hypotension; skin rashes; impaired renal function; cough.	Pregnancy; renal problems; aortic stenosis (narrowing).
Antiarrhythmics: lignocaine; verapamil; adenosine.	Restore an irregular heartbeat to normal.	Slow down the transmission of electrical impulses within the heart.	Dizziness; confusion; constipation; breathing difficulties.	Cardiac or respiratory failure; porphyria.
Anticoagulants: heparin; warfarin.	Internal blood clots—pulmonary embolus; cerebral or coronary infarcts; deep vein thrombosis.	Decrease the clotting factors in the blood.	Bleeding of the gastrointestinal tract and kidneys; bruising of the skin.	Haemophilia; high blood pressure; cerebral haemorrhage; peptic ulcers; kidney or liver failure.

Continued overleaf

Drug	Use	Action	Side effects	Contraindications
The blood and circulatory system cont.				
Antihypertensives: hydralazine; methyldopa; prazosin.	High blood pressure.	Dilate blood vessels; partially block adrenaline and noradrenaline.	Palpitations; oedema; dizziness; headaches.	Rapid heartbeat; congestive heart failure; aneurysm; depression.
Beta blockers: metoprolol; propranolol; atenolol; celiprolol; acebutolol.	High blood pressure; angina; heart attacks; arrhythmias.	Slow heart and lower blood pressure by blocking adrenaline production.	Cold extremities; general malaise; sleep disturbances; nightmares.	Asthma; chronic bronchitis; emphysema; diabetes; later stages of pregnancy.
Calcium blockers: verapamil; nifedipine; nicardipine; amlodipine; lacidipine; nimodipine; diltiazem.	High blood pressure; angina; arrhythmias; subarachnoid haemorrhage.	Relax the muscles of the heart and arteries.	Headache; oedema; fatigue; nausea; flushing; dizziness; constipation.	Heart failure; liver failure; pregnancy; heart attack; taking beta-blockers.
Diuretics: thiazides; frusemide; spironolactone; mannitol.	High blood pressure; congestive heart failure; cerebral oedema.	Cause the kidneys to excrete water and salts.	Gout; impotence; potassium deficiency.	Renal failure; pregnancy; breastfeeding; diabetes mellitus; Addison's disease.
Nitrates: glyceryl trinitrate; isosorbide dinitrate; isosorbide mononitrate.	Angina; left ventricular failure.	Widen the coronary arteries and reduce blood flow into the heart.	Headaches; flushing; dizziness.	Hypotension; narrowing of aorta; cerebral haemorrhage; head injury; glaucoma.
Statins: atorvastatin, fluvastatin, simvastatin.	High cholesterol levels, slow coronary athersclerosis, reduce risk of strokes.	Blocks production of cholesterol and use of circulating cholesterol.	Nausea; insomnia; stomach pain; muscle pain; headaches.	Severe renal condition; liver disease; pregnancy; breastfeeding.
Cardica glycosides: digoxin.	Congestive cardiac failure; atrial fibrillation.	Makes heartbeat stronger; restores normal beat.	Visual problems; weakness; headaches; depression.	Complete heart block; arrhythmia.
Aspirin.	Prevention of blood clots.	Reduces platelet stickiness.	Gastric bleeding.	Peptic ulcer; allergy to aspirin.
The respiratory system				
Decongestants, anti-tussives: triprolidine; dextro-methorphan; menthol.	Coughs; bronchial secretions.	Dry up secretions; reduce coughing.	Insomnia; tachycardia (heartbeat irregularity); restlessness; anxiety with overuse.	High blood pressure; diabetes mellitus.
Anticholinergics: ipratropium; oxitropium.	Asthma.	Relax muscles of the bronchii.	Dry mouth; constipation; difficulty in passing urine.	Glaucoma.
Antihistamines: chlorpheniramine; terfenadine; cyclizine; acrivastine; promethazine; cetirizine; loratidine.	Allergies—hayfever.	Reduce action of histamine in the body—which dilates small blood vessels, and tightens the bronchioles.	Drowsiness; rashes; dry mouth; blurred vision; palpitations.	Epilepsy; liver and kidney disorders; glaucoma; porphyria.
Bronchodilators: salbutamol; terbutaline; fenoterol; salmeterol.	Chronic obstructive pulmonary disease; asthma.	Relax the muscles of the bronchioles.	Shaking hands; headache; nervous tension; flushes; palpitations.	Hyperthyroidism; high blood pressure; arrhythmias.
Corticosteroids: prednisone; hydrocortisone; beclomethasone; . fluticasone; budesonide.	Chronic respiratory disease; asthma.	Inhibit the body's reaction to damage or disease, so reducing inflammation.	Long-term treatment—fluid retention, high blood pressure, osteoporosis, depression, diabetes; sudden cessation—rapid fall in blood pressure, shock.	Use of systemic steroids requires careful monitoring; avoid exposure to chickenpox. Inhaled steroids—oral thrush.
Montelukast; zafirlukast.	Asthma.	Leukotriene blockers (anti-inflammatory).	Gastrointestinal rashes.	Liver failure.

Drug	Use	Action	Side effects	Contraindications
The respiratory system cont.				
Decongestants: xylometazoline; ephedrine.	Hayfever; common cold.	Reduce inflammation in the nasal passages and the production of mucus.	Dryness and irritation of nose.	High blood pressure.
The digestive system				
Antacids: alginates; magnesium trisilicate; magnesium carbonate; sodium bicarbonate.	Peptic ulcers; hiatus hernia; indigestion.	Neutralize the acid in the stomach and gut so reducing inflammation.	Rare, but overuse may disturb body's fluid balance.	Antacids neutralize or react with other medications.
Anticholinergics: hyoscine; dicycloverine.	Irritable bowel syndrome; peptic ulcers.	Relax muscles of the gut, reduce gastric secretions.	Dry mouth; vision problems; difficulty in passing urine.	Glaucoma.
Antidiarrhoeals: codeine phosphate; loperamide; kaolin and morphine.	Irritable bowel syndrome; peptic ulcers.	Relax muscles of the gut, reduce gastric secretions.	Dry mouth; vision problems; difficulty in passing urine.	Glaucoma.
Antiemetics: metoclopramide; promethazine; cyclizine.	Vomiting; severe nausea; motion sickness.	Inhibits the vomit reflex at the base of the brain.	Drowsiness; dry mouth; involuntary twitches.	Kidney and liver disorders; dehydration; glaucoma.
Appetite suppressants, anti-obesity agents: methycellulose; phentermine; orlistat.	Gross obesity.	Give a feeling of fullness; dampen the appetite centre in the brain; prevent absorption of fat.	Constipation; flatulence; diarrhoea; drowsiness; dizziness; anxiety; depression.	Psychiatric disorders; drug abuse; personality disorders; pregnancy; breastfeeding; epilepsy; glaucoma.
Immunosuppressants: sulphasalazine.	Ulcerative colitis.	Suppress immune system; reduce inflammation.	Headache; rash; nausea; fever; hypersensitivity.	Blood dyscrasias; sensitivity to sulphonamides.
Laxatives: methycellulose; ispaghula; bran; lactulose; magnesium hydroxide; senna; bisacodyl.	Constipation; expulsion of parasites.	Increase the water content of the faeces; stimulate the colonic muscles to contract.	Diarrhoea; flatulence; bloating; colic pain.	Intestinal obstruction.
Replacement salts: sodium chloride; glucose; potassium chloride.	Fluid and electrolyte replacement during diarrhoea.	Replace salts and fluid.	Oedema.	Kidney and cardiovascular disorders; high blood pressure.
Corticosteroids: prednisone; dexamethasone; hydrocortisone; budesonide.	Crohn's disease.	Inhibit the body's reaction to damage or disease, so reducing inflammation.	Fluid retention, high blood pressure, osteoporosis, depression, diabetes; sudden cessation—fall in blood pressure, shock.	Use of systemic steroids requires careful monitoring; avoid exposure to chickenpox.
H2 receptor blockers: ranitidine; nizatidine; cimetidine.	Peptic ulcers; protects stomach against NSAID damage; reflux oesophagitis.	Reduce gastric acid output as a result of histamine H2 blockade.	Diarrhoea; rash; dizziness.	Some drug interractions.
Proton pump inhibitors: omeprazole; hansoprazole.	Peptic ulcers; + NSAIDS to prevent gastric side effects.	Inhibit gastric acid formation.	Diarrhoea; nausea; rash; constipation; headache.	Intestinal obstruction.
The urinary system				
Diuretics: thiazides; frusemide; spironolactone; mannitol.	Fluid retention; cirrhosis; kidney disorders.	Cause the kidneys to excrete water and salts.	Gout; impotence; potassium deficiency.	Renal failure; pregnancy; diabetes mellitus; Addison's disease.
Alkalinizing agents: potassium citrate.	Cystitis.	Decrease acidity of urine.	Gastric irritation; diarrhoea.	Bowel ulceration; renal malfunction; late pregnancy.

Continued overleaf

Drug	Use	Action	Side effects	Contraindications
The reproductive system				
Beta2 agonists: salbutamol; terbutaline.	Premature labour.	Relax uterine muscles.	Shaky hands; headache; nervous tension; flushes; palpitations.	Hyperthyroidism; high blood pressure; arrhythmias.
Antifungals: nystatin; miconazole; ketoconazole; econazole.	Yeast infection (Candidiasis).	Attack fungi.	Severe liver problems possible with ketoconazole; orally—nausea, vomiting; secondary bacterial infections.	Orally—liver disease.
Gonadotrophins and gonadotrophin–releasing hormone analogues: menotrophin; gosarelin; buseralin.	Endometriosis; infertility; excessive menstrual bleeding; PMS; uterine fibroids.	Stimulate the release of gonadotrophin.	Overstimulation of the ovaries; possible multiple pregnancy; allergic reactions.	Pregnancy; ovarian cyst; unexplained vaginal bleeding.
Hormone replacement therapy: oestrogens; progestogens.	Menopause.	Maintain the level of oestrogen.	Nausea; weight changes; oedema; depression; headaches; rashes.	Pregnancy; oestrogen-dependent cancer; deep-vein thromboses (DVTs).
Hormone: progestogens.	Painful/heavy menstruation; endometriosis; breast cancer.	Increases the level of progesterone in the body.	Nausea; fluid retention; weight gain.	Pregnancy; liver disorders; arterial disease; porphyria.
The immune system				
Antihistamines: chlorpheniramine; terfenadine; cyclizine; acrivastine; promethazine; loratacline.	Allergies—hay fever, urticaria (hives), insect stings and drugs.	Reduce the action of histamine in the body— which dilates small blood vessels, and tightens the bronchioles.	Drowsiness; rashes; dry mouth; blurred vision; palpitations.	Epilepsy; liver and kidney disorders; glaucoma; porphyria.
Immunosuppressants: cyclosporin; azathioprine; tacrolimus.	Organ transplant.	Suppress the immune system; reduce possibility of rejection of transplanted tissue.	Kidney damage; hirsutism; high or low blood pressure; nausea; susceptibility to infections.	Kidney disease (cyclosporin); pregnancy; high blood pressure; infectious disease.
The skin and senses				
Antifungals: nystatin; miconazole; ketoconazole; terbinafine; amorolfine; econazole.	Ringworm; athlete's foot; fungal nail infections.	Attack fungi.	Severe liver problems possible with ketoconazole; if taken orally—nausea, vomiting; secondary bacterial infections.	Orally—liver disease.
Corticosteroids: hydrocortisone; betamethasone; triamcinolone.	Allergies; eczema-type disorders.	Inhibit the body's reaction to damage or disease, so reducing inflammation.	Thinning of skin; worsening of infection.	Rosacea; acne; skin infections; psoriasis.
Decongestants: pseudoephedrine; xylometazoline; ephedrine.	Middle ear infections.	Dry up mucus secretions.	Dryness and irritation of nose.	High blood pressure.

DRUGS WITH GENERAL USES

Certain drugs are not formulated for a specific illness or condition but are used to treat a variety of disorders. Painkillers are the most commonly used drugs in this category. Antibiotics and antivirals are also used for a wide variety of infections to help the body's immune system fight the disease.

Drug	Use	Action	Side effects	Contraindications
Painkillers				
Opiate analgesics: morphine; diamorphine; opium; pethidine; methadone; codeine.	Severe, acute and chronic pain—heart attack, labour, cancer, kidney stones or gallstones. Moderate pain relief (eg, codeine).	Reduce the perception of pain and induce euphoria and drowsiness.	Constipation; slows breathing; nausea; lowered blood pressure; addiction.	Raised intercranial pressure; head injuries.
Simple analgesics: paracetamol.	Mild to moderate pain; fever.	Reduce the body's ability to appreciate pain; not an anti-inflammatory.	Mild skin rashes; overdose—severe liver and kidney damage.	Liver or kidney disorders.
Non-steroidal anti-inflammatories (NSAIDs): aspirin; ibuprofen; indomethacin; fenoprofen; naproxen.	Moderate pain; rheumatoid arthritis; osteoarthritis; muscular skeletal problems; gout; dysmenorrhoea; fever; headaches.	Inhibit inflammation, which irritates nerve endings and so causes pain.	Gastrointestinal disturbances; nausea; liver and kidney damage; headaches; peptic ulcers.	Peptic ulcer; asthma; blood clotting disorders; pregnancy; breastfeeding.
Fever reducers: aspirin; paracetamol.	High temperature.	Lower the body temperature by blocking the inflammatory effect of prostaglandins.	Nausea; indigestion; peptic ulcers. Aspirin may cause Reye's syndrome—do not give to children under 12 years of age.	Allergy to aspirin; liver or kidney disease; peptic ulcer; pregnancy.
Antibiotics				
Penicillins; cephalosporins; tetracyclines; sulphonamides; aminoglycosides; metronidazole.	Bacterial infections.	Find and destroy particular bacteria.	Nausea; vomiting; diarrhoea; allergic response; skin rashes; teeth stains.	Kidney problems; alcohol abuse; allergic reaction to a specific antibiotic; pregnancy (tetracyclines; sulphonamides; aminoglycosides)
Antimalaria				
Chloroquine; proguanil; pyrimethamine; mefloquine; quinine; halofantrine.	Prevention and treatment of malaria.	Seem to prevent the malaria-carrying parasite from reproducing.	Headaches; eye damage; ringing in ears. Mefloquine, rarely, headache, visual, psychiatric and neurological disturbances.	Epilepsy; early pregnancy; breastfeeding; liver or kidney disorders.
Antivirals				
Aciclovir; zidovudine; amantadine.	Cold sores; genital herpes; shingles; chickenpox; HIV; AIDS; influenza A.	Prevent the virus from multiplying.	Use on skin—slight dryness; stinging. Tablet form—nausea; headache; anaemia; insomnia; fatigue.	Anaemia; kidney and liver disorders; epilepsy; peptic ulcer.
Chemotherapy				
Cyclophosphamide; ifosfamide; vincristine; fluorouracil; etoposide; doxorubicin.	Cancers; malignancies.	Destroy cancer cells and inhibit their division; normal cells also affected.	Nausea; vomiting; hair loss; low immunity; bone marrow disturbance; sterility; life-threatening toxicity.	Pregnancy; when the severe toxic affects will not prolong or improve quality of life.

Chemotherapy

Cancer cells divide rapidly and this means that they may spread to other areas of the body via the bloodstream or lymphatic system. Chemotherapy aims to prevent this, employing "cytotoxic"—poisonous to cells—drugs that damage or kill cancerous cells. It may effect either a complete cure or a remission. Since cytotoxic drugs are not specific to cancer cells, and may affect non-cancerous cells, you need to know what to expect from a course of chemotherapy and how to deal with it.

Cancer cells are not the only fast-growing cells in your body. The cells of the blood-producing tissues in the bone marrow, the hair follicles, the digestive tract and the reproductive system all multiply rapidly. Most of the side effects of chemotherapy are caused by damage to cells in these areas. Other, less common, side effects may include diarrhoea, constipation, neuromuscular problems or kidney and bladder problems. The side effects, however, are mostly temporary and stop after the course.

COPING WITH CHEMOTHERAPY

Since chemotherapy has to be planned carefully so that it progressively destroys the cancer, but not the normal cells and tissue, the drugs are given over several weeks, with breaks in-between. Depending on the drug or drugs chosen, treatment will be divided into sessions, and each one can last from a few hours to a few days. Sometimes you may have to spend one or more nights in hospital.

During this extended period, it is important to try and minimize the disruption to your life and give yourself the best possible chance for the chemotherapy to succeed. To contend with fatigue, and feelings of lethargy and weakness—all common side effects—make sure you have plenty of rest at night and take time for short naps during the day. Arrange for help with household chores and childcare, and cut back on activities that could tire you.

You may feel faint and weak—chemotherapy reduces the production of red blood cells in

HOW THE TREATMENT IS DONE

Chemotherapy uses "cytotoxic" drugs to stop cancerous cells growing or multiplying. These are given in various ways: intravenously (injected into a vein); directly into a specific area through a catheter (a fixed line); orally (as pills, although not all drugs have an oral form).

The method chosen depends on the type and stage of cancer, the drugs prescribed, your age and general health. If you are not given oral drugs to be taken at home, you may have to attend a special outpatient clinic, or go into hospital if you need intensive treatment. The treatment is usually given in bursts to minimize the side effects and because normal cells have better recuperative powers than cancer cells. Intermittent courses of cytotoxic drugs allow normal cells such recovery time.

The best outcome (treatment success rates and happy patients) is found at centres specializing in cancer treatment, rather than district general hospitals where doctors may only treat a few cases a year.

The length of treatment and the dosages vary from person to person. An oral course may last one to two weeks, while intravenous injections may be once every three to four weeks.

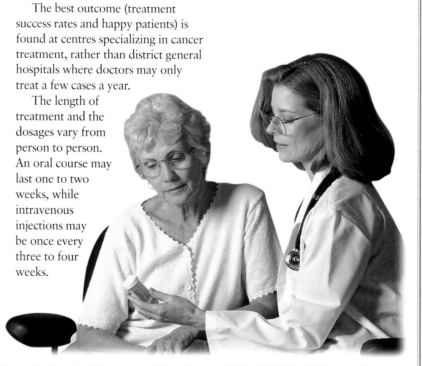

the bone marrow, which transport oxygen. A lack of these cells results in anaemia and low blood pressure. Make sure that your bath or shower is not too hot, and get in and out of it slowly. Take time to get up from a chair or out of bed.

Nausea and vomiting are the most common side effects of chemotherapy and your doctor may prescribe antinausea pills to minimize them. Although you may not want to eat, your body needs the nourishment of a balanced diet, rich in fresh fruit, vegetables and iron. Eat small amounts through the day rather than large meals and avoid takeaways, spicy or fatty foods. Drink plenty of fluids but not when eating, and don't eat before treatment.

If after a session you have an attack of vomiting, don't eat for a few hours and instead drink plenty of fluids in small amounts. Stay away from places where odours are strong—restaurants and perfume counters, for example—and use relaxation techniques to remove thoughts of nausea from your mind.

FIGHTING INFECTION

Chemotherapy drugs interfere with the production of the body's infection-fighting white cells. Your blood is monitored during treatment and if your white blood cell count falls too low, chemotherapy may be suspended or reduced to allow the bone marrow to recover.

Help your immune system by maintaining strict personal hygiene, and avoid animals, crowds and people who are ill with colds or flu or have recently been immunized. You should report any sign of an infection to your doctor immediately—fever, sweating, inflammation of the skin, sore throat, cough, vaginal discharge or itching. Cuts and abrasions are sites for infection so wear protective gloves when doing dirty chores, housework or gardening to prevent damage to your skin. The drugs can make your skin sensitive to sun, so cover up well.

Your mouth, gums and throat can be susceptible to sores that can become infected and bleed. Your mouth may feel dry and there is an increased risk that your teeth may develop cavities. Be strict with teeth cleaning, using a very soft toothbrush, and avoid commercial mouthwashes—many contain alcohol that makes the mouth even drier. Keep your mouth moist by eating chunks of fresh pineapple, or pineapple canned in fruit juice. Avoid tomatoes, oranges and grapefruit—they are too acidic.

HAIR LOSS

Certain anticancer drugs can temporarily damage the hair follicles, causing hair loss all over the body. The colour and structure of your hair may also change. Before treatment starts, have your hair cut short so it is easier to manage. Use a soft brush and mild shampoos to prevent scalp damage, avoid heated curlers and tongs, and use your hairdryer on its lowest setting. Your hair will grow back, but you can disguise its absence with a wig, a hat or scarf.

SIGNS TO WATCH FOR

Some chemotherapy drugs affect the bone marrow's ability to make platelets, the cells that help the blood to clot. During treatment you may bruise easily and a small cut may bleed profusely. Report to your doctor immediately signs such as nosebleeds that will not stop, a black colouring to the stools, blood in the urine or red spots under the skin. A blood transfusion may be needed if the platelet count drops too low. Do not take any over-the-counter medicines without checking with your doctor—many, such as aspirin, ibuprofen and paracetamol, affect platelet function.

FERTILITY PROBLEMS

Chemotherapy drugs can cause infertility in men and women. In women, they can damage the ovaries and affect the menstrual cycle. Fertility may return to normal after the treatment is stopped, but it may not. Before treatment starts you should know your options—for example, storing your eggs if you and your partner want to have a child after you have recovered. If you are having infertility treatment, it should be postponed until the chemotherapy course is completed. The drugs can also cause menopausal symptoms, such as hot flushes and vaginal dryness.

Anticancer drugs are also unsafe for a developing foetus. Always use contraception during chemotherapy. If you are pregnant, you will want to know what the implications are before starting chemotherapy, and what postponement might mean.

> ## ! Caution
>
> Do not take any other medicines at all during chemotherapy treatment unless they have been approved by your doctor, because they may clash with cytotoxic drugs. Report any severe or unexpected side effects to your doctor. Follow instructions precisely for taking oral therapy, and make sure that you do not miss a treatment session or doctor's appointment.

> ## Helping yourself
>
> Having cancer and being treated for it are both difficult. But there is much that you can do to help yourself—not only to cope with cancer but to put yourself in the best physical and mental shape to defeat it. Here are some suggestions:
>
> ♀ Try to keep a positive mental approach—cancer can be defeated in many cases.
>
> ♀ Practise relaxation techniques, such as deep breathing, meditation or visualization.
>
> ♀ Maintain your social life, but be careful not to exhaust yourself.
>
> ♀ Learn to say "no" to protect your energy levels.
>
> ♀ Continue to work if possible—or negotiate part-time hours for the course of your treatment.
>
> ♀ Keep time for and confide in your family, partner and friends.
>
> ♀ Join a self-help group for moral support.

Radiotherapy

Radiotherapy uses high-energy radiation (radioactivity) to attack malignant growths. Unlike chemotherapy, which affects the whole body, radiotherapy is a precise form of treatment that can be aimed specifically at the growth. Today, however, radiotherapy also encompasses electron-beam therapy and neutron therapy.

THE EFFECT ON CELLS

Radiotherapy is used to kill cancer cells while causing as little damage as possible to neighbouring normal cells. Cancer cells are particularly sensitive to radiation because they divide and grow quickly and, while normal cells are also affected by it, they have greater recuperative powers, so that many recover between treatments. Nevertheless, the damage inflicted on normal cells causes side effects, although the treatment itself is painless.

Radiotherapy is often used in conjunction with surgery or chemotherapy. It may be used before surgery or chemotherapy to shrink a tumour so that surgery can be less radical and chemotherapy more effective. After surgery or chemotherapy, it may be used to destroy any cancer cells that remain. Sometimes, you may be given radiotherapy during an operation or while receiving chemotherapy. Radiotherapy may also be given to ease the symptoms of advanced cancer, such as pain. How radiotherapy is used depends on the assessment of your condition and the treatment plan.

COPING WITH SIDE EFFECTS

The side effects of radiotherapy vary from person to person and also depend on which area is being treated: they can range from the mild to the acutely unpleasant. The most common are fatigue, loss of appetite, skin irritation over

WHAT TO EXPECT FROM A COURSE OF RADIOTHERAPY

A specialist doctor—a radiologist or radiation oncologist—decides on the type and dose of radiation and the precise area of the body to be treated. Most patients receive external radiation therapy: the waves of radiation are emitted from a machine and pass through

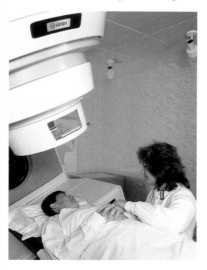

the skin to the site of the tumour. In some cases, an implant of radioactive material is positioned at the site of the tumour or you may be given a course of external radiation and then an implant.

External radiation treatment The first phase is a pre-treatment session, which can last anything from half an hour to three hours. The medical team works out exactly at what point, or port, the beam of radiation should enter the body, at what depth and for how long. Each port is recorded on your skin with an indelible marker, and sometimes a cast is made so that your body is in exactly the same position for each treatment session.

Treatment is usually given as an outpatient, every day for six to eight weeks, except weekends when the normal cells are left to recover. Shorter, more intensive courses, however, have been trialled recently

and found to be equally effective in some tumours. Areas of your body may be covered with protective shields. The session lasts up to an hour, although the radiation beam is only on for a few minutes.

Internal implant radiation treatment Implant therapy allows a high dose to be given to a limited area in a shorter time. Radioactive material is implanted, under general anaesthetic, into or close to the tumour. Alternatively, a radioactive substance is injected into the blood stream or a body cavity. While radiation is emitted you have to stay in a single room in hospital so that others are not exposed to it. However, the stay only lasts for a few days as the implant gradually loses its potency.

An implant may be kept in place for anything from a few minutes to a few days. Small implants may be left in place after you leave hospital.

the treatment area and emotional stress. There may also be local side effects—for example, radiotherapy to the head may cause hair loss on the scalp, but it will not cause other body hair to fall out; and treatment for breast cancer can cause a stiff shoulder, breast and nipple soreness and an increase or decrease in breast size.

HOW TO DEAL WITH FATIGUE

Most radiotherapy patients experience tiredness and a lack of energy. During radiotherapy, the body uses energy in the attempt to fight off the radiation and heal itself. At the same time, symptoms of the cancer, such as pain, a loss of appetite and stress compound the problem. However, much of the feeling of exhaustion fades at the end of treatment.

To help matters, have plenty of rest night and day. Cut out household chores. Ask for and accept help from friends and family. Take moderate exercise. Accept only those social engagements that you want to. Inform your employer of your treatment and choose whether to work full- or part-time or to take time off.

LOSS OF APPETITE

People undergoing radiotherapy tend to lose their appetite and with it a significant amount of weight each week. The problem is made worse if the cancer is in the digestive system as it may be difficult to chew, swallow or digest food. Your weight will be monitored during treatment and any difficulties with eating, or nausea, vomiting, constipation or diarrhoea should be reported to the medical team. It is important that you try to eat well, because studies have shown that people who maintain an adequate intake of food seem to cope better, both with the cancer and its treatment.

Eat small amounts often throughout the day rather than just at mealtimes. Maintain a well-balanced, varied diet—the dietician will tell you if you need to follow a special one. Add extra cream, cheese and butter to your food. Liquidize your food if swallowing is hard. Buy liquid diet supplements to increase your protein intake. Cook and store meals in the freezer (or get others to do so for you) so that you can eat whenever hunger strikes. Keep nibbles by your side—while watching television, for example. Cheer up meals with a glass of wine, but only with your doctor's permission.

SKIN CHANGES AND CARE

External radiation can make the skin red and sore as if after sunburn. After a few treatments it can feel dry and itchy. Any moistness should be reported to the medical team, because open sores could develop without treatment. You will be given guidelines about skincare and it is important that you follow these, because the skin becomes sensitive and fragile and susceptible to damage and infection.

Ask your doctor what products—talc, creams, sunblock and so on—you can use. Avoid stiff, tight clothing—soft, loose cotton is best. Do not scrub, scratch, rub or put a plaster on the affected area. Bathe in lukewarm water and avoid extremes of heat or cold. Keep the area out of the sun—wear a loose scarf or soft-based wig over the head. Continue with the same skincare regime after the treatment until your doctor tells you that you can change.

HANDLING EMOTIONAL STRESS

Being diagnosed with cancer and undergoing radiotherapy is frightening as you have to face the unpleasant side effects of treatment, the symptoms of the cancer itself and fear of the unknown. Make sure you keep informed about the nature of your disease, your treatment and its progress. Write down any questions that you want answered and take the list with you to your medical appointments. Join a self-help group of cancer sufferers or talk over concerns with someone you trust. Relaxation techniques can also help.

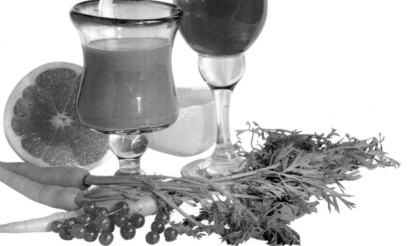

HEALTHY EATING
If swallowing is painful, liquidize fresh fruit and vegetables to make a delicious and revitalizing drink that you can sip.

Mental health therapies

There may be times in a woman's life when she needs extensive help and advice, for a long-term problem such as depression or addiction, or a crisis such as having a miscarriage or stillbirth, or being involved in a traumatic incident such as a train crash. The support of friends and family is invaluable in these situations, but sometimes it is important to seek out professional help.

There are many reasons why a professional can be the right answer for certain problems. A professional has been trained to listen, to be more objective than family or friends can be, which can give wider scope for discussion. He or she will probably have encountered your type of problem before and be able to use the experience to help you, as well as offering a repertoire of exercises and techniques to support you through difficult times.

HOW PSYCHOLOGICAL THERAPY CAN HELP

Psychological therapy and similar techniques are not only applicable to overtly mental distress. It is now widely recognized that the mind and body interact and that many disorders that manifest through physical symptoms have their primary cause in some psychological problem. This is the case with many stress-related disorders, such as irritable bowel syndrome (IBS) and anorexia. Equally, many physical disorders create mental distress, worry or fear, and the treatment of cancer, heart disease or chronic conditions such as lupus should include counselling from a professional. Finally, counselling should be available for those caring for others, for example coping with a family member with a terminal illness. It is vital that they should be able to talk to someone who is not involved.

PSYCHOLOGICAL THERAPY APPROACHES

Psychological therapy is a blanket term encompassing many approaches. Some of the most common are described below. Your doctor will be able to advise you on what may be the best for you and help you to find a therapist.

Psychoanalysis Based on exploration of the unconscious and childhood experiences, it is usually a long-term commitment. It aims to uncover the causes of the person's perceived inability to lead her life successfully.

Cognitive therapy This addresses your mental slant—the perceptions of yourself, your life and your beliefs (p. 46), and helps to restructure your thinking about them.

Behavioural therapy This is based on an analysis of behavioural patterns and on

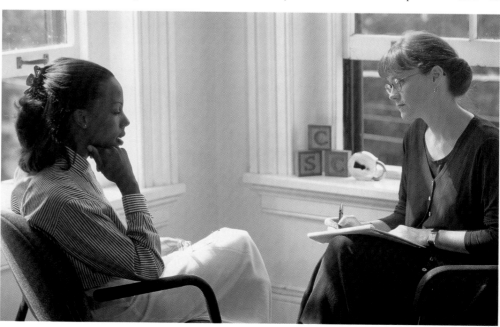

A THERAPY SESSION
The therapist gives you the time and a supportive space in which to explore and express emotions or discuss experiences that are causing you to feel depressed or anxious.

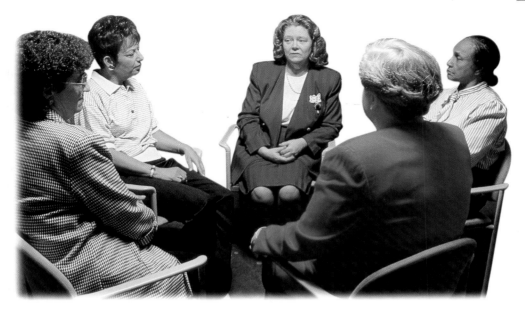

Group sessions are usually facilitated by a trained counsellor. It can be less stressful to be part of a group of people who have similar problems and can provide an environment of mutual support .

replacing those that are destructive with ones that are positive and purposeful.

Group therapies These include gestalt (focusing on the "here and now"), cognitive, behavioural, psychodrama, transactional analysis and encounter, which involves acting out current emotional conflicts and can be confrontational. Creative and movement therapies may be used in conjunction with other therapies. Creative therapies, either as part of a group or individually based, include music, dance (p. 296), drama and art. Through physical involvement in these pursuits, participants are encouraged to express themselves freely as part of healing.

Counselling Usually aimed at a particular cause of distress, such as losing a loved one or having a sexual problem, this is conducted through sessions of talking and listening. Many organizations such as colleges, hospitals, churches and charities may offer counselling, often without any charge. Counselling qualifications can vary, as can its application.

ONE-TO-ONE OR GROUP?

In addition to the different therapies available, therapists work in different ways—one-to-one, couple counselling, family counselling or in groups. One-to-one is best if you have a specific problem and need close personal attention from an individual session with the therapist. Couples and families often find that talking things through together can resolve difficult situations, although the process can be painful.

Some counsellors have specific training in dealing with particular problems, or special knowledge that can enable you to make difficult decisions. Areas covered include bereavement, rape, finances, dealing with children, physical and mental abuse, assertiveness, drugs and addiction, problems with study or work and medical issues such as infertility or cancer.

Counsellors will not tell you what to do or be judgmental. They aim to give you support and to provide pertinent information and helpful techniques that will give you the confidence to deal with your problem yourself. Many people find the presence of others with similar problems in group therapy supportive, especially in treating addictions or, for example, at Alcoholics Anonymous meetings.

HYPNOTHERAPY

Hypnotherapy (which uses hypnosis to "reprogramme" you through relaxation and concentration) and hypnoanalysis (a longer-term version that involves you recalling and releasing painful events from the past) can be useful for physical and mental problems. These include pain control (for example, when giving birth), weight control, migraines, blood pressure disorders, depression, skin complaints and addictions. Hypnosis may also be used for nausea control before chemotherapy.

Treating mental illness

Psychiatry and clinical psychology are medical treatments for mental illness. Many psychoanalysts train first in psychiatry.

Psychology is the scientific study of the mind. Researchers work in a wide variety of fields, including child development and human behaviour.

Serious mental illness such as schizophrenia, suicidal depression and mania are usually best treated initially with psychiatry. Psychiatrists can prescribe drugs; psychologists can't.

Mind and body medicine

Physical, emotional and mental life are inseparable and influence each other. Recognition of this has led to the development of a mind and body approach which can help women with their most common health concerns.

Combined with traditional medicine, the approach focuses on the whole person rather than simply the specific part that needs healing. Therapeutic programmes provide the psychological medicine that helps women cope with their anxiety, feelings of isolation and lack of control. Powerful techniques can be learnt to enable women to relax, to transform negative thought patterns and express their emotions. They are also encouraged to develop strong sources of social support in their communities.

WOMEN AND STRESS

Women are particularly vulnerable to a range of illnesses and conditions that stem from the reproductive system and can have an adverse effect on their way of life and relationships. It appears that the release of the stress hormone noradrenaline is interrelated with the release and activity of the sex hormones. So during those times when the body is undergoing hormonal changes, it may be particularly vulnerable.

Women with severe PMS have found that taking a serotonin reuptake inhibitor (for example, Prozac) can relieve feelings of stress. With the mind and body approach, the use of relaxation techniques taught by a therapist can do it as well, without the continuous use of a drug. The relaxation exercises apparently reduce the body's sensitivity to the action of noradrenaline. Similarly, the symptoms of the menopause such as hot flushes and low moods can be significantly relieved by relaxation, which again may be better for the body in the long term than HRT. Mind and body programmes have also been found effective in dealing with the anxiety and stress of infertility. Moreover, a significant proportion of women are able to become pregnant afterwards.

SOME WAYS TO START RELAXING

There are many different ways to help yourself relax. Here are five to try when sitting comfortably in a quiet place where you won't be interrupted. It takes from 15 to 25 minutes to appreciate the benefits.

1. As you breathe in, imagine the oxygen-rich air bringing the new to all parts of your body. As you breathe out, think of letting go of the old waste-filled air.

2. Place your feet flat on the ground. Concentrate on your feet and imagine them growing roots right down into the centre of the earth. As you breathe in draw up strength from the ground. As you breathe out send all the unhappiness in your life back down into the earth where it can be transformed into good energy. This takes your focus of attention out of your head so that your mind can rest.

3. Think of an inspiring word—like peace, love, trust, joy or pleasure—and repeat the word to yourself as you breathe in and out.

4. Imagine yourself in a beautiful place and try to sense everything about it—the sounds, smells, textures and sights.

5. Imagine yourself encased from head to toe in a sphere of sparkling white light, which protects and heals you.

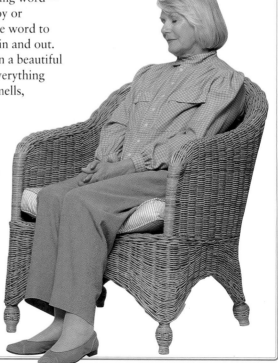

How to practise breath focus

This is the quickest way to bring about relaxation when you are facing a difficult situation or in an anxious frame of mind. The whole sequence takes about 20 minutes to complete.

♀ Take a normal breath. Don't change any aspect of how you breathe, but simply take note of your breathing.

♀ Now take a deep slow breath. Let the air come in through your nose and move deeply into your body. Take note of how the belly expands and don't try to stop it.

♀ Now breathe out through your mouth. (This is not a rigid rule. Breathe in whatever way is comfortable for you. If you find yourself getting anxious about the air in your lungs, stop the exercise for a minute or two and then try again.)

♀ Take one normal breath, and follow it with one deep, abdominal breath. Do this several times and note the differences between them, whether one makes you feel more relaxed than the other. Now take time to practise deep breathing, letting your belly expand with each inhalation.

♀ Then, on a long, slow exhalation, allow yourself to sigh. Repeat for several minutes then begin to imagine that with each out-breath all the tension and anxiety in your body go with it.

♀ Say to yourself: on inhalation, "I'm breathing in peace and calm"; on exhalation, "I'm breathing out tension and anxiety".

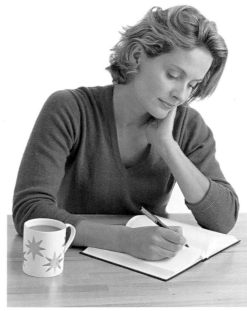

"Journalling" is one of the most powerful elements of mind and body medicine. Writing down your deepest thoughts and feelings about a traumatic event releases the stress that may otherwise provoke a physical illness.

RANGE OF OPTIONS

There are many different approaches to mind and body medicine. The one you take depends on what you are trying to solve and what suits you. Learning some of the easy physical positions and breathing exercises of yoga can help, maybe even cure, conditions such as PMS or anxiety-related disorders.

But if you have suffered a trauma such as a spinal injury, or are facing a major operation such as a hysterectomy, the answer may be more complex. Learning coping skills—such as self-nurturing or "journalling" (see above)—may only be part of your healing programme. Assertiveness training helps you to channel anger and frustration, and to transform a passive response into an assertive one (p. 47). Such training gives you communication skills to empower you to develop and sustain a rewarding network of relationships which may contribute to the recovery process. Mind and body medicine provides you with the tools to influence or change stressful situations.

BEHAVIOURAL THERAPIES

The idea of behavioural therapies derives from work on animals and the observation that animals can be persuaded to types of behaviour by rewards and dissuaded from others by negative stimuli. It is successfully applied to human problems when they involve self-destructive or antisocial behaviour—such as eating disorders, addictions, phobias and certain sexual habits.

The treatment involves gradually teaching the patient to stop automatically responding to their trigger in a particular and undesirable way—for example, an arachnophobe learns to stop going into an automatic flight response at the sight of a spider, the focus of her terror. Counter-conditioning links the stimulus to another—unpleasant—response. For example, the alcoholic can be given Antabuse, so she learns to associate alcohol with feelings of nausea.

Phobias can also be approached via systematic desensitization. For example, an arachnophobe may be confronted with a picture of a spider and will be encouraged to practise relaxation techniques (see opposite). She is then asked to assess her response to each successive stage of stimulation and relaxation.

! Caution

Don't be tempted to describe your emotions as "bad" or "good". If you find yourself being destructive with others because of your emotions, accept that you may need help to express yourself constructively. Expressing your emotions in this way benefits your mental and physical health.

Healing therapies

Hands-on healing is one of the oldest forms of treatment and is valued today for its role in mind and body medicine. Self-esteem, self-acceptance and self-worth are known to have parts to play in the healing process and a healer may bolster these in someone whose illness is traumatic or chronic. Spiritual healing, as it is called, may be available in hospitals, hospices and certain religious establishments.

Healers believe that when they place their hands on or just above the body of someone they can channel healing energy from its spiritual source to bring about subtle but profound changes. This charge of energy which comes not from but through the healer helps to restore the body's balance, activating the healing mechanism that the illness has disabled. This may not affect the actual physical problem, but it can increase the person's ability to cope with it.

SEEING A HEALER

Healing can be described as spiritual, faith, psychic and psi (parapsychological). Healers may be Christians or Buddhists, or they may have individual spiritual beliefs which you don't have to subscribe to. However, being open-minded and receptive to whatever is happening may provide the bridge you need between the problems you have and traditional treatment. You may feel worse before you feel better because pain and trauma that have been buried for years are coming to the surface before being released.

You may be asked to take your shoes off but otherwise you remain fully clothed. Some healers work with you lying down, with others you remain seated. They may work with crystals or colour (for example, bottles of coloured liquid or light boxes) as well as their hands.

You may feel nothing at all when receiving healing or you may experience sensations of warmth or pins and needles. After a session you can feel a little disoriented and it is generally recommended that you sit quietly with your eyes closed for a few minutes.

Many healers ask for donations only, others make a living from healing. Beware of anyone who charges high fees or guarantees a cure. Do not stop taking any prescribed medication.

REIKI

An ancient Tibetan Buddhist therapy, reiki (meaning "universal life energy") was rediscovered by the Japanese scholar Mikao Usui in the 19th century. The healing touch is passed from teacher to pupil in three degrees of training or "initiation", each of which involves you receiving "attunements" that enable you to use healing power. This power works via the chakras and can be transmitted to yourself or to others, even at a distance.

SHAMANISM

The most ancient form of human religious experience, shamanism is practised by indigenous peoples all over the world. Through such means as

---

CHAKRAS—HUMAN ENERGY WHEELS

Ancient Indian writings tell of points on the body where we take in and give out universal energy. In Sanskrit these are called "chakras" (pronounced "sharkrers"), which means "wheels", as the energy is sucked into the body spirally—rather like water going down the plughole.

Each chakra seems to relate to a gland of the endocrine system linking directly to the activities of hormones and different organs. As well, each chakra is associated with a layer of the aura and has physical, emotional, mental or spiritual aspects. In the healing process, each chakra is opened slowly by increasing the energy flow through it, but allowing time for whatever is released to be understood before moving on to the next.

The more energy that flows, the healthier the body. During meditation and visualization you can imagine drawing energy in through the chakras and sending accumulated debris flying out as your body is washed with light.

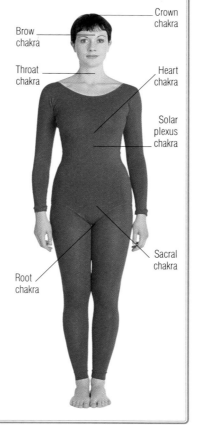

Crown chakra
Brow chakra
Throat chakra
Heart chakra
Solar plexus chakra
Sacral chakra
Root chakra

---

drumming, dancing, singing, isolation, fasting, sacred herbs or being in powerful places, the aim is to reach altered states of consciousness or trance and to heal yourself at a very deep level, by retrieving lost parts of your psyche or discovering your reason for being here. This type of healing has a particular appeal for older women who respond to sharing experiences.

SELF-HEALING

Self-healing uses the imaginative, creative and spiritual part of your nature through affirmation, visualization, prayer and meditation.

Affirmation means reprogramming yourself by turning negative thought patterns into positive ones. For example, if you constantly have the feeling that you are not good enough, your affirmation might be "I am perfect as I am". Write your affirmation on a piece of paper and carry it around with you, reading it and saying it out aloud to yourself whenever possible. Repeat it to yourself (out loud) while meditating or write it out repeatedly in regular sessions.

Visualization means using your imagination to create what you want in life. You turn your life into a story and work out what is stopping you being happy. Then you can rewrite the story so that it has a happy ending. Affirmation and visualization may be taught by counsellors and psychotherapists.

Prayer, because it is something you do by yourself at a quiet time and which occupies your mind, is a powerful way of centring yourself. You can consciously think of the good things you have in your life, and send love to yourself and to others who may need it.

THE AURA—HUMAN ENERGY FIELDS

According to Eastern tradition, the body is surrounded by layers of multi-coloured energy which can extend a few centimetres or even metres. Some healers can see the whole aura, up to seven or more layers. Most people can see the first layer, which is a narrow band of white light following the outline of the body. Try this experiment: hold two of your fingers a few centimetres apart against a plain surface and concentrate on the gap between. You may be able to see what appears to be a fine line outlining each finger. Pull your fingers gently apart and you can see the joined aura layers stretching.

Injuries, tension or pain, and emotional, mental or spiritual disharmony can be seen as dark spots or "blocks" in the aura, the layers of which relate in turn to the chakras.

There is another element to the aura. A vertical flow of energy travels up and down the spinal cord, extending well above the head and below the coccyx, like electrical power.

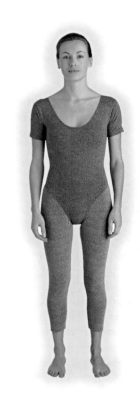

Biodynamic therapy

This form of healing works on both mind and body. It was developed by the Norwegian therapist Gerda Boyesen, who discovered the close connection in her patients between stress and the digestive system. The body cleanses itself through the digestive system but in times of stress this process is inhibited, causing both intestinal discomfort or pain and allowing the stress itself to be bottled up. The therapist works on two levels: by counselling (discussing your problems with you) and using massage (trying literally to eliminate the cause of the stress or blockage).

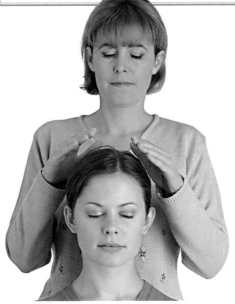

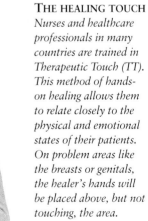

THE HEALING TOUCH
Nurses and healthcare professionals in many countries are trained in Therapeutic Touch (TT). This method of hands-on healing allows them to relate closely to the physical and emotional states of their patients. On problem areas like the breasts or genitals, the healer's hands will be placed above, but not touching, the area.

287

Physical therapies

The role of a physical therapist varies depending on what is to be remedied. A physiotherapist, for example, may work with various doctors to ease damaged joints or muscles. Therapists trained in massage techniques can assist the process of self-healing.

PHYSIOTHERAPY

A trained physiotherapist corrects or anticipates problems that arise from the body being put under pressure. Pregnancy, stroke and sports injuries are all areas of interest to a physiotherapist as are children suffering from cystic fibrosis or mobility disorders and women with some stress incontinence.

A physiotherapist knows the way the structures of the body are supposed to work and has various techniques available to either prevent or treat known disorders. The understanding of the vital role the muscles play in a women's reproductive system has helped the development of urogynaecology. For example, a pregnant woman, a new mother and a menopausal woman may all be referred by their doctor or by a hospital to a gynaecological physiotherapist for exercises to improve the tone of pelvic floor muscles and stop bladder leakage.

Physiotherapists work via manipulation (passive exercise) and taking the patient through exercises they can do themselves at home. Parents of children with cystic fibrosis will be taught by a physiotherapist how to clear their child's lungs of accumulating mucus, as will people with respiratory problems, such as chronic bronchitis or emphysema. In stroke treatment and hip or knee replacement the early involvement of a physiotherapist is essential, as it is post-operatively to help restore normal body function.

Other treatments include heat or ultrasound applied to damaged tissues such as strained ligaments, cold packs to reduce inflammation, and hydrotherapy in which patients with back or limb problems may move or be manipulated in a pool of warm water. This puts less pressure on their joints and supports their weight thus making movement and manipulation easier.

EXERCISE PHYSIOLOGIST

While a physiotherapist will treat sports injuries, an exercise physiologist aims to prevent them occurring. As a personal trainer, or advisor at a gym, a physiologist devises and supervises exercise regimes that meet the needs of the person—to lose weight, tone muscles, build stamina, for example—without causing harm. A physiologist will teach warm up and cool down stretches to prepare the body for the activities to come and to prevent lactic acid, a by-product of exercise, accumulating in the muscles after you stop your workout.

MASSAGE

As a conjunct to medical treatment or an exercise regime, massage has emotional as well as physical benefits. Massage therapists study anatomy and physiology as part of their training and use a range of hand movements to improve the circulation and flow of lymph to aid the immune system, tone muscles and smooth out knots in connective tissue. The main purpose

AROMATHERAPY AND SELF-HELP

Aromatic "essential oils", extracted from all the different parts of plants, have been used in the East for thousands of years. In the West aromatherapy, which means treatment with scents, uses these oils therapeutically to relieve stress-related complaints. A session takes about an hour and the therapist will ask you about your medical history, medicines you are taking, your lifestyle and smells you like or dislike. The purpose is to choose oils that are individual to you—each has a unique aroma and healing property— and to apply them into the skin with gentle massage. The healing characteristics of the oils can also be obtained through inhalation.

Inhalation A home remedy for coughs, colds, sinus problems.

♀ Fill a bowl with hot water, add four drops of essential oil (eucalyptus, lemon, lavender), cover your head with a towel and inhale for a few minutes at a time for up to 10 minutes.
♀ Put one or two drops on to a handkerchief or tissue and inhale when required.
Baths Add five drops of essential oil: lavender or ylang ylang to relax, basil or rosemary to stimulate, geranium to lift your spirits, clary sage to soothe emotions.

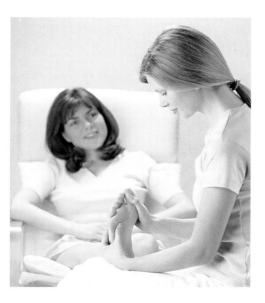

PROMOTING ENERGY FLOW
Massage of the hands and feet relates directly to the rest of the body through zones of energy similar to the channels or meridians of Eastern therapies. It is gentle and relaxing and can release blocked emotions.

is therapeutic, to encourage self-healing. It is relaxing and comforting and eases tension. The different types of massage are described right.

REFLEXOLOGY

Reflexologists use massage of the hands and feet to stimulate and balance energy flow through the body. Finger and thumb pressure on the points which reflect the body's 10 pathways or "zones" work directly on the body's organs. Reflexology has been found effective for stress, insomnia, headaches, back, neck and shoulder pain, bowel conditions, hayfever and asthma. Menstrual problems also respond well and it can help in childbirth, positioning the baby and speeding labour, and relieving anxiety, for example, in infertility or pre-operatively.

Your first visit should take about an hour. You take off only your shoes and socks and may sit or lie down. You may feel tenderness in certain spots—an indication of imbalance in the corresponding area of the body—but the treatment is quite gentle and very restful.

Vacuflex is a version of reflexology that uses felt boots and suction pads. The air is drawn out of the boots to create a vacuum, which gives the feet an all-over "squeeze" to stimulate circulation. The suction pads then apply pressure to reflex points on the feet, legs, arms and hands.

MASSAGE METHODS

Different types of massage may be called "body work", which involves touch, pressure and manipulation to restore the balance of mind and body and give a feeling of well-being.

Swedish massage

Classic Western massage, developed in the 19th century in Sweden. Therapeutic and good for relieving stiffness and tension.

Shiatsu

Japanese holistic massage applying pressure to points along the body's energy meridians. Called acupuncture without needles.

Rolfing

Originated in the US, it improves posture by stretching and pressing connective tissue and muscles. Can be quite intense.

Looyenwork

Deep precise pressure is used to stretch and lengthen muscles, allowing body to return to its natural balanced state.

Trager

A Western bodywork system using stretching, compression and rocking to release deep-seated emotional and physical tension.

Hellerwork

Of US origin, it uses manipulation and movement re-education to release tension, restore balance and improve vitality.

Thai (marma)

Rigorous treatment of the body's energy system with the therapist applying pressure with hands, elbows, knees and feet.

Tui na

Intense massage of neck, arms, hands or back from Chinese medicine. Good for neck, shoulder and back pain and migraine.

Indian head massage

Gentle treatment on upper back and arms, shoulders, neck, face and head. Improves hair and scalp condition and relieves tension.

Osteopathy and chiropractic

These two therapies concentrate on the musculoskeletal system but use different methods to relieve problems related to the spine, joints and muscles. They may both be used in conjunction with other treatment.

Osteopaths and chiropractors believe that bones can move out of position through misuse or injury. As a result of ageing or because we do not use our bodies enough, connective tissue (muscles, ligaments and tendons) can become weak or inflexible, upsetting the skeletal system. The most immediate effect is pain as muscles try to compensate and nerves are irritated. However, because the proper functioning of our body depends on the supportive framework provided by bones, the effects of these problems can be much wider.

Although both these therapies can help conditions seemingly unrelated to the musculoskeletal system, most people choose them for back and neck pain.

CHOOSING A PRACTITIONER

Osteopaths and chiropractors must have professional qualifications to practise. They diagnose as well as treat—which means that if they don't think they can help you and that you would be better off with a different sort of practitioner, they will say so. Although treatment is purely manual—no drugs or surgery are involved—some of the diagnostic techniques are similar to those of a conventional doctor. You should advise your doctor if you are interested in being treated by an osteopath or chiropractor and discuss any possible risks.

OSTEOPATHY

This treatment was developed in America at the end of the 19th century. Practitioners use various techniques of which the most important is deep tissue massage. This can be combined with manipulation and "thrusts"—sudden movements that click bones back into place. It should not be painful though you may feel stiff for a time after a session. Another gentle technique, cranial osteopathy (see box, right), is used on children or people who are frail.

Osteopaths can treat soreness and stiffness as well as severe pain, and acute as well as chronic cases. You can also see an osteopath for a regular check-up. It is a recognized therapy and you can be referred by your doctor. Even if an osteopath can't cure a problem (for example, rheumatoid arthritis which is a disease of the immune system) osteopathic treatment may reduce pain and, in time, increase your range of movement.

As well as the back and neck, osteopaths treat other areas of the body such as the feet, knees, hips, hands and arms—for example, they will try to relieve the pain of tennis elbow or repetitive strain injury and advise on preventing recurrence. They will treat acute injuries such as those from sports or car accidents (whiplash). Headaches may be helped as they can result from muscular tension and bad posture. Pregnancy, childbirth and carrying around a baby or toddler can place a lot of strain on the back and joints and osteopathy can be beneficial. In addition, osteopaths say a range of other problems may respond to osteopathy treatment: premenstrual syndrome (PMS), dizziness, recurrent sinusitis, asthma, digestive problems and glue ear (in children).

CHIROPRACTIC

Unlike osteopathy, chiropractic treatment largely concentrates on the spine and makes greater use of manipulation and thrusts in order to

GENTLE MANIPULATION
An osteopath's treatment is based on massaging deep tissue in the muscles, using hands and fingers, and manipulating the joints which are not working as they should.

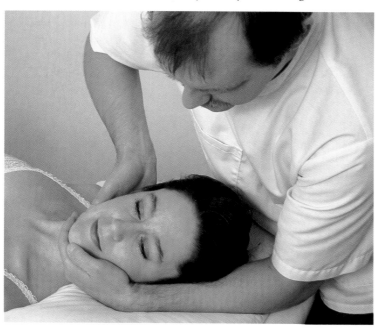

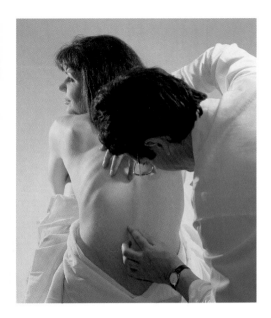

FUNCTION AND BALANCE
Chiropractic was developed at the end of the 19th century by a Canadian healer who believed the body will heal itself if attention is paid to the functioning of the nervous system. Now it is an established medical therapy in many parts of the world.

bring the body back to its proper balance. Chiropractors must complete a five-year medical training before they can practise.

They use conventional diagnostic techniques and many have X-ray machines on site (though X-rays are not taken if a woman is pregnant). Visits tend to be short (45 minutes for a first visit, 20 minutes for later ones) and treatment may not begin until the second appppointment. Basic to treatment is the chiropractic couch which can be placed at different angles to increase the effectiveness of treatment. The practitioner will decide how many treatments will be needed; the average is five.

WHAT YOU CAN EXPECT

At your first visit you will be asked about your symptoms, medical history, as well as details of your daily life—whether you drive a lot or sit at a desk all day, how much you exercise. The practitioner will want to see the way you stand and move, and may test some of your reflexes. An important part of diagnosis is examination by touch—feeling your muscles, ligaments and range of movement. An X-ray, blood test or urine analysis may be suggested. You may be asked to undress down to your underwear, but

RELATED PHYSICAL THERAPIES

There are other types of physical manipulation or massage that work on different conditions. You should check out qualifications before agreeing to a course of therapy.

Cranial osteopathy

A combination of extremely gentle touch and massage on the bones of the skull. It can be done in conjunction with osteopathy.

Sacrocranial osteopathy

The therapist focuses on the pulsations within the fluid which cushions the brain and the spinal cord, feeling for them and working on them by placing her hands on or just above the surface of your body. It is good for sensitive or painful conditions.

Zero balancing

A deeply relaxing technique developed by an osteopath/acupuncturist which uses gentle finger pressure and held stretches to enable you to release physical and emotional tension.

Polarity therapy

An amalgam of Ayurvedic and Western ideas, using manipulation, touch, stretching postures, diet and counselling. It is a gentle therapy with many women practitioners.

Bowen technique

A modern therapy developed by an Australian osteopath which uses rolling-type moves with fingers and thumbs to work on the body's soft tissue (muscles, ligaments) and the energy pathways. It is fast acting. Therapists may treat respiratory conditions, chronic fatigue, hayfever, headaches, kidney problems and lymphatic drainage as well as musculoskeletal problems.

McTimoney and McTimoney-Corley

Gentle, more holistic forms of chiropractic. They are named after their British originators and treat the whole body, using light rapid tapping movements instead of manipulation. X-rays are not used.

a gown should be offered. You may feel sore or stiff after a session as parts of the body are brought back into use, and you may find pain increases for a day or two. In acute cases you may need several weekly sessions and you may be given exercises to do between treatments.

COMPLEMENTARY THERAPIES

There may be a need, at different times and stages of your life, to discover ways of getting in touch with the inner person, to be able to use the strength of your mind to improve your physical health and well-being. In some instances it may enhance conventional treatment.

Relaxation and guided imagery

Two techniques to use together, relaxation and guided imagery help you to calm tension in your body while you conjure up attractive images to still worries in your mind. Once learnt, they enable you to counter the stress you feel, get things in proportion and remain confidant despite setbacks. They are "mindful" techniques that stop you carrying tension without realizing it, that make you aware of the present and the pleasures it holds.

Relaxation is an acquired skill that you can call on in any situation which stresses you. The methods you use will be the ones you find easiest to do (p. 284). You may choose breath focus, for example, in which you pay attention to your breathing while concentrating on muscle tension in those parts of the body where stress shows—such as the forehead, the jaw, the neck, back, shoulders and stomach. Think of the muscle as you inhale, let go of the tension in it as you exhale. As the frown lines go, the jaw unclenches, the neck relaxes and you start to feel the effects. It may be something to practise as you go to sleep.

Progressive muscle relaxation (PMR) is similar, but you increase the degree of muscular tension before you relax and let go. It is particularly helpful for women who have hyperactive minds, who are showing stress from too much happening in their lives, or women who

have wide mood swings from premenstrual syndrome (PMS). But you need to take time to practise it. After a few minutes of deep breathing, you focus on each muscle in your body, starting from the top and working down (or down, and working up if you prefer) and deliberately stay there mentally until you feel relaxed in that part. It may be a way to prepare yourself for meditation which can lead to a profound sense of calmness in mind and body.

Body-oriented methods of relaxation might not suit women with eating disorders or with chronic pain (from endometriosis, migraine or skeletal problems), as they focus your attention too closely on the source of the pain or physical distress and therefore may be counterproductive. However, guided imagery may provide the answer.

It involves you taking time out in an imaginary place, applying mindfulness—raised awareness—to sights, sounds and colours you "see" there. You can feel the warmth on your skin, smell the flowers, appreciate the hues of a sunset or the gentle lapping of waves on the sand. You close your eyes, see the image and become calm.

Another image encourages you to see your medication at work in the body destroying the disease—acting like a machine gun on a tumour, for example, or imagining the drug as an army attacking a mass of abnormal cells.

LEARN TO RELAX
By using your muscles and your mind you can let the tension in your body go and be replaced by calmness and a sense of inner peace.

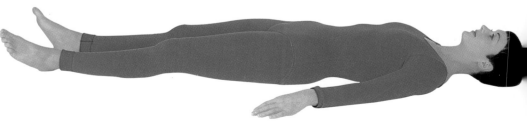

Yoga and visualization

A gentle, noncompetitive form of physical and mental exercise which is suitable for all ages and levels of fitness, yoga originated in India at the same time as Ayurvedic medicine. It has many strands—Hatha, Raja, Ashtanga, Kundalini, Tantric—all of which encourage full use of your lungs so that energy, vitality and blood circulation are improved. The form of yoga best known in the West is Hatha, which consists of asayanas (physical postures), pranayamas (breathing techniques) and relaxation or meditation that leaves you feeling revitalized. It works on every single part of the body, including internal organs, and aims to create suppleness rather than stamina and promote a balanced mental outlook.

It is ideal for people already suffering from physical problems or just starting to exercise, as each works at her own pace and the postures range from the extremely simple to the more demanding. With your doctor's consent, it is perfectly safe in pregnancy—in fact in the third trimester it may be of great use in cases where the baby is breech, encouraging flexibility in the muscles and relaxation in the mother (so the baby may find the room to turn). Yoga breathing prepares the body for pain control during contractions and keeps muscles toned for pelvic floor exercises after birth.

TAKING UP YOGA

It is best to learn yoga from an experienced teacher initially as it can be difficult to understand the postures from a book. A teacher will be able to gauge your level of fitness and stop you undertaking anything that might cause a strain. It is important to learn to relax properly at the end of a session, for example, something you might be tempted to skip unless you understand more fully what yoga is about. To gain the full benefits it is best to practise a little at least every other day, but even a weekly class can make a difference.

No special clothes are needed—just wear something you can bend and stretch in, leggings for instance, and a T-shirt. A mat is necessary—special nonslip yoga mats are available, but a rug or blanket is fine to start with. Leave an hour or two between a meal and starting a yoga session and don't drink immediately before.

Alpha-wave biofeedback

In biofeedback a person with an illness is linked to monitors which translate their heart rate, blood pressure, muscle tension or brainwave activity into sounds or video images that can be easily interpreted. The biofeedback therapist teaches the patient to use mental means to have some degree of control over previously unconscious processes—by helping them to recognize the subtle shifts in brain alpha waves, heart rate and electrical activity on the skin. It is especially useful in relaxation training as the patient can learn to control these factors without being linked to the machines. Biofeedback sessions may benefit people with eating disorders, hypertension, migraine headaches, addictions related to anxiety, and spinal injuries.

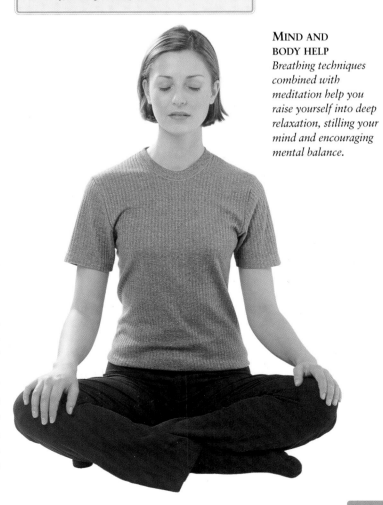

MIND AND BODY HELP
Breathing techniques combined with meditation help you raise yourself into deep relaxation, stilling your mind and encouraging mental balance.

Postural therapies

Alexander Technique, the Feldenkrais Method and Pilates (pronounced *pilartis*) are all concerned with posture. Often recommended by doctors for people with bad backs, these therapies are also excellent for preventive health care, confidence and relaxation.

THE ALEXANDER TECHNIQUE

This therapy teaches people to be aware of the way they use or misuse their bodies so that they can avoid habitual tension and move in an effortless, graceful way.

Frederick Alexander was an Australian actor who started to lose his voice during performances. When doctors were unable to uncover the cause, he decided to observe himself in the mirror while reciting and noticed that he habitually tensed his neck muscles. This affected his breathing and consequently his voice. By constantly checking and correcting himself, he was able to perform in a more natural way, and began to teach others to do the same.

We develop physical tension for several reasons. As children we pick up bad postural habits from slouching or from sitting for long periods at badly designed desks. We breathe shallowly, rather than using the entire extent of our lungs. Many of us have jobs that force us to spend many hours in positions contrary to the natural shape and movement of the body. As a result, we may lose touch with our bodies and fail to recognize the stress we are placing on them.

SEEING A TEACHER

In an Alexander Technique lesson your teacher assesses how you are misusing your body and will gently encourage it to assume the correct position. At first you may find the natural position much more difficult to sustain than the tense one. Among our common bad habits is tilting one way or the other, or holding the head too far forward. As the teacher corrects this you may feel you have tilted the other way or that your head is thrust back. You are in the process of being reeducated. Emphasis is placed on the position of the head, neck and spine as Alexander felt that if these are positioned correctly, everything else follows naturally.

BENDING AND LIFTING
At home or at work, even young and fit people can get aching bones and muscles from lifting and bending incorrectly. Here, correctly, the back is kept straight while the push is exerted by the legs.

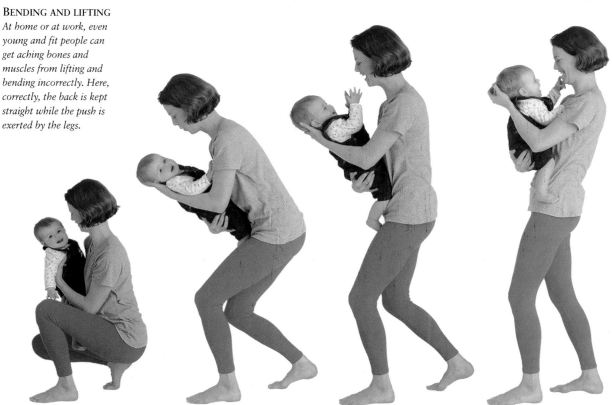

Reeducating the body takes time. The recommended number of Alexander Technique lessons is at least 10 and preferably as many as 30. Lessons are one-to-one and last about 45 minutes. They start with simple movements such as walking, sitting and lying down and progress to more complicated ones.

Instruction is a combination of demonstration by the teacher of what you are doing, discussion between the two of you and gentle guidance by the teacher with her hands. You remain fully clothed but take your shoes off. You should wear your normal clothes because this gives the best picture of your everyday range and type of movement.

WHO IT CAN BENEFIT

Anyone can benefit from Alexander Technique lessons as we all hold tension in our bodies, even if we think we have good posture. Being tense uses up energy and releasing tension can give you new vitality and a sense of lightness.

Many people find they grow taller as they stop "crunching" their spines, or wider as their shoulders stop hunching forward and their ribcage expands to its proper shape. The technique is popular with musicians, actors and athletes for enhancing performance and reducing fatigue. Musicians in particular spend many hours with their bodies twisted out of alignment as they play their instruments, and can be shown ways of minimizing this distortion and restoring their posture. Singers and actors who have to project their voices need to feel that their chests and neck muscles are relaxed rather than tense.

Alexander Technique is best known as a cure for back and neck pain but can help other joint pain, headaches and migraines. People with respiratory disorders such as asthma, digestive disorders like irritable bowel syndrome, and high blood pressure may benefit from a course of Alexander lessons. The technique can also relieve mental and emotional problems like anxiety or depression. The Alexander Technique does not aim to be a quick fix. The intention is to give you good habits to last a lifetime and help you cure your own problems.

THE FELDENKRAIS METHOD

Moshe Feldenkrais was a physicist and judo expert who taught himself to walk again after crippling knee injuries. His experience led him

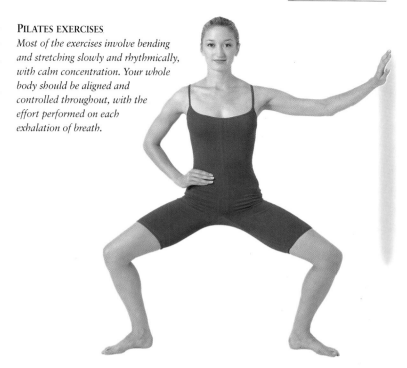

PILATES EXERCISES
Most of the exercises involve bending and stretching slowly and rhythmically, with calm concentration. Your whole body should be aligned and controlled throughout, with the effort performed on each exhalation of breath.

to develop a method to help anyone with movement difficulties. While the Alexander Technique uses an external ideal of posture, the Feldenkrais Method puts you in touch with your nervous system to find the best posture for you. It does not emphasize the head/neck/spine relationship of the Alexander Technique, but seeks to discover the imbalance upsetting the rest of the body and teaching you how to adapt. Teaching is in groups or individually.

Like the Alexander Technique, Feldenkrais is helpful for joint pain, but can also be effective in dealing with central nervous system conditions such as multiple sclerosis, cerebral palsy and stroke. The purpose of training is to show you how to expand your options, to find new ways of moving and breathing so you can live more fully, efficiently and comfortably.

PRACTISING PILATES

Pilates grows ever more popular because its exercises help you develop a leaner, longer line by strengthening the deep postural, abdominal muscles. The exercises are performed following the six principles of concentration, breathing, control, centring, flowing movement and precision. Like the Alexander Technique, Pilates is much used by dancers because it promotes graceful and balanced movement.

> **! Caution**
>
> To avoid strain and injury, try to change position frequently. If you have to stand for long periods of time, position one leg behind the other with the feet at about 45 degrees to each other and your body weight resting mostly on the rear leg. Try to keep in contact with the ground through all three points of balance on the feet: the heel, the ball and the big toe.
>
> When sitting, keep your feet in contact with the ground. If you have to lean forward, do it from the hips so that your back and shoulders are straight. Get up from time to time and move around.

Movement therapies

SLOW MOVEMENT
*Gradually and with
concentration, you can
balance the flow of
energy and achieve
equanimity with t'ai chi.*

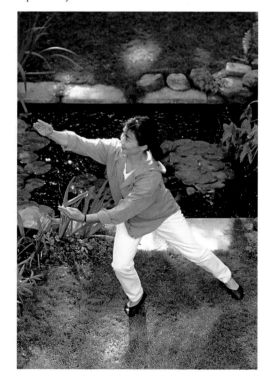

Self-help exercise systems from Asia work on your "vital energy"—chi—and its pathways in your body, seeking to find natural harmony around and within you and harnessing it.

Movement therapies originating in the Western world can help women with medical conditions express emotions such as anger, which can aid the healing process. These therapies do not need any knowledge of dance and can be adapted to varying levels of fitness or special needs. All movement therapies seek to release stress and harmonize mind and body.

T'AI CHI CHU'AN

More commonly known as t'ai chi (pronounced *tie chee*), this therapy consists of a series of movements linked together into one flowing sequence. It can be performed by people of all ages and levels of fitness.

T'ai chi was originally developed in China in the 11th century to mitigate the aggressive nature of martial arts. It aims to harmonize your yin and yang (feminine and masculine qualities) and balance the flow of energy through the body. The graceful actions do not require strength and are performed fairly slowly. This, combined with the concentration needed to remember each movement, helps take your mind off your problems. It is a calming antidote to stress and stress-related illness, helping to clear mental blocks.

You need to learn t'ai chi in a class. It may take six months of classes to learn the movements, but you will start to feel the benefits immediately because the sequences affect every muscle, tendon and joint. You should practise for at least 10 minutes a day at home. It does not increase your heart rate or make you breathless, but you may sweat from the heat your chi is generating. You will feel your posture, balance, breathing and circulation improve.

CHI KUNG

Also written "qigong", and pronounced *chee goong*, this ancient practice is gaining in popularity over t'ai chi because it is simpler to learn. There are many exercises, all of which involve meditation, controlled breathing (see box, opposite), deceptively simple postures and movements and visualization of chi as it moves in the body. It was developed specifically for healing and in China today is often included in hospital aftercare to speed recovery and to help patients whose illnesses may not have responded to other forms of medicine.

DANCE MOVEMENT THERAPY

Dance movement is a nonverbal form of psychotherapy which helps a wide variety of people, some simply interested in self-development, others who are emotionally disturbed or who have physical and mental illness. The therapy can work on an individual or group level; either way you will probably see the therapist on your own to start with. Therapists work both privately and within health, education and social services departments.

Dance movement therapy is particularly helpful for people with severe behavioural problems or for those whose feelings are too deep or complicated to put into words. It can be useful for those who are blind or deaf or have learning disabilities. It may also be beneficial for stress-related physical illness.

GABRIELLE ROTH'S FIVE RHYTHMS

Gabrielle Roth is a proponent of experimental dance and theatre working in the United States. The key to her work is spontaneity—in workshops using her methods you are encouraged to express yourself freely through dance. The goal is to put you back in touch with your body and to liberate your natural creativity and joy.

Five different types of music or rhythms are used. These are flowing, staccato, chaotic, lyrical and still. Workshops may last for one day or consist of a course performed in groups.

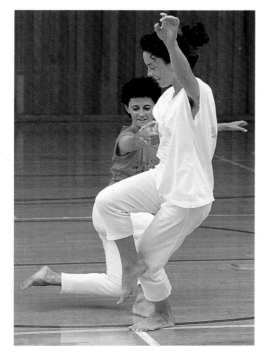

EXPRESS YOURSELF
The enjoyment of music and rhythm can unlock energy while stimulating and balancing the body. Dance movement *therapy is a valuable treatment for a range of conditions, physical or mental, and can provide relaxation for women of all ages.*

Additional workshops may offer spontaneous poetry writing, painting or drama.

BIODANZA

This dance therapy comes from South America where it was developed by a professor of medicine to help people emotionally and physically. Work is done in groups because improving your relationship with other people is part of the therapy. Dance exercises focus on five basic modes of living: your integrity and vitality; sensuality and sexuality; creativity and your ability to change; affectivity or your capacity to love; and finally transcendence—the expansion of consciousness and sense of ecstasy.

MEDAU

The aim of this dance therapy is to produce a strong, lithe body at ease and in harmony with itself. The movements are rhythmic and dynamic, without jerky repetitions or overstretching. Medau has been adapted to help problems such as back pain, arthritis, Parkinson's disease, high blood pressure, heart and psychiatric disorders.

LEARN TO STAND AND RELAX

Standing with good, relaxed posture is at the heart of chi kung (qigong). By "centring" your weight on your frame and calming yourself with breathing you won't waste energy by holding unnecessary tension inside. Once learned, it helps you carry out actions using energy economically while gaining access to the unlimited source of energy within. Begin by doing the exercise for a few minutes at a time.

Imagine you are hanging from the crown of your head like a puppet on a string and that all your tension is sinking downward and going out through your feet. Concentrate on each of the elements shown below until they become second nature.

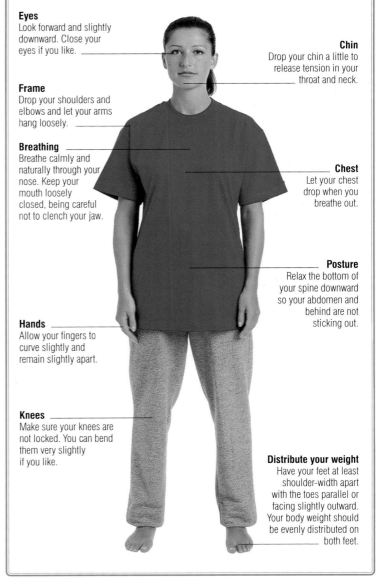

Eyes
Look forward and slightly downward. Close your eyes if you like.

Frame
Drop your shoulders and elbows and let your arms hang loosely.

Breathing
Breathe calmly and naturally through your nose. Keep your mouth loosely closed, being careful not to clench your jaw.

Hands
Allow your fingers to curve slightly and remain slightly apart.

Knees
Make sure your knees are not locked. You can bend them very slightly if you like.

Chin
Drop your chin a little to release tension in your throat and neck.

Chest
Let your chest drop when you breathe out.

Posture
Relax the bottom of your spine downward so your abdomen and behind are not sticking out.

Distribute your weight
Have your feet at least shoulder-width apart with the toes parallel or facing slightly outward. Your body weight should be evenly distributed on both feet.

ALTERNATIVE MEDICINE

Different systems of diagnosis and care have been practised around the world for centuries. They embrace different approaches to healing the body and maintaining health. Generally their aim is holistic— to treat the whole person as an individual, and not just her symptoms.

Herbal medicine

Herbal medicine is the oldest form of medicine known. More than 80 percent of the world's population has used herbs for health. In properly qualified hands, herbalism can be a safe and effective therapy.

However, it is often not known why a particular herb produces its effect and some should not be used in pregnancy or given to children. You should consult your doctor as well as a herbalist practitioner before trying herbs.

Herbal medicine uses plant material from around the world in the treatment of ailments. All parts of the plant—stems, leaves, roots and seeds—may be used by herbal practitioners, who regard the active ingredients of each as useful in preventing or treating illness. Medical herbalists always look at the patient's habits, lifestyle and overall well-being to find and treat the underlying cause of any problem, not just the symptoms. Remedies are tailored to the individual rather than the disease, so no two prescriptions are likely to be the same.

> **Caution**
> Over-the-counter herbal remedies can be taken for minor complaints for short periods of time. Never treat yourself if you are pregnant or breastfeeding. Read any instructions or warnings on the packaging to ensure that the remedy is not counterproductive. Never self-prescribe herbal remedies.

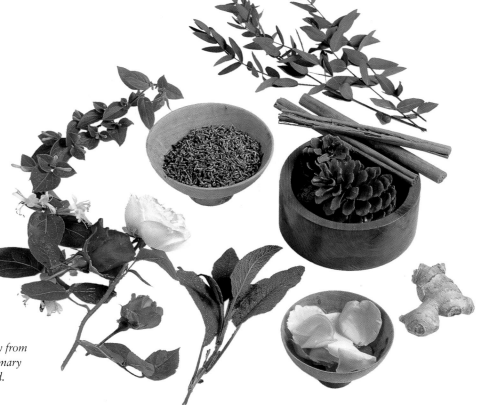

THE OLDEST MEDICINE
Herbs have been used medicinally from ancient times and are still the primary source in many parts of the world.

THE WONDER OF PLANTS

Many pharmaceutical drugs are extracted from plants or contain synthesized versions of substances found naturally in plants. However, herbalists believe that giving the whole plant is safer and more effective than prescribing an isolated chemical.

Plants contain other substances apart from the active one and these either enhance its action or prevent side effects. For example, the drug ephedrine, used in conventional medicine to treat asthma, also raises blood pressure. But the plant from which it comes contains a substance which prevents a rise in blood pressure. Herbalists believe the digestive system has evolved to cope with plants, and introducing an artificial substance to a sick body increases the stress it is under. This can in turn weaken the person and lead to more illness later.

WHAT THEY CAN TREAT

Herbs can be used to treat almost any condition, acute or chronic. Complaints commonly taken to herbalists include skin problems such as psoriasis, acne and eczema, and digestive problems such as ulcers, colitis, irritable bowel syndrome (IBS) and indigestion.

They can also treat hormonal and gynaecological disorders—premenstrual syndrome (PMS), endometriosis, infertility or problems connected with the menopause, pregnancy problems and postnatal depression—and circulation disorders such as varicose veins or hypertension. Be careful about what you take since some herbs decrease fertility. Other conditions they can help include arthritis, migraine, headaches, hayfever, asthma, insomnia and stress, and infections such as flu and tonsillitis.

SEEING A HERBALIST

Your first visit to a herbalist may take at least an hour. He or she will want to find out all about your symptoms and state of mind as well as what you eat and the sort of life you lead. You may also be given a physical examination, similar to that conducted by a family doctor, to obtain a blood pressure reading, to test your reflexes or to assess the condition of your heart or lungs.

Treatment can take a variety of forms. The most common is a tincture, which is a herbal extract preserved in alcohol which you take as drops. You may be given dried herbs which you

FLOWER REMEDIES

These are diluted infusions of wild plants for the self-treatment of emotional symptoms. They are safe to take and can be used by children as well as adults. You will find flower remedies in natural health stores.

The original and best known remedies are those developed by the English doctor and homeopath Edward Bach (pronounced *batch*) in the 1930s, but there are now some two dozen producers of infusions worldwide.

The following are examples of Bach Flower Remedies:
Rescue Remedy A combination of five remedies for treating shock or to comfort and calm at times of particular stress (it is also available as a cream).

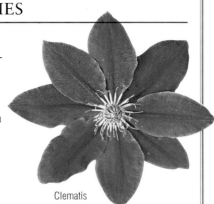

Clematis

Clematis For inattention, dreaminess, absent-mindedness or mental escapism.
Elm For when you feel overwhelmed by inadequacy and responsibility.
Larch For lack of self-confidence, feelings of inferiority and fear of failure.
Walnut Assists during adjustment to change such as the menopause or divorce.

brew in the same way as tea to make an infusion or you may be asked to make a decoction, in which you boil tough material such as roots and bark and then strain and drink the liquid. Infusions and decoctions can taste very strange. Tablets, suppositories, creams or ointments may also be prescribed.

HEALING TOGETHER

You may be asked to change your diet or to make some adjustments to your lifestyle, such as getting more exercise or giving yourself time to relax. As with all alternative medicine, healing is a matter of teamwork between you, the therapist and the treatment. The aim is to restore the body's natural balance, which is called homeostasis.

The follow-up appointment will be shorter and may occur two weeks later, with further visits at monthly intervals, if they are necessary. You can often combine herbal treatment with conventional drugs, but make certain that both your doctor and your herbalist know that you are doing this.

Homeopathy

> **! Caution**
> While being treated it is best not to eat or drink strong-tasting substances such as chilli, coffee or peppermint, or to have alcohol or take any other medication, because all can interfere with the remedy's effect. Special types of toothpaste are available in natural health shops for use while receiving homeopathic treatment.

In use for more than 200 years, homeopathy is still one of the more popular alternative medicine approaches. It can be used to treat people of all ages. Many homeopaths are conventional family doctors who also offer regular holistic healthcare.

Homeopathy is based on the principle that "like cures like". In other words, something that causes symptoms in a well person can also cure the same symptoms in someone who is sick. This is somewhat similar to the principle behind vaccinations. However, because of the way they are prepared, homeopathic remedies are so greatly diluted they contain no chemical trace whatsoever of the active substance and are therefore safe. They were developed at the end of the 18th century by a German doctor, Samuel Hahnemann, after he became disillusioned with the medical practices of his time.

HOMEOPATHIC REMEDIES

Remedies are prepared from plants, minerals and animal substances (such as insects, snake venom and cuttlefish bone). The substances are steeped in liquid which is then drained off and diluted many times until there is so little left of the original substance that it is not detectable scientifically. With each dilution the liquid is "succussed"—shaken vigorously—which causes an "energy imprint" of the original substance

to be left in it. This imprint works on the body's own energy system, boosting its natural healing responses.

There are about 3,000 remedies and finding the correct one can be complicated. Remedies are chosen because the substances in large doses would cause precisely the sort of symptoms from which you are suffering. The practitioner will need to take into account the nature of all your symptoms, physical and emotional.

He or she will also need to find out all about you and your personality and may prescribe a "constitutional" remedy, which is geared specifically to your particular physical and mental constitution and designed to give you an overall boost. Usually a homeopath prescribes one remedy at a time.

TAKING THE REMEDIES

Remedies are generally given as pills, which are allowed to dissolve on or under the tongue. You should not touch the pills with your fingers but put them directly on your tongue from the packet or tip them into your mouth from the lid and then suck them. You should not eat or drink for 15 minutes before and 15 minutes after taking the remedies.

Sometimes your symptoms will worsen for a short period of time when you start the remedies. In homeopathic terms, this indicates that

BIOCHEMICAL TISSUE SALTS

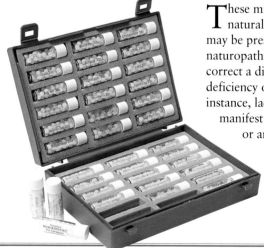

These mineral salts, found naturally in the human body, may be prescribed by homeopaths, naturopaths and herbalists to correct a disease caused by deficiency of one of them. For instance, lack of calc phos can manifest itself as teeth problems or an inability to absorb nutrients. There are 12 biochemical tissue salts, taken in highly diluted combinations of two or more.

calc fluor (*calcium fluoride*)
calc phos (*calcerea phosphorica*)
calc sulph (*calcium sulphate*)
ferr phos (*iron phosphate*)
kali mur (*potassium chloride*)
kali phos (*potassium phosphate*)
kali sulph (*potassium sulphate*)
mag phos (*magnesium phosphate*)
nat mur (*natrium muriaticum/
    sodium chloride*)
nat phos (*natrium/sodium phosphate*)
nat sulph (*natrium/sodium sulphate*)
silicea (*silica*)

your body's defences are being stimulated. Homeopathy works from the inside out, and often external symptoms—such as those involved in a skin complaint—can be the last to clear up. You may even find that your symptoms reverse themselves. For example, if your hayfever started as itchy eyes, proceeded to sneezing and then attacked your chest, the symptoms may recur in reverse order as you start to get better.

If you are taking any form of conventional medicine, make sure that you tell your doctor and your homeopath about treatments in case of possible interactions.

SOME COMPLAINTS AND THEIR REMEDIES

Homeopaths maintain special pharmacies which provide over-the-counter remedies to help people with certain symptoms. In homeopathy, symptom analysis is key to successful prescription. Talk with the pharmacist about your choices and the dilutions recommended, and follow instructions precisely.

Symptoms	Remedy
Obesity	
Fearful and depressed, slightly obsessional, cold but sweaty, lack of energy, indigestion, recurrent infections	calcerea
Moody, anxious, depressed, tendency to wake and worry in the early hours of the morning	kali phos
Constant eating but never feel satisfied, talk too much but do too little, diarrhoea, indigestion, flatulence	sulphur
Smoking	
Dry smoker's cough, usually worse in morning	bryonia
Trying to quit smoking	tabacum
Restlessness, low body weight, pale, chest weakness	tuberculinum
Cystitis	
Continuous passing of urine	belladonna
Urine feels hot and is passed in drops with violent burning pain	cantharis

Symptoms	Remedy
Colds and hayfever	
Violent sneezing, dry cough	aconite
Throbbing headache, obstructed nose, pain in throat	chamomilla
Sore runny nose, mouth dry, eyes irritated, feverish	arsenicum album
Much sneezing, runny nose, dry hacking cough	allium cepa
Eyes worse than nose, sneezing with streaming eyes first thing in morning	euphrasia
Nose blocked at night, sneezing in morning, sensitivity to light, itching in ears	nux vomica
Menstrual problems	
Irregular periods, heavy painful periods coming on too soon	belladonna
Painful periods	mag phos
Irregular periods, spasmodic period pains especially in lower back, irritability	nux vomica
Irregular or absent periods, heavy or late periods with pain on left	pulsatilla

Ayurvedic medicine

See also:

1/BEING A WELL WOMAN
Essentials of good health
pp. 16–19

3/GENERAL HEALTH ISSUES
Women and heart disease p. 132

5/ILLNESSES & EMERGENCIES
Digestive system problems
p. 192; p. 198; pp. 202–203

Ayurveda (which means "science of life") is a complete healthcare system that originated in India about 3,000 years ago. There, and in Sri Lanka, it is a mainstream form of treatment, practised alongside Western-style medicine. It is rapidly gaining popularity in the Western world.

According to Ayurveda, the world is composed of five elements: space, air, fire, water and earth. Existence is governed by three "doshas" (energies), each made up of two of the elements. Health in general consists of finding a balance between these three energies. Each person tends to be dominated by one dosha and

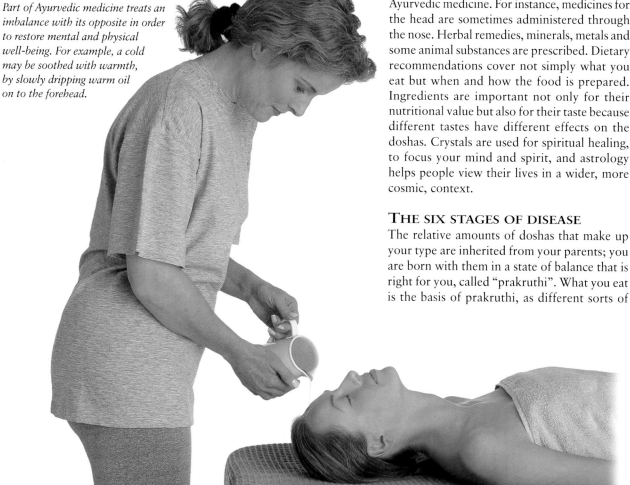

RELAXATION TECHNIQUES
Part of Ayurvedic medicine treats an imbalance with its opposite in order to restore mental and physical well-being. For example, a cold may be soothed with warmth, by slowly dripping warm oil on to the forehead.

needs to work with this energy to find the lifestyle uniquely suited to her.

Ayurvedic medicine recognizes six stages of disease and aims to intervene at the first stage, when the doshas first get out of balance. Western medicine tends to intervene only at the third or fourth, when marked symptoms appear. Health is a dynamic process which needs to take into account not just a person's constitution and age but also the seasons and climate, even the movements of the planets. Treatment is wide-ranging and may include massage, self-massage, detoxification (for example, saunas, enemas or laxatives), diet, herbal and other remedies, surgery, counselling, meditation, yoga, crystals and astrology.

Some methods of treatment are unique to Ayurvedic medicine. For instance, medicines for the head are sometimes administered through the nose. Herbal remedies, minerals, metals and some animal substances are prescribed. Dietary recommendations cover not simply what you eat but when and how the food is prepared. Ingredients are important not only for their nutritional value but also for their taste because different tastes have different effects on the doshas. Crystals are used for spiritual healing, to focus your mind and spirit, and astrology helps people view their lives in a wider, more cosmic, context.

THE SIX STAGES OF DISEASE
The relative amounts of doshas that make up your type are inherited from your parents; you are born with them in a state of balance that is right for you, called "prakruthi". What you eat is the basis of prakruthi, as different sorts of

THE DOSHAS

Ayurvedic practitioners believe that there are three kinds of energy in the body, which are called doshas, and that our constitutions are characterized by the relationships between these. One or two of these doshas will usually be dominant, and each person can be described as a pitta type or a vátha/kapha type, for example. You are born with your doshas in balance, but they may need readjusting throughout life.

Elements	Mental	Physical	Mental and physical effects of imbalance	
Vátha				
air space	creativity, energy	nervous system, processes of elimination, breathing	confusion, loss of energy, insomnia, anxiety	persistent bodily discharges, breathing disorders, intolerance of cold
Pitta				
fire water	desire, joy	memory, heat regulation, digestion, vision	irritability, feeling driven, dullness	digestive disorders, impaired vision, irregular body temperature, premature greying
Kapha				
earth water	courage, tolerance, friendship	structure of body, growth, weight	intolerance, insecurity, jealousy	sexual problems, too thin, excess mucus, muscle weakness

foods are more suited to different dosha types. Through stress, the wrong diet or injury, your constitution can become unbalanced and you enter a state called vikruthi. Practitioners do not aim to change the constitution you inherited, but to restore its original balance.

The stages of a disease build up from mild to full blown:

Accumulation Excess dosha accumulates in its natural sites in the body causing minor discomfort. Ayurvedic practitioners aim to intervene now.

Aggravation Accumulated dosha becomes irritated, producing more specific symptoms.

Dispersion Aggravated dosha spills out into the rest of the body, causing much more widespread symptoms.

Relocation Clear signs of dysfunction appear in both the original and other sites of the body. This stage corresponds with the time people in the Western world generally seek medical attention.

Manifestation The symptoms can be grouped into the specific diseases recognized by Western medicine.

Maturation The disease is fully developed. There still exists a possibility of a cure, but it becomes chronic or fatal if left untreated.

CHOOSING A PRACTITIONER

Training in Ayurvedic medicine includes five years in medical school and one in hospital practice. There are currently only a few schools outside India offering the full training and not enough trained practitioners to meet the demand for treatment. You can locate your nearest practitioner through the Ayurveda Institute (address p. 312).

Traditional Chinese medicine

Like Ayurvedic medicine (pp. 302–303), this complete and ancient healthcare system is still a mainstream form of medicine in its country of origin. It is widely available and also well established in the Western world.

Traditional Chinese medicine (TCM) has three main components—herbal medicine (pp. 298–299), massage (tui na, p. 289) and acupuncture (pp. 306–307). It is said that the best results come from using two or more of the components at the same time.

As with Ayurvedic medicine, TCM's theoretical basis is completely different from that of Western science. In holistic terms, illness of all kinds, whether physical, emotional, mental or spiritual, is the result of an imbalance in our vital energy known as qi or chi (pronounced *chee*). An imbalance can be caused by internal factors such as heredity and emotions, and external factors such as the weather, pollution, infection, injury and drugs. TCM treatment aims to restore the balance.

THE FLOW OF ENERGY

Chi, the source of all the body's activity and maintenance, is in a constant state of flux. It is divided into two complementary forces called yin and yang, and manifested in five interrelated elements: wood, fire, earth, metal and water. These elements both nourish and control each other—for example, water nourishes wood (trees) but controls fire.

These forces and elements are related to parts of the body, functions and emotions and the practitioner uses these connections to assess exactly where an imbalance might be and what is causing it.

In TCM, prevention is as important as a cure, and is recommended as a way of maintaining equilibrium—called homeostasis. Balance is particularly important at times of change or stress as well as for a wide variety of conditions, both physical and mental.

YIN AND YANG

The balance of yin and yang is key to the flow of chi and so to health and well-being in TCM. Traditionally, yin is associated with the female characteristics, and with shade, passivity and softness. Yin governs the front of the body, the interior organs and the muscles. Yang is associated with the masculine traits, with the

THE CHANNELS OF CHI

The channels along which the energy called chi flows are known as meridians. The meridians correspond to yin and yang organs:
♀ Arm tai yin (lung, or Lu).
♀ Leg tai yin (spleen, or Sp).
♀ Arm shao yin (heart, or He).
♀ Leg shao yin (kidney, or Kid).
♀ Arm jue yin (pericardium, or Per).
♀ Leg jue yin (liver, or Liv).
♀ Arm yang ming (large intestine, or LI).
♀ Leg yang ming (stomach, or St).
♀ Arm tai yang (small intestine, or SI).
♀ Leg tai yang (bladder, or Bl).
♀ Arm shao yang (san jiao, or SJ).
♀ Leg shao yang (gallbladder, or GB).

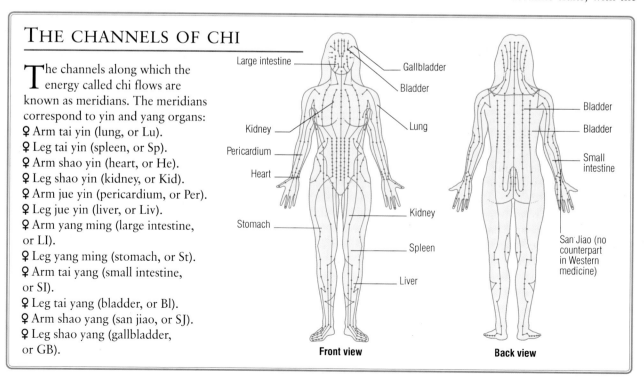

Front view   **Back view**

THE FIVE ELEMENTS

The ideas behind Chinese medicine have grown out of close observation of the natural world. In the philosophy of TCM, the ways in which nature deals with or meets changes—called dynamic processes—are translated to the functioning of the body. The five elements have individual characteristics. Wood is growing, flexible, rooted. Fire is dry, hot, ascending, moving. Earth is productive, fertile, has potential for growth. Metal is cutting, hard, conducting. Water is wet, cool, descending, flowing, yielding. All have yin and yang aspects, and all five elements support each other. The aim of TCM is to apply the elements to the health of the body and to discover what it is that is causing disharmony.

Parts of body	Sense organ	Emotion	External symptoms
Wood			
liver, gallbladder, tendons	eyes	anger	in nails
Fire			
heart, small intestine, blood vessels	tongue	joy	in complexion
Earth			
spleen, stomach, muscles	mouth	worry	in lips
Metal			
lungs, large intestine, skin	nose	grief, melancholy	in body hair
Water			
kidneys, bladder, bones	ears	fear	in head and hair

sun and vitality, and governs the back of the body and the skin.

An imbalance of too much yin can lead to physical symptoms of chronic disease, diarrhoea, and to feeling cold and sleepy. Mental symptoms include being too submissive, impractical, overly sensitive and lacking conviction. Too much yang leads to the opposite: acute disease, constipation and feeling hot and restless. Mentally, an imbalance of yang makes people domineering, insensitive, dogmatic and overly materialistic.

SEEING A PRACTITIONER

As in Ayurvedic medicine, detailed advice on diet and lifestyle is an integral part of the treatment. You will be asked when and how you eat, the taste of the food, the time you get up, exercise or go to bed—since all are deemed relevant to your health and well-being. As well as finding out all about you and your life, in much the same way as a doctor does, a practitioner of TCM will take your pulse in six places on each wrist and examine the state of your tongue, nails, skin and hair.

Remedies may contain animal parts such as powdered deer horn or insect skin. If you do not want these particular remedies because you suspect that they may be prepared from endangered species, you should say so and the practitioner can avoid them.

Make sure you see a reputable practitioner who uses a proper supplier because standards on imported herbal remedies are not as stringent as those on ones produced domestically. Practitioners should be registered. Check that language is not a barrier to communication with your practitioner.

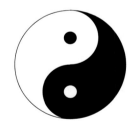

YIN AND YANG
The t'ai chi symbol illustrates how yin and yang are balanced and interlinked but opposite.

Acupuncture

The philosophy behind traditional Chinese medicine is to avoid pain, keep illness and disability at bay and to lead a healthy and fulfilling life. Acupuncture—the use of needles to stimulate the flow of qi or chi (energy) in the body—is as much a method of achieving these ends as is the use of herbal remedies. Its practice has evolved over many thousands of years and today in Western countries qualified and experienced practitioners offer acupuncture treatment for many conditions. It is also regarded as preventive, for ongoing well-being.

Fully registered acupuncturists have completed a recognized training in Chinese medicine, meet the Western standards of anatomy, physiology and pathology, and understand conditions in the same medical terms as a conventional doctor, although do not offer treatment in that way. They use the letters CA (Certified Acupuncturist) after their names.

In acupuncture terms, a condition shows that there is disharmony in the body caused by a deficiency or excess of the yin and/or yang energy (p. 305) or the presence of a pathogen which may be either superficial or has penetrated internal tissue. Other considerations are how long the pathogen has been there and what it may have affected in that time.

The use of needles is completely safe; strict hygiene is standard practice, with rigorous sterilization procedures. Made of stainless steel (some have copper-coil handles), the needles vary in lengths and thicknesses—the most commonly used are fine and between 1.25 cm (½ in) and 7.5 cm (3 in) long.

METHODS OF DIAGNOSIS

In a typical first session, which may last from 30 minutes to an hour, an acupuncturist will take a personal history, in a similar way to a conventional doctor. He or she will ask you to describe in your own words the problem you have. After this, diagnosis is made on the basis of four examinations.

The first, looking, is an assessment of your physical appearance, your skin colour and tone, and your tongue. The second, hearing and smelling, may be done so discreetly it may not even be obvious to you, and the intention is to find clues to deficiency or excess. Next comes questioning, when the acupuncturist seeks more information about you which may have a bearing on the fuller picture of your disharmony. The final part is touching, during which the practitioner will gain understanding of your painful areas by examination (not internal), feel your skin to assess its temperature and condition, and take your pulse in more than one place (the wrist and neck, for example).

The information gathered enables the acupuncturist to identify the type of disharmony you have and how it is affecting you before deciding on and explaining the treatment. It is rare that one treatment will resolve a problem; many over several months may be needed for chronic and longstanding conditions. Progress may be slow if acupuncture is sought as a last resort, as it commonly is.

Acupuncture is contraindicated in someone with a blood condition, high fever or a severe psychotic condition. It is only used in pregnancy in the third trimester when the foetus is breech, or for labour pains. In this case, moxabustion (the burning of small mugwort cones) may be recommended by a midwife.

A treatment should not be given if you have recently been drinking alcohol or taken drugs (although acupuncture is known for its successful use in alcohol and drug rehabilitation). When trying to quit smoking, acupuncture can help withdrawal symptoms but is not advised at the same time as using nicotine patches or gum.

PLACING THE NEEDLES
The acupuncturist treats conditions by placing needles so that harmony is restored to the body. The needles are round-ended and rarely draw blood but may cause a tingling feeling.

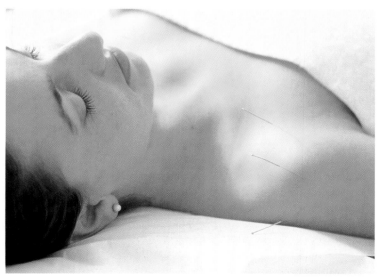

NEEDLES AND FINGER PRESSURE

The 14 meridians of the body, known as energy pathways, have over 350 acupoints which acupuncturists categorize according to the effects they are believed to have on the body's organs.

The acupuncturist will insert needles to stimulate or calm, or use acupressure—fingertip or nail massage—on those acupoints related to your condition. The insertion and manipulation of needles to achieve the desired therapeutic effect usually causes little pain, although there may a tingling sensation. This is called "deqi", literally acquiring the qi (chi or energy).

Acupuncturists may also use moxabustion, the application of heat above an acupoint. The heat comes from tiny cones of smouldering mugwort leaves (*Artemesia vulgaris*, known as moxa), which burn down until the skin turns red. The musky odour of moxa may remain on clothing and hair for a time after the session.

Moxa may be used with needles on an acupuncture point or in a special box which allows a larger area—such as the kidneys—to be warmed. To turn a baby from its breech position, a cone is burnt on the little toe, on alternate sides, until the heat is felt. The number of sessions needed varies.

ACUPOINTS AND PAIN RELIEF

There is much documentation to show that acupuncture and acupressure can relieve physical pain—they release the body's natural painkillers, endorphins, and other neurotransmitters. Both may provide symptomatic relief in stroke rehabilitation and in relieving nausea, for example. The basis of a TENS machine, used widely during labour and in chronic physical conditions such as arthritis, is the application of a mild electric current to stimulate the nerves along which pain travels.

PAIN RELIEF WITH TENS

Transcutaneous electrical nerve stimulation (TENS) stimulates the body to release its own pain-relieving chemicals. It is a completely safe method of pain control and can also be used in conjunction with pain-relieving drugs such as anti-inflammatories. However the effects vary from person to person; it doesn't always work and just occasionally it can make pain worse. If this happens you should discuss it with your doctor.

TENS machines can be worn under clothes and consist of small battery-operated units attached by wires to pads containing electrodes which you stick to your skin. The current is tiny and feels like tingling or buzzing. You adjust the level yourself. TENS machines are used in hospitals to relieve the pain of injuries, during labour and after operations. You can also use them at home for all types of pain, such as that of shingles or a torn muscle or ligament. The machines may be hired or bought.

HAND-HELD CONTROL
TENS machines are easily transported and allow you to feel more in control of your pain. The pads and electrodes are placed on the pathways along which your particular pain travels.

> **! Caution**
> **Do not use a TENS machine:**
> ♀ On undiagnosed pain.
> ♀ In the first three months of pregnancy.
> ♀ On the abdomen during the whole of pregnancy.
> ♀ If you wear a heart pacemaker or have serious heart rhythm problems.
> ♀ Near vital organs (follow instructions carefully as to where you can place the pads).

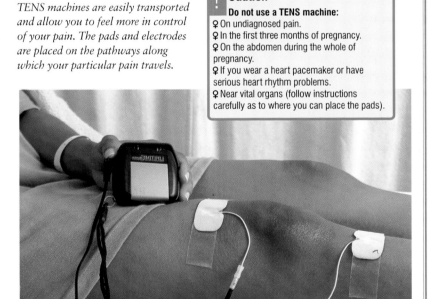

Naturopathy

Naturopaths are the family doctors of holistic medicine, and the practice goes back to ancient times. To them, disease is something that happens naturally when an organism is not functioning as it should and their aim is to discover the best way of fighting it. They use a variety of therapies to support the body's own natural healing powers to restore wellness.

The principles of naturopathy maintain that the body has the ability to heal itself and that symptoms of disease are the body's attempts to right itself and should not be suppressed. Treatment should not inflict further harm and is tailored to the individual not the disease. The long-term aim of treatment is to reeducate the patients so that they can take care of their health for themselves.

WAYS OF HEALING

According to naturopaths, the fundamental requirements for good health are fresh air, clean water, gentle exercise, relaxation and a good diet. The causes of disease can be chemical, mechanical or psychological.

A naturopath may use therapies such as iridology (below) and kinesiology (p. 310) to provide further insight into your problem. The two treatments you are most likely to receive from a naturopath are hydrotherapy and nutritional therapy. Nutritional therapy uses fasting, special diets, the elimination of certain foods, and infusions, which together allow the body to rest and detoxify. These measures are only temporary but long-term dietary changes may be recommended too. Nutritional supplements and herbal or homeopathic remedies may also be prescribed.

Naturopaths treat physical and mobility problems using therapies like osteopathy, chiropractic and the Alexander Technique. They are skilled in special soft-tissue techniques which can relieve muscular tension, decongest and free movement in any part of the body, not just the joints. They may advise you on exercises to do at home. Counselling may be given or meditation and relaxation techniques taught to help your psychological outlook.

SEEING A NATUROPATH

Naturopaths use conventional medical techniques for diagnosis, such as blood and urine tests, and alternative ones such as iridology (study of the iris, see box left).

In addition, like all alternative medicine practitioners, they will want details of your medical history, an indepth view of your lifestyle and an understanding of your current state of mind.

During treatment you may undergo a "healing crisis", which makes your symptoms temporarily worsen. In naturopathic terms, this is a good sign because it shows that the treatment is working. You may also find that old symptoms return, usually in the reverse order of their appearance (as in homeopathy, pp. 300–301).

As you get better, the symptoms should progress from the deeper tissues to the more superficial and from the more vital organs to the less vital.

Naturopathy can benefit anyone, whatever their age and complaint, and can also be used preventively. It is worth considering for chronic conditions such as chronic fatigue syndrome, allergies, hayfever, asthma and migraine headaches, and can speed recovery from an infection or injury.

IRIDOLOGY

This therapy may be used in conjunction with others to detect a tendency to disease—which can be seen in the iris. Practitioners look for a range of signs indicating poor health by study of the colour, texture and markings of the iris. There is, however, no scientific proof that this procedure works.

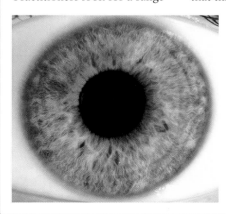

A MAP OF THE BODY
Iridologists believe that the iris maps the human glands, organs and body systems, so that flecks, streaks or other marks in the eye all have a counterpart in different areas or functions of the body. A special magnifying camera can make a slide for enlarged viewing and assessing.

Hydrotherapy

The medium of water, used either at different temperatures or with added minerals or herbs, may heal all kinds of disease. It is sometimes employed by osteopaths and physiotherapists and is a staple of naturopathy.

Modern hydrotherapy started in the 18th and 19th centuries in Germany and led to the establishment in Europe of hydrotherapy hotels or "hydros", many of which are still in existence and offer a wide range of healing and treatments. Similarly, "spas" use naturally warm mineral-rich spring waters for internal and external medical treatment. Thalassotherapy involves the use of seawater in the same way.

HOW IT WORKS

Hot water brings blood to the skin and takes it away from internal organs. This has a sedative effect on the body as a whole, relieves pain and stimulates the elimination of toxins through sweat. Cold water has the opposite effect. It increases blood flow to internal organs thereby stimulating the body as a whole, and reduces inflammation in outer organs. Water sprays and jets massage the body and may give pain relief by stimulating the nerves in the same way that TENS machines do (p. 307).

OTHER WATER THERAPIES

Water is also used in other therapies:

Colonic irrigation A stream of fresh water is passed around the colon through the rectum for about half an hour to clean out accumulated waste matter. Usually, several treatments are needed. Practitioners believe that a modern diet high in processed foods damages the health of the intestines, which leads to toxins accumulating rather than being broken down and eliminated. These are then reabsorbed by the body and can lead to a range of health problems. This treatment may be harmful if it is done too often.

Water birth Being in warm water during labour is relaxing and can help to relieve pain. Many believe it is also a more soothing way for the baby to be born, as long as care is taken and proper professional guidance given on safety and scrupulous hygiene. Some hospitals have birthing pools or you may be able to rent one.

Flotation This involves floating in warm water filled with mineral salts to make you com-

See also:

1/BEING A WELL WOMAN
Healthy body systems pp. 30-43

3/GENERAL HEALTH ISSUES
Skeletal system problems pp. 78–91
Problems of the mind pp. 94–115
Blood and the circulation pp. 116–124

4/HORMONAL HEALTH
Endocrine system problems pp. 136–143
Reproductive problems pp. 146–149

5/ILLNESSES & EMERGENCIES
Body system problems pp. 188–249

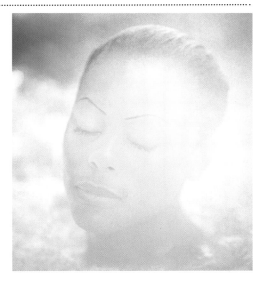

STEAMING
Steam-bath cabinets enclose the entire body except the head and cause profuse sweating. Saunas are less humid. At home, a towel over a bowl of hot water can direct steam to the head or any part of the body.

pletely buoyant in an enclosed compartment. In the darkness and silence, with no need to use your muscles, you reach a state of profound relaxation. The therapy is thought to help ease pain or stress-related conditions, as well as strengthen the immune system. Some places offer movies or music to aid relaxation.

Sprays and affusions (pouring) These combine jets of hot or cold water directed at parts of the body to ease pain and to aid relaxation.

WRAPPING OR SWATHING
Damp sheets are used to wrap around the whole body or parts of it to help eliminate toxins.

Nutritional therapy

A combination of special diets and nutritional and herbal supplements is used by nutritional therapists to treat an enormous number of ailments. Nutritional therapists consider many of today's diseases to be the result of poor nutrition or improperly absorbed nutrients from bad eating habits, apathy, lack of money, lack of time or constant dieting. As well as nutritional deficiencies, food allergies and toxic overload can cause persistent tiredness and lead to disease besides such dramatic and immediate symptoms such as vomiting.

Pollutants in food, water and the environment increase our need for nutrients yet we get fewer from foods because of the non-organic and chemical methods of growth or processing. Over time, environmental stress and malnutrition can damage your ability to absorb food, creating a vicious circle of ill-health.

WHO IT CAN HELP

Nutritional therapists treat problems clearly connected to food such as weight, eating disorders (people with eating disorders may need psychiatric help or counselling), food allergies and intolerances and digestive disorders. The therapy may help with hormonal problems such as PMS or polycystic ovaries and with menopausal symptoms.

Nutritional therapy may be used preventively, for instance to reduce the risk of heart disease, breast cancer or osteoporosis later in life. Preconceptional nutritional therapy for both partners may reduce the risk of miscarriage and birth defects and may help prevent your children from developing allergies. It has achieved success with problems with a mental link such as insomnia, anxiety, addictions, depression, learning difficulties and attention deficit hyperactivity disorder in children.

FORMING A DIAGNOSIS

Therapists start by taking a detailed medical history. They will ask about your everyday diet and habits such as drinking alcohol and smoking. They also discuss what exercise you regularly take, your emotional state and what medication, if any, you are on and any side effects you are experiencing.

The therapist may also use diagnostic tests such as hair analysis—which assesses the state of health of the body—and kinesiology. Developed by a chiropractor in the United States in the 1960s, kinesiology draws from Chinese medicine in that it is based on energy flow and the body imbalances that disrupt it.

A kinesiologist uses muscle testing to detect those changes that occur when a person comes into contact with something to which he or she is allergic. The practitioner places a food or chemical—for instance, a piece of toast if wheat allergy is suspected—in the patient's hand or under the tongue and then checks to see if the muscles linked by a meridian (energy channel) have weakened. Kinesiology is most often used for allergies and allergic conditions such as rhinitis, hayfever and asthma, as well as migraines, but practitioners also treat muscular sports injuries, chronic fatigue and stress. It is excellent for picking up niggling digestive and other problems, to correct them before they become an illness.

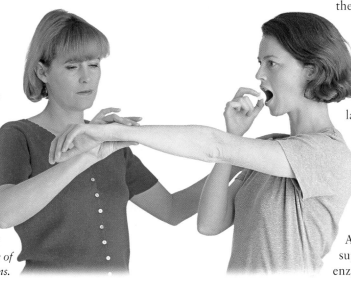

MUSCLE TESTING
A kinesiologist works on your energy flow. If the flow is blocked it indicates weakness in an organ and this registers in related muscles. Muscle-strength tests are painless and seek to find the cause of minor health problems.

PRESCRIBING A PROGRAMME

A nutritional therapist may prescribe supplements—vitamins, minerals, enzymes, amino acids, essential fatty acids and fibre—in megadoses depending on the person's needs, although some vitamins, such as B$_6$, should not be taken in excess of the recommended daily allowance unless medically supervised. Diets are short term and advice is given on menu planning and food preparation. A basic diagnostic diet, which usually lasts for two weeks, excludes those foods which most commonly cause allergies. Eating the same foods too often may overload the body's detoxification pathways and a rotation diet ensures that each foodstuff is eaten only at intervals of four days or more. Raw food, juice-only diets and fasting cleanse the body of toxins and give the digestive system a rest.

Nutritional therapists recommend a varied wholefood diet of fresh food and minimal animal fats and protein. You may be advised on exercise and relaxation to encourage a normal eating pattern again. It is important not to confuse nutritional therapists with dieticians, who are trained in nutritional science and work with doctors to provide diets for specific conditions such as obesity, diabetes and coeliac disease.

UNDERSTANDING BLOOD SUGAR

Maintaining a stable level of blood sugar is important to health. Foods are turned into sugar at different speeds. To find the correct balance for your needs, use the glycaemic index. Foods that are digested rapidly have a very high or high index; those that are digested slowly have a moderate to very low index.

Indications of hypoglycaemia (an imbalance) are fluctuating energy, fatigue (especially on waking and mid-afternoon), cravings for sweet foods such as cakes, irritability and lack of concentration. You may feel weak, light-headed or irritable if you skip a meal or it is delayed.

COMBATING LOW BLOOD SUGAR

If you have symptoms of low blood sugar levels, you should eat mostly those foods with a low glycaemic index. Avoid high index foods as they tend to cause low blood sugar, even if you have an initial burst of energy after eating. Combine a high index food with one of a lower rating: for example, baked potato with cheese, vegetables or chicken. Eat regularly, little and often, with no more than three to four hours between food. Snack on fresh fruit rather than biscuits in between meals. Other healthy snacks based on natural foods include unsalted and

GLYCAEMIC INDEX

Foods with a high glycaemic index may give an initial surge of energy but this is often followed by a slump. Foods low on the index release energy slowly.

Very high

Cornflakes, glucose, maltose, puffed rice, rice cakes, white bread*

High

Bananas, brown rice, carrots, corn, corn chips, mangoes, muesli, oat bran, parsnips, potatoes, raisins, rye crackers, white rice, wholegrain bread

Moderate

Kidney beans (cooked or canned), lactose, oranges, peas, potato crisps, pumpernickel bread, sucrose, white and wholewheat pasta

Low

Apples, barley, chickpeas, lentils, milk, peaches, pears, wholegrain rye bread, yogurt

Very low

Fish, fructose, grapefruit, green vegetables, meat, peanuts, plums, seafood, soya beans

Foods with a high glycaemic index are generally those that are high in refined carbohydrates and sugar

unsweetened popcorn, plain yogurt, crispbreads, nuts, raw vegetable sticks and dried fruit such as apricots or figs.

Starchy foods can encourage the body to produce hormones that make you sleepy. This can account for a mid-afternoon slump, especially if your lunch consists of a sandwich, pasta salad, baked potato or crisps. Try instead to lunch on a salad with protein such as hard-boiled eggs, chicken or fish, or a sustaining and nutritious soup, and save your carbohydrate-based meals for breakfast or the evening.

Dehydration prevents the body from absorbing essential nutrients and energy. So drink plenty of water, especially if you also drink strong coffee and tea in quantity.

> **! Caution**
> Some conditions such as diabetes mellitus, anaemia and low thyroid function have lack of energy and fatigue as symptoms. Always consult your doctor if you are persistently tired..
> The dietary guidelines for a non-insulin dependent diabetic are the same as those for someone with hypoglycaemia: eat low index foods and take meals at regular intervals.

Directory of women's health sources

Organizations are listed alphabetically by medical condition or by the service they provide.

A

BRITISH ACUPUNCTURE COUNCIL
63 Jeddo Road
London W12 9HQ
020 8735 0400
email: info@acupuncture.org.uk
www.acupuncture.org.uk

AFTER ADOPTION
12-14 Chapel Street
Greater Manchester M3 7NN
0161 839 4930

AGE CONCERN
Astral House, 1268 London Road
London SW16 4ER
0808 808 6060
www.ageconcern.org.uk

POSITIVELY WOMEN (AIDS AND HIV)
347-349 City Road
London EC1V 1LR
020 7713 0222
email: poswomen@dircom.co.uk

TERENCE HIGGINS TRUST (AIDS)
52-54 Grays Inn Road
London WC1X 8JU
020 7242 1010
email: info@tht.org.uk

AL-ANON FAMILY GROUPS (FOR THOSE WHO ARE
AFFECTED BY SOMEONE ELSE'S DRINKING)
ALATEEN (PART OF AL-ANON FOR AGES 12-20)
61 Dover Street
London SE1 4YF
020 7403 0888
email: alanonuk@aol.com
www.hexnet.co.uk/alanon

ALCOHOLICS ANONYMOUS
PO Box 1, Stonebow House
Stonebow
York YO1 7NJ
01904 644 026
www.alcoholics-anonymous.org.uk

ALCOHOL COUNSELLING & PREVENTION SERVICES
34 Electric Lane
London SW9 8JT
020 7737 3579
email: info@acaps.co.uk
www.acaps.co.uk

SOCIETY OF TEACHERS OF THE ALEXANDER
TECHNIQUE
129 Camden Mews
London NW1 9AH
email: enquiries@stat.org.uk
020 7351 0828

BRITISH ALLERGY FOUNDATION
Deepdene House, 30 Bellegrove Road
Welling
Kent DA16 3PY
020 8303 8525
email: allergybas@compuserve.com

ALZHEIMER'S DISEASE SOCIETY
Gordon House
10 Greencoat Place
London SW1P 1PH
020 7306 0606
email: 101762.422@compuserve.com
www.alzheimers.org.uk

ALZHEIMER'S SCOTLAND - ACTION ON DEMENTIA
22 Drumsheugh Gardens
Edinburgh EH3 0XS
0800 317 817
email: alzheimers@alzscot.org

ANOREXIA NERVOSA *SEE* EATING DISORDERS

FIRST STEPS TO FREEDOM (ANXIETY DISORDERS)
7 Avon Court
Park Road
Kenilworth
Warwickshire CVV8 2GX
01926 851 608
email: firststepstofreedom@compuserve.com
www.firststeps.demon.co.uk

AROMATHERAPY ORGANIZATIONS COUNCIL
3 Latymer Close
Braybrooke
Market Harborough
Leicestershire LE16 8LN
01858 434242

ARTHRITIC ASSOCIATION
First Floor Suite
2 Hyde Gardens
Eastbourne
East Sussex BN21 4PN
01323 416 550
email: info@arthriticassociation.org.uk

ARTHRITIS & RHEUMATISM COUNCIL
St Mary's Gate
Chesterfield
Derbyshire S41 7TD
01246 558 033
email: info@arc.org.uk

NATIONAL ASTHMA CAMPAIGN
Providence House
Providence Place
London N1 0NT
08457 010203
www.asthma.org.uk

NATIONAL ASTHMA & RESPIRATORY TRAINING
CENTRE
The Athenaeum
10 Church Street
Warwick CV34 4AB
01926 493313
email: enquiries@nartc.org.uk

AYURVEDIC COMPANY OF GREAT BRITAIN
81 Wimpole Street
London W1G NRF
www. unifiedherbal.com

B

BREAST CANCER CARE
Kiln House
210 New Kings Road
London SW6 4NZ
0808 800 6000
email: bcc@breastcancercare.org.uk
www.breastcancercare.org.uk

LA LECHE LEAGUE (BREASTFEEDING INFORMATION)
BM 3424
London WC1N 3XX
020 7242 1278

THE BREASTFEEDING NETWORK
PO Box 11126
Paisley
Scotland PA2 8YB
0870 900 8787
email: broadfoot@btinternet.com

BULIMIA *SEE* EATING DISORDERS

C

CANCER BACUP (BRITISH ASSOCIATION OF CANCER
UNITED PATIENTS)
3 Bath Place, Rivington Road
London EC2A 3DR
020 7613 2121 (London)
0800 181199 (outside London)

CANCERLINK
11-21 Northdown Street
London N1 9BN
0808 808 0000
email: cancerlink@canlink.demon.co.uk
www.cancerlink.org

MACMILLAN CANCER RELIEF
89 Albert Embankment
London SE1 7HQ
020 7840 7840
email: postmaster@macmillan.org.uk

CARERS NATIONAL ASSOCIATION
20-25 Glasshouse Yard
London EC1A 4JT
020 7490 8818
email: info@ukcarers.org

NATIONAL CHILDBIRTH TRUST
Alexandra House, Oldham Terrace
London W3 6NH
020 8992 2616
email: nationalchildbirthtrust@lineone.net

CHILDLINE
Freepost 1111
London N1 0BR
0800 11 11
www.childline.org.uk

BRITISH CHIROPRACTIC ASSOCIATION
Blagrave House, 17 Blagrave Street
Reading
Berkshire RG1 1QB
0118 950 5950
email: enquiries@chiropractic-uk.co.uk
www.chiropractic-uk.co.uk

NACC (COLITIS AND CROHNS DISEASE)
4 Beaumont House
Sutton Road
St Albans
Herts AL1 5HH
01727 844 296
email: nacc@nacc.org.uk

COELIAC SOCIETY OF UK
PO Box 220
High Wycombe
Bucks HP11 2HY
Tel: 01494 437 278
www. coeliac.co.uk

INSTITUTE FOR COMPLEMENTARY MEDICINE
PO Box 194
London SE16 1QZ
020 7237 5165

THE CONTINENCE FOUNDATION
307 Hatton Square
16 Baldwin Gardens
London EC1N 7RJ
020 7831 9831
email: continence.foundation@dial.pipex.com
www.continence-foundation.org.uk

CYSTIC FIBROSIS TRUST
11 London Road
Bromley, Kent BR1 1BY
020 8464 7211;
out-of-hours 020 8464 0623
www.cftrust.org.uk

D
DEPRESSION ALLIANCE
35 Westminster Bridge Road
London SE1 7JB
020 7633 0557
email: information@depressionalliance.org
www.depressionalliance.org

BRITISH ASSOCIATION OF DERMATOLOGISTS
19 Fitzroy Square
London W1T 6EH
020 7383 0266
email: admin@bad.org.uk

DIABETES UK
10 Queen Anne Street
London W1M 0BD
020 7636 6112
email: bda@diabetes.org.uk
www.diabetes.org.uk

INSULIN DEPENDENT DIABETES TRUST
PO Box 294
Northampton NN3 2BN
01604 721 325

DIGESTIVE DISORDERS FOUNDATION
PO Box 251
Edgeware
Middlesex HA8 6HG

DRUGS AID
16 Clive Street, Caerphilly
Wales CF83 1GE
029 2088 1000
email: drugaid@talk21.com

BRITISH DYSLEXIA ASSOCIATION
98 London Road
Reading RG1 5AU
0118 966 2677
email: bda-dyslexia.demon.co.uk

E
EATING DISORDERS ASSOCIATION
1st Floor, Wensum House
103 Prince of Wales Road
Norwich, Norfolk NR1 1DW
01603 621 414 (adult - weekdays 9-6)
01603 765 050 (youth - weekdays 4-6)
email: info@edauk.com
www.edauk.com

NATIONAL ECZEMA SOCIETY
163 Eversholt Street
London NW1 1BU
0870 241 3604

NATIONAL ENDROMETRIOSIS SOCIETY
50 Westminster Palace Gardens
Artillery Row
London SW1P 1RL
020 7222 2776
email: Endonifo@compuserve.com
www.Endo.org.uk

BRITISH EPILEPSY ASSOCIATION
New Anstey House, Gateway Drive
Yeadon
Leeds
West Yorkshire LS19 7XY
0808 8005050

THE EYECARE INFORMATION SERVICE
P.O. Box 131
Market Rasen
Lincolnshire LN8 5TS
01673 857 847
www.eye-care.org.uk

F
FAMILY PLANNING ASSOCIATION
2-12 Pentonville Road
London N1 9FP
020 7837 5432
www.fpa.org.uk

ISSUE (NATIONAL FERTILITY ASSOCIATION)
114 Lichfield Street
Walsall
West Midlands WS1 1SZ
01922 722 888
email: webmaster@issue.co.uk
www.issue.co.uk

G
GENERAL INFORMATION
www.netdoctor.co.uk

INTERNATIONAL GLAUCOMA ASSOCIATION
108c Warner Road
London SE5 9HQ
020 7737 3265

H
BRITISH HEART FOUNDATION
14 Fitzhardinge Street
London W1H 6DH
020 7935 0185
heartline 0990 200 656
www.bhf.org.uk

HERPES VIRUS ASSOCIATION
41 North Road
London N7 9DD
020 7609 9061

FACULTY OF HOMEOPATHY
15 Clerkenwell Close
London EC1R 0AA
020 7566 7800
email: info@trusthomeopathy.org.uk
www.trusthomeopathy.org.uk

I
PRIMARY IMMUNODEFICIENCY ASSOCIATION
Alliance House, 12 Caxton Street
London SW1H 0QS
020 7976 7640
email: pimmune@dial.pipex.com
www.pia.org.uk

CHILD (THE NATIONAL INFERTILITY SUPPORT NETWORK)
Charter House, 43 St Leonards Road
Bexhill-on-Sea
East Sussex TN40 1JA
01424 732 361
email: office@child.org.uk
www.child.org.uk

K
NATIONAL KIDNEY FEDERATION
6 Stanley Street
Worksop, Notts S81 7HX
01909 487 795
email: natkidney@compuserve.com
www.kidney.org.uk

L
LEUKAEMIA CARE SOCIETY
2 Shrubbery Avenue
Worcester WR1 1QH
01905 330 003
email: leukaemiacare@ukonline.co.uk
www.leukaemiacare.org

LONG-TERM MEDICAL CONDITIONS ALLIANCE
Unit 212, 16 Baldwin Gardens
London EC1N 7RJ
020 7813 3637
email: alliance@imca.demon.co.uk

BRITISH LUNG FOUNDATION
78 Hatton Garden
London EC1N 8LD
020 7831 5831
email: blf@britishlungfoundation.com
www.lunguk.org

LUPUS UK
St James' House
Eastern Road
Romford
Essex RM1 3NH
01708 731 251

M

NATIONAL MENINGITIS TRUST
Fern House, Bath Road
Stroud
Gloucestershire GL5 3TJ
01453 768 000
email: support@meningitis-trust.org.uk
www.meningitis-trust.org.uk

WOMEN'S HEALTH CONCERN PUBLICATIONS
(MENOPAUSE, HRT)
Wellwood, North Farm Road
Tunbridge Wells TN2 3DR
020 8780 3007

MIND (MENTAL HEALTH)
15-19 Broadway
Stratford
London E15 4BQ
020 8519 2122

MIGRAINE ACTION ASSOCIATION
178a High Road
Byfleet
West Byfleet
Surrey KT14 7ED
01932 352 468
email: info@migraine.org.uk
www.migraine.org.uk

MISCARRIAGE ASSOCIATION
Clayton Hospital
Northgate
Wakefield
West Yorkshire WF1 3JS
01924 200 799
www.miscarriageassociation.org.uk

MULTIPLE SCLEROSIS SOCIETY
MS National Centre
372 Edgware Road
London NW2 6ND
020 8438 0700
email: info@mssociety.org.uk
www.mssociety.org.uk

MUSCULAR DYSTROPHY GROUP OF GREAT BRITIAN
& NORTHERN IRELAND
7-11 Prescott Place
London SW4 6BS
020 7720 8055
email: info@musculardystrophy.org
www.musculardystrophy.org

MYASTHENIA GRAVIS ASSOCIATION
Keynes House
Chester Park
Alfreton Road
Derby DE21 4AS
01332 290 219
www.crabby.demon.co.uk

N

BRITISH COLLEGE OF NATUROPATHY
& OSTEOPATHY
Frazer House
6 Netherall Gardens
London NW3 5RR
020 7435 7830
www.bcno.org.uk

O

OBESITY ADVICE
01279 866 010

OSTEOPATHIC INFORMATION SERVICE
Premier House
10 Graycoat Place
London SW1P 1SP
020 7235 5231

NATIONAL OSTEOPOROSIS SOCIETY
PO Box 10
Radstock
Bath BA3 3YB
01761 472 721
email: info@nos.org.uk
www.nos.org.uk

P

PAIN SOCIETY
9 Bedford Square
London WC1B 3RE
020 7636 2750
email: painsoc@compuserve.com
www.staff.nco.ac.uk/r.j.hays/painsoc.html

THE PITUITARY FOUNDATION
PO Box 1944
Bristol BS99 2UB
email: helpline@pitpat.demon.co.uk
www.pituitary.org.uk

ASSOCIATION FOR POSTNATAL ILLNESS
25 Jerdan Place
London SW6 1BE
020 7386 0868

NATIONAL ASSOCIATION FOR PRE-MENSTRUAL
SYNDROME (NAPS)
7 Swift Court, High Street
Seal
Kent TN15 0EG
01732 760011
email: contact@pms.org.uk
www.pms.org.uk

BRITISH PREGNANCY ADVISORY SERVICE
Head Office, Austy Manor
Wootton Wawen
Solihull
West Midlands B95 6BX
01564 793 225
Actionline: 08457 30 40 30
email: comm@bpas.org
www.bpas.org

PSORIASIS ARTHROPATHY ALLIANCE
PO Box 111
St Albans AL2 3JQ
01923 672 837
email: info@paalliance.org
www.paalliance.org

R

BRITISH REFLEXOLOGY ASSOCIATION
Monks Orchard
Whitbourne
Worcester WR6 5RB
01886 821207
email: bra@britreflex.co.uk
www.britreflex.co.uk

RELATE (RELATIONSHIP COUNSELLING)
Herbert Gray College
Little Church Street
Rugby
Warwickshire CV21 3AP
01788 565675

REPETITIVE STRAIN INJURY ASSOCIATION
380-384 Harrow Road
London W9 2HU
020 7266 2000
email: rsia@dial.pipex.com

S

NATIONAL SCHIZOPHRENIA FELLOWSHIP
28 Castle Street
Kingston-upon-Thames
Surrey KT1 1SS
020 8974 6814

INSTITUTE OF PSYCHOSEXUAL MEDICINE (SEXUAL
HEALTH)
12 Chandos Street
Cavendish Square
London W1G 9DR
020 7580 0631
email: ipm@telinco.co.uk
www.ipm.org.uk

QUIT (SMOKING)
Victory House
170 Tottenham Court Road
London W1T 7NR
0800 002 200
www.quit.org.uk

NHS SMOKERS HELPLINE
0800 169 0169

SHEFFIELD SPEECH & LANGUAGE THERAPISTS
AGENCY
Fulwood House
Old Fulwood Road
Sheffield
South Yorkshire S10 3TH
0114 271 6765

SPINAL INJURIES ASSOCIATION
Newpoint House
76 St James' Lane
London N10 3DF
020 8883 4296

STROKE ASSOCIATION
Stroke House
Whitecross Street
London EC1Y 8JJ
020 7490 7999
email: stroke@stroke.org.uk
www.stroke.org.uk

T

TWINS & MULTIPLE BIRTH ASSOCIATION
(TAMBA)
Harnott House
309 Chester Road
Little Sutton
Ellesmere Port CH66 1QQ
0870 121 4000
email: tamba@information4u.com
www.tamba.org.uk

Y

BRITISH WHEEL OF YOGA
Central Office
25 German Street
Sleaford
Lincolnshire NG34 7RU
01529 303233

Index

glaucoma 241
glucose 275
gluten intolerance 201
glycaemic index 311
glyceryl trinitrate 274
goitre 139
gold 272
gonadotrophins 276
gonorrhoea 74, 164
gosarelin 275
gout 81
Grave's disease 139
group therapies 282
guided imagery 292
gums 175, 239
gynaecological physiotherapy 188
gynaecologist 268

H

haematologist 268
haemorrhage 120
haemorrhoids 123, 175, 196, 201
hair disorders 234
hair removal treatment 235
hallucinogens 100
halofantrine 277
haloperidol 273
hands 80
hangover 96
Hashimoto's thyroiditis 139
hay fever 205, 239, 301
hazardous substances 28
headaches 79, 113-15
healing 286-7
health and safety issues 28-9
healthy eating see nutrition
hearing 43, 236
heart attack 128, 131, 255, 271
heart disease 126-33
heart rate 22, 126
heartburn 175, 191
Heimlich manoeuvre 256
heparin 273
hepatitis 73, 192, 270
herbal medicine 141, 225, 227, 298-9
herpes virus 247
  see also genital herpes
hiatus hernia 191
hip replacement 81
hirsutism 235
HIV (human immunodeficiency virus) 73, 208-9
hives see urticaria
Hodgkin's disease 125
Holmes and Rahe life change index 109
homeopathy 300-1
hormone birth control methods 60-1
hormone deficiencies 90
hormone therapy 156, 166
hormones 126, 135, 220, 273, 276
HRT (hormone replacement therapy) 144-5, 272, 273, 276
human papillomavirus 158
hydralazine 274

hydrocortisone 273, 274, 275, 276
hydrotherapy 308, 309
hygiene 197
hymen 38
hyoscine 275
hypercholesterolaemia 133
hyperlipidaemia 133, 137
hypermetropia see long-sightedness
hyperparathyroidism 91
hypertension see blood pressure
hyperthyroidism 139
hyperventilation 45
hypnosis 107, 237
hypnotherapy 283
hypnotic drugs 273
hypochondriasis 106
hypothalmus 33
hypothermia 257
hypothyroidism 87, 138, 234
hysterectomy 161, 164-5
hysteria see dissociative disorder
hysterosalpingogram 264
hysteroscopy 264

I

ibuprofen 277
ifosfamide 277
illegal substances 100
imipranine 272
immune system 40-1, 163, 204-9
  drugs 276
immune-linked arthritis 82-3
immunization see vaccination
immunoassay 264
immunologist 268
immunosuppressants 272, 275, 276
immunotherapy 204
Implanon 61
incontinence 37, 188-9
indigestion 128, 175
indomethacin 277
infants 271
infections 258
  acute 244-51
  sexual 72-5
infertility 162, 168, 182-3
inflammatory bowel disease 201, 202
influenza 214
inoculation see vaccination
insomnia 25
insulin 137, 273
intercourse 69, 179, 208
intestines 36
intimacy 58-9
intravenous pyelogram see pyelogram
investigative tests 263-5
ipratropium 274
iridology 308
iritis 247
iron 18, 117, 195
irritable bowel syndrome 200-1, 282
isocarboxazid 272
isosorbide dinitrate 274
isosorbide mononitrate 274

ispaghula 275
itching 136, 193
IUD (intrauterine device) 64, 148, 149, 164

J

jaw ache 79
jet lag 271
  see also flying
joints 31, 78-9
journalling 47, 285
juvenile rheumatoid arthritis 82

K

kaolin and morphine 275
ketocanazole 276
kidney disorders 137, 245
kinesiology 310
knees 79
kyphosis 84

L

labour 176-7
labyrinthitis 236
lacidipine 274
lactulose 275
laparoscopy 167, 182, 264
laparotomy 167, 264
large cell carcinoma 221
laryngitis 249
laughter 44
laxatives 196, 199, 275
lerbutaline 276
lesbians 55
leukaemia 125
libido 70
life change index 109
life cycle 12-15, 27, 38-9
lifestyle 77, 84, 114, 154, 196
ligaments 78, 79, 88
lignocaine 273
liquids 18
lithotripsy 194
liver disease 193, 201
liver spots 228
long-sightedness 240
loperamide 275
lordosis 84
lubrication 69
lumbar puncture 250, 265
lumpectomy 155
lung diseases 213, 215
  cancer 220-1
lung function test 265
lungs 35
lupus 206
lupus erythematosus 82
lymph cancers 125
lymph circulation 40
lymph gland removal 155
lymph nodes 40, 156
lymphocytes 41
lymphodema 156
lymphoma 125

M

McTimoney and McTimoney-Corley technique 291
macular degeneration 242
magnesium hydroxide 275

malaria prophylaxis 271
malignant melanoma 233
mammograph 265
mammography 153
mannitol 274, 275
massage 141, 288-9
mastectomy 155
mastitis 151, 179
mastoiditis 236
masturbation 54
maturity 27
ME (myalgic encephalomyelitis) see chronic fatigue syndrome
measles 271
medau 297
Medic-Alert 254
medical personnel 266-8
medical records 262
meditation 45
Mediterranean diet 19
mefloquine 277
melanocytes 228
melanoma 233
men, sexual problems 69
menarche 38
Ménière's disease 237
meningitis 87, 237, 250-1
meningococcal septicemia 251
menopause 14, 142-3, 154, 191
  premature 133, 168
menorrhagia 149
menotrophin 276
menstrual cycle 146-7
menstrual disorders 22, 146-9, 301
menstruation 95, 117
mental health 67, 282-3
mental illness 105
menthol 274
metabolism 191
methadone 101, 277
methotrexate 272
methycellulose 275
methyldopa 274
metoprolol 273
metronidazole 277
miconazole 276
midwife 268
migraine headaches 107, 114-15, 241
milk 93, 219
mind 44-9, 94-103, 284-5
minerals 19, 141
mirena 64
miscarriage 180-1
mites 218
mitral valve prolapse 131
moiré shadow photography 265
moisture levels 18
monilia see thrush
monoamine oxidase inhibitors 272
mood swings 140
morning-after pill 63, 66
morphine 277
motherhood 13, 178-9
motion sickness 237
motor neurone disease 32, 211
mouth problems 239, 258

Acknowledgments

IF THE PUBLISHERS HAVE UNWITTINGLY INFRINGED COPYRIGHT IN ANY ILLUSTRATION REPRODUCED, THEY WOULD PAY AN APPROPRIATE FEE ON BEING SATISFIED TO THE OWNER'S TITLE.

T=TOP; B=BOTTOM; L=LEFT; C=CENTRE; R=RIGHT

1 ALAN BECKER/THE IMAGE BANK; 2 LAURA WICKENDEN, 3TL CORBIS, 3TR, BL THE PHOTOGRAPHERS LIBRARY, 3BR IMAGES COLOUR LIBRARY; 5 LAURA WICKENDEN; 6L STEVE PREZANT/THE STOCK MARKET, 6R ANTHONY SNYDER/CORBIS, 7L THE STOCK MARKET, 7R BENELUX/POWERSTOCK/ZEFA; 8 DAVID MADISON/GETTYONE STONE, 9L ROBERT HARDING PICTURE LIBRARY, 9R J. L. PALAEZ/THE STOCK MARKET; 10/11 LAURA WICKENDEN; 12 ED BOCK/THE STOCK MARKET, 13T SUPERSTOCK, 13B LAURA WICKENDEN; 14T LORI ADAMSKI PEEK/GETTYONE STONE, 14B ROB LEWINE/THE STOCK MARKET, 15T WALTER HODGES/GETTYONE STONE, 15B ELIE BERNAGER/GETTYONE STONE; 16, 18, 20 LAURA WICKENDEN, 21 T & D MCCARTHY/THE STOCK MARKET; 23L BRUCE AYRES/GETTYONE STONE, 23C DAVID MADISON/GETTYONE STONE, 23R AMWELL/GETTYONE STONE; 24 PAUL FORRESTER; 26 LAURA WICKENDEN, 27TL DALE DURFEE/GETTYONE STONE, 27TR PETER CORREZ/GETTYONE STONE, 27BL DAN BOSLER/GETTYONE STONE, 27BR ROBERT HARDING PICTURE LIBRARY; 28 STEVE ALLEN/THE IMAGE BANK, 29 JOSE L. PELAEZ/THE STOCK MARKET; 37 JOHN BARLOW; 44, 45T LAURA WICKENDEN, 45B IAIN BAGWELL; 46 BRITT ERLANSON/THE IMAGE BANK, 47 CHRIS BAKER/GETTYONE STONE; 49 JAMES DARELL/GETTYONE STONE; 50/51 LAURA WICKENDEN; 52L ROBERT HARDING PICTURE LIBRARY, 52CL JOE POLOLLIO/GETTYONE STONE, 52CR DAN BOSLER/GETTYONE STONE, 52R KEN FISHER/GETTYONE STONE; 54 DAN BOSLER/GETTYONE STONE, 55 GETTYONE STONE; 56, 57, 58, 60, 62, 64 LAURA WICKENDEN; 68 ADRIAN WEINBRECHT; 71, 76/77, 80 LAURA WICKENDEN; 81T MEHAU KULYK/SCIENCE PHOTO LIBRARY, 81B MIKE DEULIN/SCIENCE PHOTO LIBRARY; 82L ANDREW SYDENHAM, 82C DON KLUMPP/THE IMAGE BANK, 82R BRUCE PLOTKIN/GETTYONE STONE, 83, 84, 85, 86, 88 PAUL FORRESTER; 90L, R PROF. P. MOTTA/DEPT. OF ANATOMY/UNIVERSITY "LA SAPIENZA", ROME/SCIENCE PHOTO LIBRARY, 91 BSIP, LBL/SCIENCE PHOTO LIBRARY; 92 SCIENCE PHOTO LIBRARY, 93 CHRISTOPHER BISSELL/GETTYONE STONE; 95L, C LAURA WICKENDEN, 95R CHAS WILDER; 96 STEWART COHEN/GETTYONE STONE; 98 PAUL FORRESTER; 101 DAVID MADISON/GETTYONE STONE; 102L ANDREW SYDENHAM, 102C JAMES DARELL/GETTYONE STONE, 102R BRITT ERLANSON/THE IMAGE BANK; 104, 105 LAURA WICKENDEN; 106 WALTER HODGES/GETTYONE STONE, 107 JOHN HENLEY/THE STOCK MARKET; 108 LAURA WICKENDEN; 110 POWERSTOCK/ZEFA; 112 ADRIAN SYDENHAM, 113 LAURA WICKENDEN; 114, 115, 117 PAUL FORRESTER; 119TL, TC, TR ANDREW SYDENHAM, 119B MATT MEADOWS/SCIENCE PHOTO LIBRARY; 120L SIMON FRASER/ROYAL VICTORIA INFIRMARY, NEWCASTLE UPON TYNE/SCIENCE PHOTO LIBRARY, 120R RICHARD SHOCK/GETTYONE STONE; 123 PAUL FORRESTER; 124T DUSTY WILLISON/ROBERT HARDING PICTURE LIBRARY, 124B KEN FISHER/GETTYONE STONE; 127L RB STUDIO 97/THE STOCK MARKET, 127CL BARRY YEE/GETTYONE STONE, 127CR THE STOCK MARKET, 127R RICK GOMEZ/THE STOCK MARKET; 132, 134/135 LAURA WICKENDEN; 136L DALE DURFEE/GETTYONE STONE, 136CL POWERSTOCK/ZEFA, 136CR ROBERT HARDING PICTURE LIBRARY, 136R IAN O'LEARY/GETTYONE STONE, 137T ROBERT HARDING PICTURE LIBRARY, 137B IAIN BAGWELL; 139L FRANK SITEMAN/GETTYONE STONE, 139C GEORGE SHELLEY/THE STOCK MARKET, 139R JEFF BLANTON/GETTYONE STONE; 140 MICHAEL A. KELLER STUDIO/THE STOCK MARKET; 142 ARIEL SKELLEY/THE STOCK MARKET, 143 LAURA WICKENDEN; 147L LARRY WILLIAMS/THE STOCK MARKET, 147CL JAMES DARELL/GETTYONE STONE, 147CR JOSE L. PELAEZ/THE STOCK MARKET, 147L THE PHOTOGRAPHERS LIBRARY; 148 HENRY ARDEN; 152 IAIN BAGWELL; 157 LAURA WICKENDEN; 158 THE WELLCOME PHOTOLIBRARY, 159 DR E. WALKER/SCIENCE PHOTO LIBRARY; 160 LAURA WICKENDEN; 169 MARTYN F. CHILLMAID/SCIENCE PHOTO LIBRARY; 171 GIOVANNI LUNARDI/ROBERT HARDING PICTURE LIBRARY; 172 ROBERT HARDING PICTURE LIBRARY, 173 NORBERT SCHAFER/THE STOCK MARKET; 179 ADRIAN WEINBRECHT, 182 JO FOORD; 184 CHAS WILDER, 185L JAMES KING-HOLMES/SCIENCE PHOTO LIBRARY; 186/187 LAURA WICKENDEN; 194 QUEST/SCIENCE PHOTO LIBRARY; 196 PAUL FORRESTER, 197 LAURA WICKENDEN; 202 ROMILLY LOCKYER/THE IMAGE BANK, 203 LAURA WICKENDEN; 204 PAUL FORRESTER; 207 LAURA WICKENDEN; 208 ROMILLY LOCKYER/THE IMAGE BANK; 214 THE STOCK MARKET; 216 IAIN BAGWELL, 217 ANDREW SYDENHAM; 218T HARRY SMITH COLLECTION, 218B EYE OF SCIENCE/SCIENCE PHOTO LIBRARY, 219 ANDREW SYDENHAM; 221 SCOTT CAMAZINE/SCIENCE PHOTO LIBRARY; 224 LAURA WICKENDEN, 225T ANDREW SYDENHAM, 225B DAVID JORDAN; 228TL SCIENCE PHOTO LIBRARY, 228TR JANE SHEMILT, COSINE GRAPHICS/SCIENCE PHOTO LIBRARY, 228BL, BC, BR DR P. MARAZZI/SCIENCE PHOTO LIBRARY, 229 TONY LATHAM; 230 ARIEL SKELLEY/THE STOCK MARKET, 231 LAURA WICKENDEN; 232 DR P. MARAZZI/SCIENCE PHOTO LIBRARY, 233 BSIP LAURENT H. AMERICAIN/SCIENCE PHOTO LIBRARY; 234 LAURA WICKENDEN, 235 COURTESY OF SHEILA GODFREY CLINIC; 237 LAURA WICKENDEN, 239 PAUL FORRESTER; 243 ROSENFELD IMAGES /SCIENCE PHOTO LIBRARY; 245T LAURA WICKENDEN, 245B SCIENCE PHOTO LIBRARY; 246 ROBERT HARDING PICTURE LIBRARY, 247 CLAIRE PAXTON & JACQUI FARROW/SCIENCE PHOTO LIBRARY; 251 LAURA WICKENDEN; 252, 253, 254, 255, 256, 257, 258, 259 PAUL FORRESTER; 260/261 LAURA WICKENDEN; 271 JON FEINGERSH/THE STOCK MARKET, 271 JOHN BARLOW; 278 ROBERT HARDING PICTURE LIBRARY; 280 LARRY MULVEHILL/SCIENCE PHOTO LIBRARY, 281 ANDREW SYDENHAM; 282 SCOTT BARROW/ROBERT HARDING PICTURE LIBRARY, 283 JOHN GREIM/SCIENCE PHOTO LIBRARY; 284 LAURA WICKENDEN, 285 CHAS WILDER; 286/287 LAURA WICKENDEN; 288 IAIN BAGWELL, 289 TONY LATHAM; 290 HATTIE YOUNG/SCIENCE PHOTO LIBRARY, 291 BSIP, ROUX/SCIENCE PHOTO LIBRARY; 292 LAURA WICKENDEN, 293 IAIN BAGWELL; 294 LAURA WICKENDEN, 295 PAUL FORRESTER, 296 IMAGES COLOUR LIBRARY; 297T JOHN WALMSLEY, 297B PAUL FORRESTER; 298 ANDREW SYDENHAM, 299 IAN GOWLAND/A-Z BOTANICAL COLLECTION; 300 PAUL FORRESTER; 302 LAURA WICKENDEN; 306 STRAUSS/CURTIS/THE STOCK MARKET, 307 FAYE NORMAN/SCIENCE PHOTO LIBRARY; 308 ELLEN MARTORELLI/GETTYONE STONE, 309T DAVID STEWART/GETTYONE STONE, 309B; 310 LAURA WICKENDEN.

THE 'WHEN YOU QUIT SMOKING' CHART IS TAKEN FROM *THE NEW LIVING HEART* BY MICHAEL E. DEBAKEY, MD & ANTONIO M. GOTTO, JR., MD, PUBLISHED BY ADAMS MEDIA COROPORATION, HOLBROOK, MASSACHUSETTS, USA, 1997.